D0071272

Enhancing Communication Skills of Deaf & Hard of Hearing Children in the Mainstream

James J. Mahshie, PhD
Professor
Department of Hearing, Speech, and Language Sciences
Gallaudet University, Washington DC

Mary June Moseley, PhD
Professor
Department of Hearing, Speech, and Language Sciences
Gallaudet University, Washington DC

Susanne M. Scott, MS, CCC-A
Cochlear Implant Education Center
Laurent Clerc National Deaf Education Center
Gallaudet University, Washington DC

James Lee, MS
Clinical Supervisor
Department of Hearing, Speech, and Language Sciences
Gallaudet University, Washington DC

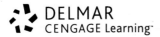

DELMAR
CENGAGE Learning

Australia • Brazil • Japan • Korea • Mexico • Singapore • Spain • United Kingdom • United States

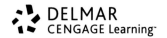

**Enhancing Communication
Skills of Deaf & Hard
of Hearing Children
in the Mainstream**
James J. Mahshie, Mary June
Moseley, Susanne M. Scott,
James Lee

Vice President, Health Care
  Business Unit: William
  Brottmiller

Editorial Director: Cathy
  L. Esperti

Acquisitions Editor: Kalen
  Conerly

Developmental Editor: Juliet
  Steiner

Editorial Assistant: Molly
  Belmont

Marketing Director: Jennifer
  McAvey

Marketing Coordinator: Chris
  Manion

Production Editor: John
  Mickelbank

Art and Design Specialist: Bob
  Plante

*HV
2471
.M34
2005
C,2*

For product information and
technology assistance, contact us at **Cengage Learning
Customer & Sales Support, 1-800-354-9706**
For permission to use material from this text or product,
submit all requests online at **www.cengage.com/permissions**
Further permissions questions can be emailed to
permissionrequest@cengage.com

Library of Congress Control Number: 2005014924

ISBN-13: 978-0-7693-0099-3

ISBN-10: 0-7693-0099-5

Delmar
Executive Woods
5 Maxwell Drive
Clifton Park, NY 12065
USA

Cengage Learning is a leading provider of customized learning
solutions with office locations around the globe, including
Singapore, the United Kingdom, Australia, Mexico, Brazil, and Japan.
Locate your local office at **international.cengage.com/region**

Cengage Learning products are represented in Canada by
Nelson Education, Ltd.

For your lifelong learning solutions, visit **delmar.cengage.com**

Visit our corporate website at **www.cengage.com**

Notice to the Reader
Publisher does not warrant or guarantee any of the products described herein or perform any independent analysis in connection with any of
the product information contained herein. Publisher does not assume, and expressly disclaims, any obligation to obtain and include information other than that provided to it by the manufacturer. The reader is expressly warned to consider and adopt all safety precautions that might
be indicated by the activities described herein and to avoid all potential hazards. By following the instructions contained herein, the reader
willingly assumes all risks in connection with such instructions. The publisher makes no representations or warranties of any kind, including
but not limited to, the warranties of fitness for particular purpose or merchantability, nor are any such representations implied with respect to
the material set forth herein, and the publisher takes no responsibility with respect to such material. The publisher shall not be liable for any
special, consequential, or exemplary damages resulting, in whole or part, from the readers' use of, or reliance upon, this material.

Printed in the United States of America
  4 5 6 7 8   14 13 12 11 10

ED170

Contents

Preface

In the United States today, there is a strong impetus toward educating children with various disabilities in mainstream settings rather than in isolated schools or classrooms. The "inclusion" of deaf and hard of hearing children in mainstream settings has added new challenges to clinicians whose caseload in the past would probably not have included these children. Few professional training programs offer more than basic information about working with students with hearing loss. A significant reason for writing this book was to address a need for a concise source of information for clinicians with limited experience with deaf clients. Of the approximately 10 million deaf or hard of hearing school-aged children in the United States, only 65,000 are in educational settings specifically designed for deaf children. Thus, the vast majority of these children are in mainstream settings. Moreover, although there are large numbers of deaf or hard of hearing children throughout the United States, they are often dispersed throughout large geographic areas, resulting in many deaf and hard of hearing children being found in settings in which the child is either alone or in schools with only a few other children with hearing loss. (In a recent survey conducted by the Research Institute at Gallaudet University, the 6,470 students who completed the survey reported that they are the ONLY deaf students in their building.)

Although clinicians typically are comfortable with the variety of language, fluency, and articulation cases that comprise the typical case load, many speech-language clinicians working with deaf or hard of hearing children experience uncertainty about how and where to begin. Are there norm-referenced tests that should be used to assess deaf or hard of hearing children? Can I use the familiar standardized tests with my deaf client? What can I do to maximize this child's communication in the classroom? How can I develop a therapy plan that will lead to appreciable gains when I have such limited opportunity to work with these children? What is the prognosis for spoken language development? What can be done to help the deaf or hard of hearing child in a mainstream school to have confidence about his or her communication abilities and to be accepted despite his or her obvious differences from others in the class?

This book is aimed at clinicians in mainstream settings who have posed these questions to the authors over the years. More and more children with hearing loss are being educated in mainstream schools, yet in many cases the professionals providing speech and language services to these children have received only limited training related to those with hearing loss.

In particular, this text is aimed at speech-language pathologists (and other professionals advocating for improving the communication skills of children who are deaf or hard of hearing) in mainstream settings who have a relatively large case load, with a minority of cases involving hearing loss. The text further assumes that although clinicians are interested in improving the quality of the clinical services they provide to the deaf and hard of hearing children they serve, they must balance this desire with the likelihood that the incidence of these cases in their overall case load will be low.

This text takes a holistic view of deaf and hard of hearing children. Although the emphasis is on development of effective communication skills by these children, the focus is not exclusively on the "ears" of the child, nor is it on speech alone, rather it is on the total child as communicator. The emphasis is not only on the specific skills needed but also on the environment and context in which communication occurs.

The text also addresses the advocacy role of clinicians in mainstream settings. In many cases, the speech-language pathologist or educational audiologist is the sole professional concerned with the deaf or hard of hearing child's communication. Issues involved with deaf or hard of hearing children's communication in mainstream settings and the role that clinicians can play in maximizing acceptance and optimal communication environments will be described.

This book further examines some of the difficult dilemmas that confront those concerned with education of deaf and hard of hearing children in the mainstream. For example, although many children with hearing loss will be using sign language to some extent, the majority of clinicians will probably have limited sign language proficiency. This text will present issues related to such situations while also providing useful guidance to clinicians about how to proceed despite what may be less than optimal circumstances. Finally, the book provides a useful framework for viewing and assessing the communication abilities and goals for children ranging from those with emerging language to those in high school. The framework is both comprehensive and specific, providing a set of skills and abilities and attitudes and incentives that need to be considered in working with children for whom hearing loss is the primary concern. The first section of the book examines overall factors important for working with deaf and hard of hearing children, and the second part of the book will look at various ages and levels of knowledge and discuss assessment and intervention techniques through the presentation of case studies.

We appreciate the support and help of many people during the development of this book. The idea originated with a series of lectures provided to various speech and hearing professionals in Dublin, Ireland, during the first author's sabbatical. Thanks to Margaret Leahy and those in the Department of Clinical Speech and Language Studies at Trinity College, Dublin, for the opportunity to begin exploring this area through these lectures.

We also thank the many colleagues and student assistants who have helped with various aspects of this book: Antoinette Allen, Fred Brandt, Laura Chetwynd, Melanie Coll, Laura O'Brien, Robin Goffen, Colleen Maloney-Mercier, Rala Stone, Scott Bally, and Mary Pat Wilson. We are also indebted to Juliet Steiner for her editorial assistance, along with the helpful comments from two anonymous reviewers.

The authors have found the writing of this text to be both a rewarding and a challenging task, as they articulated the various strategies and approaches for working with deaf and hard of heading children that have resulted from their collective experience. We are grateful to those children who we have been fortunate to work with over the years (including our own) and from whom we have learned so much. It is our hope that the result of our efforts will be a useful text that will support clinicians working with deaf and hard of hearing children.

James Mahshie
Mary June Moseley
Susanne Scott
James Lee

About the Authors

James J. Mahshie is Professor in the Department of Hearing, Speech, and Language Sciences at Gallaudet University. He received his MS and PhD from Syracuse University. His research has focused on both better understanding of the speech production patterns of deaf individuals and the development of effective computer-based strategies for speech improvement. Dr. Mahshie has extensive teaching and clinical experience related to spoken language production of deaf and hard of hearing individuals.

Mary June Moseley is a Professor in the Department of Hearing, Speech, and Language Sciences at Gallaudet University. She received her MA and PhD from Kent State University. Dr. Moseley has considerable teaching and clinical experience in language development/refinement with preschoolers through adolescents and has published and presented at conferences on those topics.

Susanne M. Scott, MS, CCC-A, has worked at Gallaudet University for 24 years. She has extensive experience in working with deaf and hard of hearing individuals from birth through adults. She has done numerous presentations at national conventions/conferences and has written articles and books related to habilitation with deaf and hard of hearing individuals. Ms. Scott has supervised and taught graduate students in the Department of Hearing, Speech, and Language Sciences at Gallaudet University in the area of aural rehabilitation. Currently she is an outreach specialist in the Cochlear Implant Education Center at the Laurent Clerc National Deaf Education Center at Gallaudet.

James Lee is a Clinical Supervisor in the Department of Hearing, Speech, and Language Sciences at Gallaudet University. He earned his BA from the University of Connecticut and his MS degree in Speech-Language Pathology from Gallaudet University. He has worked with deaf and hard of hearing children at Boston Children's Hospital's Center for Deaf and Hard of Hearing Children, the Fairfax County Public School System, and Kendall Demonstration Elementary School in Washington, DC.

PART I

Background

Chapters 1 through 3 of this book will examine a number of topics affecting the communication development of deaf and hard of hearing children. The first chapter addresses a number of factors that influence English language development and the interactions that occur among these factors. Central to this chapter is the notion that deaf and hard of hearing children comprise a diverse group and that it is important to consider a range of skills and abilities that will have an impact on an individual child's likelihood of successfully developing that spoken language.

Building on these concepts, the second chapter addresses a number of topics related to communication access. These topics include the assessment of the learning environment and strategies for optimizing the environment so the child with hearing loss has the most optimal access to communication possible.

Chapter 3 addresses the issues surrounding assessment of deaf and hard of hearing children's communication abilities and strategies for addressing the communication needs of these children.

Factors Influencing the Acquisition and Refinement of Communication Skills

Introduction

This chapter will discuss the speech and language skills in *hearing* children from infancy through high school. Particular emphasis will be given to how the acquisition and refinement of these different skills may be impacted by hearing loss. In addition, definitions and other general issues relating to deaf and hard of hearing children will be presented.

CHILDREN WITH HEARING LOSS

Children with hearing loss are those children whose hearing is different from what would be considered "normal" on an audiogram. This would include hearing loss of any type, degree, configuration, laterality, or age of onset. Even a minimal hearing loss will prevent complete access to language and communication and can have a significant impact on how a child communicates and functions academically, socially, and emotionally.

Throughout this book the terms *deaf* and *hard of hearing* will represent the continuum of hearing loss and describe how a child accesses communication. The term *deaf* will refer to those children whose primary access to communication is through vision (e.g., speechreading or sign language). The term *hard of hearing* will refer to those children whose primary access to communication is through audition alone or audition and vision combined. Despite the label, a child's ability to access communication may change depending on the condition and the communication situation. For example, a child who uses a sensory aid (hearing aid or cochlear implant) may function as a hard of hearing communicator while using her sensory aid in a quiet environment and function as a deaf communicator when not using her sensory aid or when in a very noisy environment.

HOLISTIC APPROACH TO CHILDREN WHO ARE DEAF OR HARD OF HEARING

This book presents a number of themes that are essential to the optimal improvement of communication skills of children who are deaf or hard of hearing. Central to these themes is the notion that we are dealing with a whole child, one whose communication occurs in the context of her social environment, whose abilities will be tied to cognitive abilities and knowledge of the world, and whose cultural background will play a significant role in how she communicates. All of these factors become important in evaluating and providing services aimed to improve communication by the child who is deaf or hard of hearing.

A Deaf Child versus a Child Who Is Deaf

Although the issue of labels is often discussed in the literature, it is more than mere labels that requires us to look beyond the child's hearing loss when considering the development of communication skills. The child with a hearing loss is more than ears needing auditory training or an articulator needing therapy. She is a complex individual who needs to communicate her immediate needs as well as to further her total development. It cannot be stressed enough that subsequent delays in one or more areas of development may result from failure to facilitate age-appropriate development of communication skills. The need to communicate is not suspended because the child has a hearing loss, only the means to easily develop spoken language skills. A child with a hearing loss is first and foremost a *child* and the major aim of speech-language pathologists and audiologists is to facilitate development of as many aspects as possible of that child at age-appropriate times.

Areas such as cognitive, motor, and psychosocial development need to be considered as significant factors in the communicative development of children as well as linguistic and sensory factors. Beyond these attributes of the child, it is also important to examine the cultural and environmental conditions within which the child exists. A deaf child of deaf parents, an African-American deaf child of hearing parents, and a Latino deaf child of oral deaf parents will each present a different set of environmental attributes that will have an impact on how that child communicates. It is imperative that background attributes of the child are determined to ensure that the therapy strategies developed are appropriate and reasonable for the child and consistent with the goals and aspirations of the parents.

As children grow, they will be more and more aware of the world around them and the need to accept their own communicative strengths and weaknesses. In educational settings, a communication environment that is accepting of the differences will be nurturing to children who are deaf or hard of hearing. In addition, professionals can employ strategies to provide hearing children in mainstream environments and their teachers with information and experiences that promote a view of deafness as a difference, rather than a disorder.

FACTORS AFFECTING COMMUNICATION DEVELOPMENT

The communication skills of the young child with hearing loss are affected from the day the child is born. Linguistic, sensory, social, and cognitive information is received by the newborn from the environment immediately following birth. For the child with hearing, the foundation for language and linguistic competence begins as a neonate. The child hears the spoken language of her community from parents, interacts with parents based on sound (e.g., crying), and begins the process of learning to perceive and interpret the various sounds in the environment.

When hearing ability is reduced to any extent, multiple aspects of the child's development will be affected. In the following sections, the impact of hearing loss on numerous aspects of a child's development will be explored.

Prelanguage Communication

Several aspects of the linguistic system begin to develop from birth. The ability to perceive speech distinctions, the production of sounds, and the development of communicative intent all seem to propel the child toward production of her first volitional, meaningful utterances during the 1st year of life.

The Production and Perception of Speech

The development of speech and the ability to perceive and understand speech are intertwined. The process whereby the two systems interact with the environment is not fully understood, and there continues to be some dispute concerning the relative importance of nature versus nurture. Nonetheless, there is clearly an interaction between the innate abilities of the child to produce speech and the ability to hear and understand speech.

The hearing child begins vocalizing from birth, with these vocalizations being interpreted by the caregiver as communicative almost from the very beginning. At birth, there is a nondifferentiated birth cry that the child employs for nearly all needs—discomfort, hunger, fatigue, etc. Toward the end of the 2nd month, the child is beginning to differentiate these cries to use different cry patterns to signify different needs. Beginning in the 3rd month, the hearing child is beginning to produce "cooing" sounds that comprise predominantly back vowels and consonants. These cooing sounds gradually become more syllabic in nature, with the emergence of babbling occurring between the 3rd and 6th month (Oller, 1980).

At the same time the child is exhibiting these production characteristics, there is evidence that the hearing child as young as 1 month of age is already able to differentiate certain acoustic differences between speech segments. Eimas, Siqueland, Jusczyk, and Vigorito (1971) showed that 1-month-old infants could discriminate between [p] and [b] based on voice onset time differences. Neonates are even able to distinguish the voices of their caregivers and begin discriminating the prosodic characteristics of their environmental language. This is not surprising because there is increasing evidence that the infant's ability to perceive intonation, stress, and syllabification probably forms the basis for the earliest sound-meaning relationships (Fernald, 1991).

During the first 6 months the child does begin to clearly show preferences for the environmental language and has begun to be able to categorize many of the phonemic categories of that environmental language (see Kuhl, 1987, for a more comprehensive review of studies exploring phonemic perception by infants). There is clear evidence that by 6 months of age, hearing children are forming language-specific vowel categories.

There is also evidence of a connection between the production and perceptual abilities of very young children. This connection is perhaps best reflected in the ability of the child to imitate. Neonates are able to imitate adult facial expression and hand gestures, and children as young as 4 to 6 months of age show the ability to imitate /i/ and /a/ patterns (Kuhl and Meltshoff, 1982). There is further evidence that infants can imitate the absolute value of adult fundamental frequency at 2 to 5 months of age.

Between 3 and 6 months of age the hearing child typically begins to produce long strings of sounds and syllables. These utterances eventually include reduplication (e.g., baba or mama) that marks the beginning of babbling. Babbling is considered the precursor of actual speech development, and current views suggest that there is a strong connection between the babbling utterances of hearing children and later sound development (Vihman, 1996).

In summary, there is an appreciable body of research suggesting that very young hearing children are already beginning to exhibit elements of basic speech production and perception abilities and that the connection between these two is being established. The initiation of babbling represents the next step in the process of spoken language development, with current research suggesting a connection between babbling and later language development.

With the early importance of perceiving and producing speech (or speech-like) utterances, it would seem obvious that a child with a hearing loss would experience significant differences from her hearing peers in both the production and perception of speech. The earliest studies of vocalizations of deaf infants suggest that their vocalizations are similar to those of hearing children through the earliest babbling stages and that divergences in development of these two groups tend to occur later in the babbling stage (e.g., Mavilya, 1972). More recent research, however, suggests that there are early and significant differences in vocalizations of deaf and hearing infants (Oller, Eilers, Vull, & Carney, 1985). Given the connections that are evident between hearing and speech production, this is not a surprising situation.

Development of Turn-Taking and Communicative Intent

Development of a communication system begins from infancy through the interaction between the caregiver (frequently the mother) and the child (Haynes & Shulman, 1998). For example, during nursing mothers may be active in stroking the child and talking to the child. When the child is sucking, mothers are known to be quiet and while the child is quiet, mothers talk to the child and touch her. Interactions such as these form the basis of turn-taking involved in communication. When the child does not hear during this time, it may affect the development of the knowledge of the turn-taking system upon which language is built.

During these earliest interactions, the child's hearing loss begins to have an impact on her relationship with the caregiver. The bond between mother and child is an ongoing process that is propelled by the development of communication between the two (Haynes & Shulman, 1998). In our society, communication is the foundation upon which this and other relationships are built. However, when a child has a significant hearing loss, the communication attempts made by the mother may be unheard by the child. As a result the child may respond in less than expected ways that may then diminish the interaction for the mother. This lack of reinforcement may begin a cycle that limits or reduces the bond between mother and child. This dynamic can be true of other relationships as well, including peer relationships. The impact of these fractured relationships on the child's development (including psychosocial development, self-esteem, and progmatic skills) is an area that is becoming recognized as more and more important. (Bench, 1992).

Parents of young children (birth to 6 months) tend to interpret all sounds the child makes as *intentionally* communicative (Bates, 1976). For example, if the child burps, the mother may say, "Oh, do you have a tummy ache?" The parent constantly acts as though the young child is requesting something or communicating herself. At around 6 months, the child has truly learned to be intentional in communication and begins to expand the communicative repertoire. For example, the child will request something in the environment by gesturing (pointing to something in the environment), which is then handed to the child by her mother. During this time, the child is also expanding the number of sounds she is producing and eventually (around 1 year to 18 months) may begin her first words.

Deaf children also begin demonstrating the use of gestures for communication around 6 to 8 months. The deaf child in a verbal environment, that is, an environment in which sign language is not used, continues relying on gestures longer than the hearing child, with the system being more elaborate and highly organized (McAnally, Rose, & Quigley, 1994). This deaf child may not have first spoken words until much later than the hearing child, if at all. Deaf children with deaf parents, who are receiving American Sign Language as their primary input, develop gestural systems that then become words in sign language at a similar age as the development of first spoken words (Volterra & Erting, 1994).

During this 1st year, hearing and deaf children are developing schema for concepts about the world around them. These concepts develop through the daily activities in which the child participates, including play. For example, the child learns the routine for taking a bath:

1. Go upstairs
2. Go to the bathroom
3. Take off the baby's clothes
4. Run the water
5. Lift the baby into the water
6. Give the baby a toy to play with
7. Wash the baby
8. Remove the baby from the tub and dry her
9. Dress the baby

Eventually the child attaches language to the activity that is happening. In addition, the child's playing with various types of toys provides opportunities to learn about how things work in the world.

Deaf children experience many of the same activities but may not have the words to express their knowledge of this activity or other objects and activities around them. There has been some discussion in the literature as to whether deaf children play the same and learn the same concepts as hearing children. Because many of the research techniques require some knowledge of language by the child and some deaf children do not have the beginnings of language at an early age, the results of these studies are inconclusive. Paul and Quigley (1994) provide a clear discussion of the issues in determining the cognitive skills of deaf children and the extensive need for further research.

For deaf children with hearing parents the lack of efficient communication may continue to affect the relationship between parent and child. This dynamic, as well as its social and emotional impact on the child, has been shown to affect communication in families of children with physical problems (Rosetti, 1996). Anecdotal information suggests that this early and sometimes continued lack of an efficient communication system and common language between a child with a hearing loss and parent or family may be far more complex and have a far greater impact than initially believed. What and how parents communicate are integral components in the development of children. How children perceive themselves and their world is guided significantly by their parents through communication.

Early Language

First words are thought to develop from the child's social interactions during that 1st year. The child learns to take turns, focus on auditory input in the environment through the models she hears, increases reliance on speech for communication, and begins to experience activities that help her make sense of the world (Haynes & Shulman, 1998).

Production and Perception of Speech

The first words of hearing children are frequently represented phonologically by front consonants (especially stops), vowels, and consonant-vowel/consonant-vowel-consonant syllable structure. Thus, the child is faced with the task of learning to produce these sounds and apply them to the objects in her environment.

It is recognized that the lack of access to sound by a child with hearing loss may make the production and differentiation of sounds difficult. With no sensory input, the child has no way to evaluate her own production and refine her motor movements to match the models available. The difficulty in producing sounds may translate to difficulty in saying words, thus limiting the child's ability to easily communicate about the objects and people in her environment.

A particular deaf or hard of hearing child's acquisition of speech skills is dependent upon a number of factors, including the amount and quality of auditory input to which the child has access, the educational setting, the amount of family support, and the amount and quality of intervention provided by specialists. Although the types of speech errors may vary from child to child, there is clearly a tendency for children with hearing loss to begin showing evidence of "deaf speech" during the earliest stages of spoken language development. These include differences from normal in both the segmental and suprasegmental characteristics of speech (Hochberg, Levitt, & Osberger, 1983; Osberger &McGarr, 1982). Among prevalent suprasegmental characteristics are those affecting:

- The timing, rhythm, and syllable structure of speech
- Breath control
- Intonation patterns and overall fundamental frequency characteristics
- Nasal resonance
- Voice quality

Among the most prevalent segmental errors characterizing the speech of deaf and hard-of-hearing children are the following:

- Neutralization of all vowels
- Production errors involving diphthongs
- Voice-voiceless errors
- Fricative and affricate consonant errors
- Velopharyngeal control errors affecting the accuracy of nasal consonants

These patterns clearly form the areas most often addressed in therapy and can have an adverse affect on the overall intelligibility of the speech of children who are deaf or hard of hearing.

Language and Communication

The hearing child's acquisition of spoken language during this period expands her life exponentially. As mentioned earlier, children begin to interact with a wider and wider circle of adults and peers. The ability to communicate effectively within these contexts is essential. For the child with a hearing loss these interactions may be inefficient, facilitated by an adult (parent or interpreter) or nonexistent. These interactions and the subsequent social and linguistic skills as well as a sense of identity are critical to a child's development. Identity formation literature emphasizes the role of others in the formation of self (Longres, 1995). Although a certain amount of interaction can be achieved nonverbally, true and full interaction with others is based upon a shared language and the ability to understand and to be understood.

Hearing children typically begin to produce their first words around 12 to 18 months of age (Haynes & Shulman, 1998). These first words frequently represent things and people that are in their immediate environment. Between 18 and 24 months of age, children typically go through a period of putting two words together: learning to express specific semantic relationships in sentences. For example, many children use the word combination "more _____" (e.g., "more milk" or "more cookie") to express the recurrence of an object or person. At this early stage (preschool age) of language development, hearing children are showing the rudiments of syntactic development. As they combine two words and expand their utterances to three or more words, they begin to use nouns, verbs, some prepositions (e.g., in or on), adjectives, and other syntactic classes of words. Sentence structure tends to start with a simple subject-verb-object (SVO) word order and become increasingly complex, including subject and verb phrases, infinitive phrases, and other embedded sentences (Brown, 1973).

These first words represent the child's growing knowledge of communicative functions or how to get things accomplished in the environment. For example, the child has learned how to request action and information, give information, describe action, greet individuals (e.g., "hi" and "bye"), and generally use words, which have probably replaced many gestures (Haynes & Shulman, 1998). As the hearing child continues to develop language, she becomes able to more easily participate in conversations by verbal turn-taking, talking about a topic through several exchanges with another person and initiating and responding to a conversational exchange (Haynes & Shulman, 1998). There is evidence that older preschool children (around 4 years of age) are able to repair a conversation when it breaks down and choose words that take into account some of the information about their listener (e.g., age, role, and shared information) (Haynes & Shulman, 1998).

These skills constitute the beginnings of a more sophisticated knowledge of language that will eventually lead to easy manipulation of words and ideas. The child is becoming a sophisticated language user who is able to apply language knowledge to reading, writing, and spelling, to carry on long conversations, to understand various types of discourse structure, (e.g., narrative or expository), and to generally function as a mature language user.

Children with hearing loss tend to develop a spoken vocabulary and semantic relationships that are similar to those of their hearing peers. There is evidence, however, that they may not express these words as early as hearing children (Curtiss, Prutting, & Lowell, 1979). During this time of early communication development, if the child does not have the groundwork for communication laid at the prelinguistic level, the entire language system may be affected and may continue to lag behind that of the hearing child.

Research suggests that when a child with a significant hearing loss begins to put words together, she may not use the extensive classes of grammatical structures evident in hearing children (Kretschmer & Kretschmer, 1978; Quigley & Paul, 1984). For example, deaf children often omit function words such as articles, prepositions, and morphemes that express plurality and past tense, and other less concrete words. Sentence structure may rigidly adhere to SVO word order and tends to develop less over time than does the hearing child's sentence structure (McAnally et al., 1994).

Deaf and hard of hearing children may continue to use more gestures to express communicative functions and fewer words (Skarakis & Prutting, 1977). Although they may express some of the same communicative functions as the hearing child, because their words are limited they may have less opportunity to dialogue with peers and adults in their environment, so turn-taking skills may not develop as early. McKirdy & Blank (1982) report that deaf and hard of hearing children, aged 4.2 to 5 years, are less likely to respond appropriately in a conversational exchange than their hearing peers. As their conversational partner's initiations become more complex, deaf children tend to experience more difficulty in responding appropriately. Very little is known about young deaf children's ability to repair conversations and take the listener's perspective.

At this stage, young hearing children are using language to expand their cognitive skills, to express new ideas and to problem-solve. The exact relationship of cognition and language is disputed among scholars (e.g., see Haynes & Shulman, 1998). Some believe that at some point in the learning process, language helps advance cognitive skills by providing a means by which new knowledge can be processed and retained (Paul & Quigley, 1994). Although there is evidence that children with hearing loss develop cognitive skills appropriately for their age, the lack of a strong communicative system may make it difficult to determine the extent of cognitive knowledge and schemas.

Later Language

As the hearing child enters school, the communication system continues to develop and become refined. The advent of written language and the challenges of learning school discourse become necessary for children to continue to learn more advanced language forms and usage as well as to realize academic success.

The early elementary years have been shown to be important in language learning in many ways. The hearing child continues to develop vocabulary and grammatical sentence structures as she begins to learn new subject matter in school. In addition, this vocabulary and sentence structure become increasingly used in new types of discourse. The child must learn instructional discourse that is used by teachers in schools, which differs from conversational discourse, where children learn to carry on a dialogue. Instructional discourse is more formal (e.g., more precise articulation and more formal vocabulary), includes more questions, is decontextualized, and is group oriented instead of individually oriented (Wallach & Miller, 1988).

In addition, the child must learn different types of discourse, especially narrative and expository discourse. Narrative discourse is associated with the telling of a story and has a specific structure of its own (e.g., setting, initiating event, internal response, attempt at goal attainment, consequence, and ending) (Stein & Glenn, 1979). There is evidence that hearing children learn to use the components of narratives by the time they are around 7 years old (Applebee, 1978). This structure is used in school settings in both verbal and written modes.

During the early school years, the child is also learning expository discourse structure. Expository structure is highly fact-oriented and may take several different forms: descriptive, sequential, cause-effect, and problem solution (Wallach & Butler, 1984). Poetry and drama are also discourse types that are taught regularly in schools. The child needs to learn to manipulate these various forms of discourse, both on a verbal level and through the written mode to succeed in school.

The process of reading is described as learning to *decode* and *comprehend*, whereas literacy includes the *context* of the application of skills. Being literate may include reading and writing skills in the context of literate thought, which is the ability to engage in critical or reflective thought (Paul & Quigley, 1994). Factors that may be associated with this process are text-based factors such as vocabulary, syntax, organization of the text, and punctuation rules; reader-based factors such as motivation, prior knowledge, and metacognitive skills; and context-based factors such as the purposes of reading (poetry, expository, etc.) and the setting in which reading is accomplished, and instructional factors (Paul & Quigley, 1994). The child who must learn many of these factors *at the same time* as she is learning to read is probably at a disadvantage for developing fluent reading skills.

As the child gets into a structured school setting, learning to read, write, and spell becomes a prime part of her curriculum. It is generally understood that children through grade three learn to read and after grade three, read to learn (Paul & Quigley, 1994). Reading for new knowledge becomes the major focus of the school day beyond third grade. The amount of information that is presented and must be learned is considerably more at the upper elementary grades and through the middle and high school years. The reading process is dependent on a child's *metalinguistic* skills, learning to reflect on one's language and talk about it. Hearing children are developing these metalinguistic skills during the elementary school years.

In addition to learning to read and write, the child is refining all aspects of language during the elementary and high school years. Language, both verbal and written, is becoming much more complex. The child is learning to use advanced sentence structure (e.g., pronominalization or relativization), and her sentence structure is becoming longer and more complex. The child is also learning to use various linguistic devices to help assemble a cohesive narrative, either verbal or written. For example, the child learns to use pronouns to refer to a previously established topic:

> The boy ran up the street. *He* went into *his* friend's house.

(*He* and *his* refer to *the boy* in the previous sentence.) Cohesive devices used commonly include referential cohesion, lexical cohesion (BOY and STUDENT may refer to the same person in discourse), relative clauses, adjectives to describe, and ellipsis (Moseley & Hughes, 1990; Wallach & Miller, 1988).

The use of these cohesive devices may also help the child develop the ability to infer, a necessary part of understanding most forms of verbal and written discourse. Inference requires the ability to speculate about language, about what might happen and to use metacognitive and metalinguistic skills. The child is learning to use all aspects of nonliteral language: indirect requests, humor and satire, idioms, and other forms of figurative language. In addition, word knowledge is expanding, including knowledge of forms such as antonyms and synonyms.

All of these areas discussed earlier are expanding in both the verbal and the written mode. In addition to learning the process of identifying the written form, the child must learn to comprehend and express new language forms in this new mode.

In spoken interactions, the child is refining the ability to take turns on a topic, talking for a longer period of time while using utterances relevant to the topic. She is refining the ability to take the listener's perspective, choosing words that will reflect appropriate understanding of the age, role, and shared information with the listener. The child continues to become sensitive to the listener's needs and is more readily able to repair conversations when they break down by requesting additional information, "reading" the nonverbal signals of the listener, and employing other repair strategies to assure a smooth flow of conversation and communication.

Learning to read, write, and spell may be difficult for the deaf child who does not have a strong language base. It is well documented that the majority of 18- to 19-year-old deaf students fail to reach reading proficiency above the fourth grade level (Quigley & Paul, 1994). It has been further documented, both in the literature and anecdotally, that children with hearing loss are at higher risk for developing reading problems and for having difficulties with the more advanced aspects of language that were discussed in the preceding paragraphs. The impact of limited experience of the world, together with difficulties with reading, writing, and spelling collectively result in reduced literacy among many children who are deaf and hard of hearing.

Yoshinaga-Itano (1986) looked at the narrative structures in the writing of school-age children with hearing loss. The children in her study were less productive with respect to clauses, sentence length, and composition length; their sentences lacked complexity; and they made more grammatical errors. These findings are consistent with anecdotal comments from teachers in the field. In addition, expository structure may be a problem for children with hearing loss (deVilliers, 1995).

School-age vocabulary development for many deaf children does not parallel the knowledge of some hearing children. There is some evidence that these children exhibit fewer lexical items than their hearing peers, have decreased knowledge of common content words, and have difficulty with English function words. Other studies indicate problems with understanding and use of analogies, words with multiple meanings, synonyms and antonyms, and all aspects of nonliteral language, including common idioms and humor (McAnally et al., 1994). Semantic domains that include auditory imagery may also be problematic (e.g., *sizzle* or the bell *tolls*). These difficulties tend to be found in both spoken and written language of some children who are deaf or hard of hearing.

Quigley and Paul (1984) discussed extensive investigation of the syntactic skills of deaf and hard of hearing children. They report that the most common syntactic constructions that are problematic in the writing of deaf children are verb systems, negation, conjunction, pronominalization, complementation, relativization, question formation, and forced SVO patterns for sentence construction. The use of cohesive devices, which includes relativization and pronominalization, also may be problematic in writing narratives (Moseley & Hughes, 1990).

Hughes and James (1985) looked at the verbal language of deaf and hard of hearing students to determine whether they were able to make repairs on a conversational level when communication broke down. Their findings suggest that elementary-age children (6 to 9 years) are able to change mode of expression and revise and repeat information when the conversation breaks down, indicating knowledge of pragmatic skills that enable them to keep up with their listeners. However, teachers in schools report that many children with hearing loss need some guidance in developing repair skills (Deyo & Hallau, 1983), as well as other turn-taking skills such as topic initiation, termination, and maintenance.

Difficulty in taking the listener's perspective verbally (and sometimes in sign language) has also been documented for many deaf and hard of hearing children (Moseley & Hughes, 1990; Nichols & Moseley, 1996). Anecdotally, teachers consistently discuss this area as being problematic for their students.

Adolescent Language

During middle school and high school, language has a major role in all subjects including reading, math, history, geography, and even art. Teachers assume that by the time the student is at this stage, she has mastered language. Writing skills continue to be emphasized, and students are required to use more complex language, including an increased vocabulary, more advanced sentence structure, and different kinds of language for different situations. During high school the adolescent prepares for adult roles and responsibilities. This requires the student to adjust to increased cognitive demands and the development of expanded verbal skills. The student must be able to use abstract thinking and problem-solving and develop new verbal skills to accommodate more complex concepts and tasks.

Standardized and informal tests continue to be used to measure student performance. Often, conclusions about what students have learned in school are based on their performance on these tests (LaSasso, 1999). In addition, most states use competency tests to measure student performance. In many cases, students who perform below certain "cut levels" on these tests may actually be held back a grade or allowed to complete high school without a standard diploma (Randall, McAnnally, Rittenhouse, Russell, & Sorensen, 2000).

The adolescent with hearing loss may still be working on acquiring the necessary language skills to accommodate the demands of middle school and high school. These students may require direct speech-language intervention either on an individual or small group basis or in the classroom. In addition to working on language skills necessary to succeed academically, deaf and hard of hearing adolescents may be refining their receptive and expressive communication skills to prepare for life after high school.

It is clear that the use of language during the school years is extremely complex. The language base for these elements begins in the prelinguistic communicative period. It would seem that many children with hearing loss never quite "catch up" with language development, and the result may be a breakdown in many aspects of language comprehension and use that affect the learning process in schools. Additionally, this language delay begins to impact the whole child. Self-esteem will be affected as the child begins to perceive the gap between herself and her peers. Her ability to effectively navigate conversations with peers in group settings within the classroom or in other school environments (e.g., the cafeteria or library) may be significantly limited. The child's relationships with peers and adults may lack depth and intensity because of communication barriers. All of the above adversely impact the psychosocial development of the child.

Summary

The concepts described in this chapter have been incorporated into subsequent portions of the book. That is, the authors have emphasized that children with hearing loss are first and foremost children. Although their hearing loss can result in specific communication issues, it is important to examine both those areas that are uniquely affected by a hearing loss and those areas that are part of typical development of all children. The goal is to facilitate development of communicative abilities that are typical of all children.

References

Applebee, A. N. (1978). *The child's concept of story.* Chicago: University of Chicago Press.

Bates, E. (1976). *Language in context.* New York: Academic Press.

Bench, R. J. (1992). *Communication skills in hearing-impaired children.* Clifton Park, NY: Singular.

Brown, R. (1973). *A first language: The early stages.* Cambridge, MA: Harvard University Press.

Curtiss, S., Prutting, C., & Lowell, E. (1979). Pragmatic and semantic development in young children with impaired hearing. *Journal of Speech and Hearing Research, 22,* 534–552.

deVilliers, P. (1995, October). *"Gearing up" for literacy.* Paper presented at the Conference on Language & Deafness—A Decade in Review, Omaha, NE.

Deyo, D., & Hallau, M. (1983). *Communicate with me: Conversation strategies for deaf students.* Washington, DC: Gallaudet University Pre-College Programs.

Eimas, P. D., Siqueland, E. R., Jusczyk, P. W., & Vigorito, J. (1971). Speech perception in infants. *Science, 171,* 303–306.

Fernald, A. (1991). Prosody in speech to children: Prelinguistic and linguistic function. *Annals of Child Development, 60,* 1497–1510.

Haynes, W. O., & Shulman, B. B. (1998). *Communication development foundations, processes, and clinical applications.* Baltimore: Williams & Wilkins.

Hochberg, I., Levitt, H., & Osberger, M. J. (1983). *Speech of the hearing impaired: Research, training and personnel preparation.* Baltimore: University Park Press.

Hughes, M., & James, S. L. (1985). Deaf children's revision behaviors in conversations. *Journal of Communication Disorders, 18,* 227–243.

Kretschmer, R. R., & Kretschmer, L. W. (1978). *Language development and intervention with the hearing impaired.* Baltimore: University Park Press.

Kuhl, P. K. (1987). Perception of speech and sound in early infancy. In P. Salapatek & L. Cohen (Eds.) *Handbook of infant perception.* New York: Academic Press.

Kuhl, P. K., & Meltshoff, A. N. (1982). The bimodal perception of speech in infancy. *Science, 218,* 1138–1141.

LaSasso, C. J. (1999, May). *Reading comprehension of deaf students: Empowering parents and teachers to improve deaf students' English literacy.* Paper presented to A&S 720: Seminar in Assessment and Habilitation of Deaf and Hard of Hearing Children. Washington, DC.

Longres, J. (1995). *Human behavior in the social environment* (2nd ed.). Itasca, IL: Peacock.

McAnally, P. L., Rose, S., & Quigley, S. P. (1994). *Language learning practices with deaf children* (2nd ed.). Austin: Pro-Ed.

Mavilya, M. (1972). Spontaneous vocalization and babbling in hearing impaired infants. In G. Fant (Ed.), *Proceedings of the International Symposium on Speech Communication Ability and Profound Deafness, Stockholm, 1970.* Washington, DC: Alexander Graham Bell Association for the Deaf.

McKirdy, L., & Blank, M. (1982). Dialogue in deaf and hearing proschoolers. *Journal of Speech & Hearing Research, 25*(4), 487–499.

Moseley, M. J., & Hughes, M. (1990, April). *A descriptive pragmatic inventory for deaf adolescents/adults: Implications for intervention.* Paper presented to the Maryland Speech & Hearing Association, Ellicott City, MD.

Nichols, M., & Moseley, M.J. (1996). Language skills. In Moseley, M. J., & Bally, S. J. (1996). *Communication therapy: An integrated approach to aural rehabilitation with deaf and head of hearing adolescents and adults.* Washington: DC: Gallaudet University Press.

Oller, K. (1980). The emergence of the sounds of speech in infancy. In G. Yeni-Komshian, J. F. Kavanaugh, & C. A. Ferguson (Eds.), *Child phonology I: Production.* New York: Academic Press.

Oller, K., Eilers, R., Vull, D., & Carney, A. (1985). Prespeech vocalizations of a deaf infant: A comparison with normal metaphonological development. *Journal of Speech and Hearing Research, 28,* 47–63.

Osberger M. J., & McGarr, N. (1982). Speech production characteristics of the hearing impaired. *Speech Language, 8,* 221–283.

Paul, P. V., & Quigley, S. P. (1994). *Language and deafness* (2nd ed.). Clifton Park, NY: Singular.

Quigley, S. P., & Paul, P. V. (1984). *Language and deafness.* San Diego, CA: College Hill Press.

Randall, K., McAnally, P., Rittenhouse, B., Russell, D., & Sorensen, G. (2000). High stakes testing: what is at stake? *American Annals of the Deaf, 145*(5), 390–393.

Rosetti, L.M. (1996). *Communication intervention: Birth to three.* Clifton Park, NY: Singular.

Skarakis, E., & Prutting, C. A. (1977). Early communication: Semantic functions and communicative intentions in the communication of the preschool child with impaired hearing. *American Annals of the Deaf, 122,* 382–391.

Stein, N. L., & Glenn, C. G. (1979). An analysis of story comprehension in elementary school children. In R. O. Freedle. (1979). *New directions in discourse processing* (Vol. 2). Norwood, NJ: Ablex.

Vihman, M. M. (1996). *Phonological development: The origins of language in the child.* Cambridge, MA: Blackwell.

Volterra, V., & Erting, C. J. (Eds.). (1994). *From gesture to language in hearing and deaf children.* Washington, DC: Gallaudet University Press.

Wallach, G. P., & Butler, K. G. (1984). *Language learning disabilities in school-age children.* Baltimore: Williams & Wilkins.

Wallach, G. P., & Miller, L. (1988). *Language intervention & academic success.* Boston: College-Hill.

Yoshinaga-Itano, C. (1986). Beyond the sentence level: What's in a hearing-impaired child's story? *Topics in Language Disorders, 6*(3), 71–84.

Communication Access: Overview and Issues

Introduction

This chapter presents an overview of what the clinician needs to consider in determining a child's ability to access communication through both vision and hearing. Included is a discussion of communication access, a description of hearing and vision issues that affect communication access, and a description of various measures that can be taken to optimize communication access for a deaf or hard of hearing child. Also included is a brief discussion of communication access issues that are inherent in various educational settings.

WHAT IS COMMUNICATION ACCESS?

Communication access is defined as the means by which an individual is able to receive information for both learning and for face-to-face interactions with others. For both deaf and hearing children, access for day-to-day communication occurs primarily through both hearing and vision. While both of these modalities may be used, a significant difference exists among deaf, hard of hearing, and hearing children concerning the relative importance of one modality or the other. For a child who is deaf, there tends to be a greater reliance on vision to gain access to communication. Although a hard of hearing child may have some access to sound and hence more ability to use hearing for communication than the profoundly deaf child, there is still a greater reliance on vision for communication than is typical of hearing children.

A number of issues are related to ensuring that a child has adequate communication access. First and foremost, the child must have a minimum level of auditory and visual acuity to be able to access information for communicating. However, although acuity is necessary, it is not sufficient in and of itself to enable a deaf or hard of hearing child to effectively communicate. The child must also have linguistic knowledge of the communication form that relies on a particular auditory or visual modality. For example, although a child's vision may be "normal," without knowledge of spoken English, speechreading is not sufficient for gaining information. Inadequate or incomplete knowledge of American Sign Language (ASL) similarly limits the child's ability to have adequate access to that language form. Furthermore, the person with whom the child is communicating must also have adequate linguistic knowledge of the communication form being used by the child to ensure that communication will occur. If a visual language such as ASL is the expected form of communication, then those with whom the child is communicating must have a level of proficiency with ASL for the child to have access to appropriate linguistic context in these situations. Finally, many possible factors within the child's environment can impact the child's access to information. Things such as a noisy environment when audition is being relied upon or a visually distracting environment when the child relies on speechreading or signing can negatively impact the child's ability to access information.

HEARING CONSIDERATIONS

Working with a child with a hearing loss requires an understanding of every aspect of the child's hearing abilities. Each child will present unique hearing, listening, and understanding abilities, which in turn will determine that child's potential to access the world through hearing. It is recognized that numerous factors contribute to a child's hearing and listening development. These factors are discussed in the following section.

Age of Onset

The earlier the hearing loss occurs in the child's life, the greater is the impact on the child's development. The first 3 years in a child's life are critical for language acquisition (Hayes & Northern, 1996). Thus, the child with a profound hearing loss from birth will have different issues related to communication access than a child whose hearing loss occurs at a later age. The issue of access to both spoken and signed languages depends on the child receiving adequate input during these early years.

Age of Identification/Intervention

Until recently the average age of identification of hearing loss in the United States was 30 months (National Institutes of Health, 1993). Currently many states have implemented (or are in the process of implementing) Early Hearing Detection and Intervention programs that are identifying more babies who are deaf or hard of hearing shortly after birth (Joint Committee on Infant Hearing, 2002). Earlier identification in turn is leading to the provision of intervention services at a younger age than before. Although the full impact of early identification of children with a hearing loss is only now being realized, early identification is clearly an important step toward maximizing an individual child's access to communication. It is evident that early intervention will result in improved acquisition of language, and subsequently less negative impact of the hearing loss on the child's overall development (Yoshinago-Itano, 1999).

Type and Cause of Hearing Loss

The type and cause of a child's hearing loss will directly impact communication development. There are four types of hearing loss: conductive, sensorineural, mixed, and central (auditory processing disorder). Table 2-1 provides a description of the various types of losses, some possible causes, and the effect of each on both communication and treatment options (Rhodes, 1995).

Very different medical, educational, and habilitative concerns are associated with each of these different types of hearing loss. Knowing the type and cause of the child's hearing loss helps in determining the best possible course of action. This book specifically addresses the needs of children with conductive, sensorineural, or mixed hearing losses. There are excellent sources of information available that can assist the clinician in working with the child with central auditory difficulties (see resource list in Appendix A). Additionally, many of the principles involved in assessing and working with a child with other forms of hearing loss that are discussed in this text have value for the child with auditory processing problems.

Laterality and Symmetry of the Hearing Loss

A child can have a hearing loss in either one or both ears, and the effect on communication access is dramatically different in each case. If he has a loss in just one ear, it is referred to as a *unilateral* hearing loss; loss in both ears is referred to as *bilateral* hearing loss. If the hearing loss is similar in both ears it is called *symmetrical,* whereas a hearing loss that is different in each ear is referred to as an *asymmetrical hearing loss* (Stach, 1997).

Although a child with a unilateral hearing loss may develop spoken language normally, this is not necessarily the case. A unilateral loss may have a negative impact on a child's cognitive, academic, or social development (Culbertson & Gilbert, 1986). A recent study by Bess, Dodd-Murphy, and Parker (1998) has shown that children with minimal sensorineural hearing loss (unilateral or bilateral) typically experience more difficulty than hearing children on a series of educational and functional test measures.

It is also important to know whether the child has a symmetrical or asymmetrical hearing loss to understand the potential impact that loss may have on hearing. For example, a child with a flat moderate sensorineural hearing loss in the right ear and a severe-to-profound sensorineural hearing loss in the left ear will function quite differently from a child with a symmetrical, flat moderate sensorineural hearing loss.

Table 2-1 A Description of the Types of Hearing Loss

Type of Hearing Loss	Description	Possible Causes	Effect upon Communication	Treatment
Conductive	Hearing loss caused by a disruption of sound through the outer and/or middle ear	• Blockage of the ear canal (e.g., wax, foreign object) • Blockage of the eustachian tube opening (e.g., infection, allergy) • Damage to the eardrum • Congenital malformation of the outer and/or middle ear • Otitis media (middle ear fluid)	• Sounds seem dull or not loud enough (reduction of sounds at all frequencies) • Affects *audibility* (ability to detect the presence of speech) not *intelligibility* (ability to discriminate the word-sound distinctions of individual speech sounds (Flexer, 1999)) • Words and sentences can be heard and understood if made louder • Can result in delayed speech, language, and academic skills	Medical treatment might include: • Removing wax or foreign body • Giving medication for allergies/infection • Lancing the eardrum to drain fluid from the middle ear • Surgically repairing the damaged eardrum • Surgically replacing the middle ear bones (ossicles) • Fitting a hearing aid (possibly a bone conduction aid)
Sensorineural	Hearing loss due to sensory or nerve damage in the inner ear, the auditory nerve, and/or the brain stem	• Illness (e.g., spinal meningitis) • Heredity • Rh factor • Trauma • Exposure to extremely loud sound • Syndromes (e.g., Waardenburg) • Drugs • Prematurity	• Audibility vs. intelligibility; even if speech/sound is made loud enough it may not be intelligible (Flexer, 1999) • Not all speech sounds can be heard • Speech can be difficult or impossible to understand by listening alone	• Use of a hearing aid that will amplify the sound/speech but may not improve the quality of sound that is heard • Use of a cochlear implant that improves detection of sound, but does not guarantee recognition of speech without speechreading and training

Type	Definition	Causes	Effects/Characteristics	Interventions
Mixed	Hearing loss that occurs when both a conductive and sensorineural hearing loss are present	• Anoxia (lack of oxygen to the brain) • Same as for conductive and sensorineural; for example, a child with a sensorineural hearing loss (e.g., due to heredity) who also has otitis media will demonstrate a mixed hearing loss	• Will affect communication in the same way conductive and sensorineural hearing losses affect communication • May have an increased effect; for example, a child who is unable to use his hearing aid because of middle ear fluid	• Conductive hearing losses are treated medically • Use of hearing aid may not be possible while experiencing outer/middle ear problem
Central (auditory processing disorder)	Hearing loss due to damage of the auditory cortex and/or other parts of the brain used to process sound	• Anoxia • Prenatal infections • Birth trauma • Prematurity • Drugs • Rh factor • Brain diseases	• Poor concentration/attention span • Inconsistent response to sound • Difficulty following directions • Slow or delayed responses to verbal directions • Frequently asks for repetition • Misunderstands • Easily distracted • Difficulty listening in noise • Memory deficits • Relies on visual cues when attempting to communicate • Difficulty locating the source of sound	• Classroom accommodations • Amplification • Direct treatment • Compensatory strategies

Source: Adapted from Rhodes, L. (1995). *Introduction to deaf-blindness workshop.* Paper presented at the Central Missouri Deaf-Blind Task Force.

Stability of Hearing

A child's ability to hear may change from day to day or may show a progressive decline over time. Such fluctuations in hearing depend upon the cause of the hearing loss. A child with a conductive hearing loss due to middle ear fluid may experience hearing that *fluctuates* with the loss being greater when middle ear fluid is present. A child with a congenital *progressive* sensorineural hearing loss will experience diminishing access to spoken language as hearing sensitivity changes. Because the child's hearing acuity actually changes with time, amplification needs and requirements will also change. It is thus important to audiologically track the child with a progressive hearing loss both to monitor the change and to ensure that the child's hearing is appropriately amplified.

Audiologic Information

It is important that the professional working with the child understands the results from a recent audiologic evaluation (performed within the last 12 months). Results from the audiologic evaluation are recorded on an audiogram as depicted in Figure 2-1, which typically contains three components: pure tone testing results, speech audiometry findings, and immittance results. The audiogram provides useful information about the type, laterality, degree, and configuration of the hearing loss. The following is a description of each of the above components as well as the implications of each for a child with hearing loss.

Pure Tone Testing

The audiogram is a graph that the audiologist uses to chart what the child is able to hear. Response to frequencies/tones ranging from 250 through 8000 Hz are plotted along the horizontal axis and intensity thresholds for each frequency measured in decibels (dB hearing level [HL]) are plotted along the vertical dimension. The higher the decibel level is, the more intense the sound. The least intense sound that the child is able to hear is called the *auditory threshold* (Stach, 1997). On the audiogram all sounds that are greater in intensity than the child's threshold (toward the bottom of the graph) will be audible. Sounds with less intensity than those at the child's threshold (toward the top of the audiogram) will not be audible.

Audiologic testing is performed in a sound-isolated test booth so that the audiologist can assess the child's ability to detect very low intensity sounds without interference from environmental noise (Flexer, 1999). The audiologist uses an audiometer to present calibrated sounds to the child. Pure tone testing is done in three ways: by air conduction (AC) (testing done while the child wears headphones or ear inserts), by bone conduction (BC) (testing done using a bone vibrator placed behind the ear or on the forehead), and in sound field (SF). The child listens to various frequency tones (measured in Hertz [Hz]), and the audiologist notes the lowest decibel level at which the child is able to hear each frequency/tone presented (auditory threshold levels).

To plot the child's responses to pure tone test results on an audiogram, the audiologist uses different symbols. All audiograms have a key or legend that can

GALLAUDET UNIVERSITY AUDIOLOGY CLINIC, Mary Thornberry Building
800 Florida Avenue, NE, Washington, DC 20002-3695 (202) 651-5328 (V/TTY) (202) 651-5324 (FAX)   Audiologist: _____

Name:_____ Date:_____ Age:_____ Sex:_____   Transducer: headphones insert

DOB:_____ Referred by:_____   Response
Reliability: good   moderate   poor

AUDIOMETER:_____   IMMITTANCE METER:_____

LEGEND

	Right	Left
Air: Unmasked	○	✶
Masked	△	▢
Bone: Unmasked	◁	▷
Masked		

No Response ▼
Best Bone ▢
Vibrotactile Response ✶
Unaided Sound Field S
Narrow Band Noise
Warble Tone

AUDIOGRAM
FREQUENCY (PITCH) IN HERTZ (Hz)

125   250   500   1000   2000   4000   8000

HEARING LEVEL (LOUDNESS) IN DECIBELS (dB)   ANSI 1992

0
10
20
30
40
50
60
70
80
90
100
110
120

Air Conduction   R L R L R L R L R L R L R L
Bone Conduction

PURE TONE AVERAGE   (R: ___ L: ___)

	Right	Left
AIR	dBHL	dBHL

TYMPANOMETRY (daPa)

daPa   Right Left
C₁=
SC=

ABBREVIATIONS
C1 Canal Volume
CNA Could Not Average
CNE Could Not Establish
CNT Could Not Test
DNT Did Not Test
HL Hearing Level
MLV Monitored Live Voice
MTS Monosyllable, Troches, Spondees Test
MCL Most Comfortable Listening Level
NR No Response
PB% Word Recognition
SC Static Compliance
SDT Speech Detection Threshold
SRT Speech Recognition Threshold
S/N Signal To Noise Ratio
UCL Uncomfortable Listening Level

ACOUSTIC REFLEX MEASUREMENTS

Ear	Right				Left			
Stimulus	.5K	1K	2K	4K	.5K	1K	2K	4K
Contra (HL)								
Decay								
Ipsi (HL) (SPL)								

SPEECH AUDIOMETRY (dBHL)   MLV ☐   RECORDED ☐   LIST: _____

	SDT	SRT	MCL	UCL	PB% / HL	PB% / HL	PB% / HL	SIGNAL NOISE / HL	MTS Categ% / Recog%
R					/	/	/	%	/
L					/	/	/	%	/
SF UNAIDED					/	/	/	%	/
AIDED					/	/	/	%	/

TEST INTERPRETATION:

TYPE: R   L
☐ No Hearing Loss ___   ___
☐ Conductive   ___   ___
☐ Mixed   ___   ___
☐ Sensorineural   ___   ___

DEGREE
R: _____

L: _____

RECOMMENDATION(S)
☐ Medical Referral
☐ Recheck Following Consultation
☐ Special Tests_____
☐ Hearing Aid Evaluation

COMMENTS:_____

☐ New earmold(s)
☐ Hearing Aid Check
☐ See Hearing Aid Worksheet
☐ Annual Reevaluation
☐ Other (Specify): _____

_____   _____
Supervising Audiologist, CCC-A   Graduate Clinician

98-290M

Figure 2-1.   Gallaudet University Audiogram

Source: Courtesy of Gallaudet University, Department of Audiology and Speech-Language Pathology.

be used to understand the symbols (Table 2-2). On most audiograms AC test results are plotted using O's to indicate the right ear responses and X's to indicate the left ear responses. BC results are plotted using an arrow opening to the left for the left ear and opening to the right for the right ear. Because a sound presented

Table 2-2.	Symbols and Terms Used to Describe Pure Tone Thresholds under Various Conditions	

Abbreviation	Meaning	Symbol
AC	Air conduction threshold	X (left ear); O (right ear)
BC	Bone conduction threshold	> (left ear); < (right ear)
SF	Sound field threshold	A (with amplification) C (with cochlear implants) S (unaided)
	Masked bone threshold	] (left ear); [(right ear)
	Masked air conduction thresholds	□ (left ear tested); △ (right ear tested)

by BC can be detected by both the ear being tested and the contralateral, nontest ear, it is sometimes necessary to present noise to the ear not being tested to isolate hearing results to the test ear. This is known as *masking*. Masked BC threshold results are plotted on the audiogram using rectangles open on one side (to the left for the left ear and to the right for the right ear). If masking is used during AC testing, a triangle is used when the right ear is the test ear and the left ear is masked (noise presented through the left headphone), and an open box is used when the left ear is the test ear and the right ear is masked. If the child is tested in SF, the symbol "S" is used to plot results. If testing is done in SF while the child is using a hearing aid(s), often the symbol "A" is used to plot the results ("C" may indicate results with a cochlear implant).

Typically the frequencies/tones presented during an audiologic evaluation are spaced in octave intervals from 250 through 8000 Hz. These frequencies are used because, collectively, they comprise speech sounds. For example, if a child is only able to detect the low frequencies (250 to 500 Hz), then he is only able to hear oral-nasal differences, some vowel sounds, and the prosody of speech. If he is able to detect frequencies through 2000 Hz, then most vowels and consonants (except /s/ and /z/) would be audible (Flexer, 1999).

The *pure tone average* refers to the average of the three speech frequencies (500, 1000, and 2000 Hz). It can be calculated for AC, BC, and SF responses. These three frequencies are used because it is believed that they carry most of the information necessary for understanding speech. This is because much of the information contained in the speech signal is in the high frequencies. When pure tone thresholds fall sharply in the high frequencies, the three-frequency average may lead to overestimation of the child's threshold level for hearing speech. In such cases, the pure tone average is calculated using the best two of the three speech frequencies (Lloyd & Kaplan, 1993). Whether using two or three frequencies for the child with a sensorineural hearing loss, one expects that the pure tone average threshold will approximate the child's speech recognition threshold (to be described later).

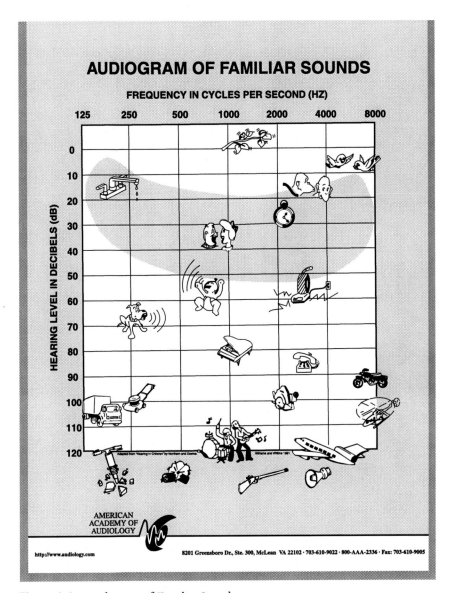

Figure 2-2. Audiogram of Familiar Sounds

Source: Courtesy of the American Academy of Audiology.

Figure 2-2 is an audiogram with various speech sounds and familiar environmental sounds superimposed. The shaded area is known as the *speech banana*. The speech banana indicates the approximate frequency and intensity levels of conversational speech. The child's pure tone responses and aided responses should be plotted on this type of audiogram to determine which speech and environmental sounds the child has the potential to access given that the speaker is

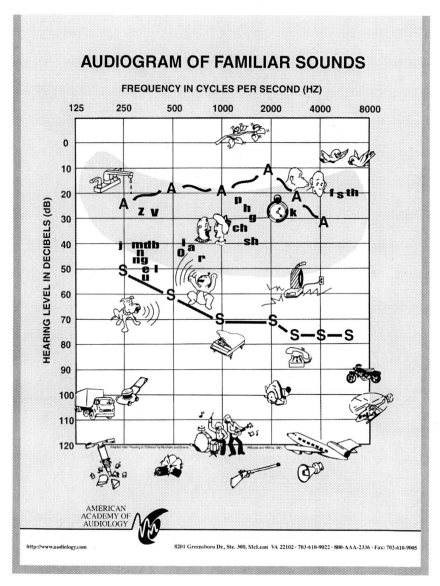

Figure 2-3. Audiogram of Familiar Sounds with Aided and Unaided Responses
Plotted

Source: Courtesy of the American Academy of Audiology.

close to the child, the environment is quiet, and the child is attending (Flexer,
1999). Figure 2-3 shows a sample audiogram of a child tested in SF in the aided
(A) and unaided conditions (S). Results are plotted on the audiogram of familiar
sounds. Note that without amplification conversational speech is not audible, but
many environmental sounds are. With amplification the child has the acuity

Table 2-3 Degree of Hearing Loss and Impact upon Communication

Hearing Levels (dB HL)	Classification (Degree)	Communicative Effect
10 to 10	Normal	None
11 to 25	Minimal	Difficulty hearing quiet speech in the presence of noise
25 to 40	Mild	Difficulty hearing quiet or distant speech, even in quiet
40 to 55	Moderate	Conversational speech is audible if at a close distance
55 to 70	Moderately severe	Loud conversational speech is audible
70 to 90	Severe	Conversational speech is not audible
>90	Profound	Loud sounds may be audible

Source: Stach, B. A. (1998). *Clinical audiology: An introduction.* Clifton Park, NY: Singular.

needed to access speech sounds during conversational speech. It should be noted, however, that even with acuity, or the ability to detect or sense sounds at a particular frequency, the child may still have difficulty interpreting speech sounds in that frequency range.

Degree of Hearing Loss

Table 2-3 depicts a classification system used to describe the decibel levels associated with varying degrees of hearing loss. This system applies to both pure tone and speech results. To estimate the communicative effect or degree, the mean of the three speech frequencies (500, 1000, and 2000 Hz) for the better ear is established (Lloyd & Kaplan, 1993). If there is a sharply sloping configuration, it is more appropriate to use the best two of the speech frequencies. This classification system is also used to describe hearing levels at various frequency ranges in one or both ears. For example, a child may exhibit a moderate hearing loss in the right ear and a severe to profound hearing loss with no responses (at equipment limits) beyond 3000 Hz in the left ear.

Whereas the categorization system is often used to describe the *communicative* effect of a hearing loss, the system can often be less than adequate for characterizing a child's access to speech. Those working with children who are deaf or hard of hearing often encounter children whose audiograms might suggest a level of functioning that differs considerably from the way the child is actually communicating. Two children might have pure tone thresholds that are identical and hence have identical descriptions of their degree of loss, yet one child might have greater or lesser access to speech than the thresholds suggest. It is important to look beyond the audiogram to develop an accurate picture of how useful hearing can be for communication by an individual child.

Table 2-4. Configuration of Hearing Loss	
Term Used to Describe Configuration	*Description of Configuration**
Flat	Thresholds are within 20 dB of each other across frequency range
Rising	Thresholds for low frequencies are at least 20 dB poorer than those for high frequencies
Sloping	Thresholds for high frequencies are at least 20 dB poorer than those for lower frequencies
Low frequency	Hearing loss is restricted to the low-frequency area on the audiogram
High-frequency	Hearing loss is restricted to the high-frequency area on the audiogram
Precipitous	Steeply sloping high-frequency hearing loss of at least 20 dB per octave
Trough "cookie bite" (Lloyd & Kaplan, 1993)	20 dB or greater loss at 1000 Hz or 2000 Hz than at 500 and 4000 Hz or both

*The primary frequencies considered in describing the audiometric configuration are 500 to 4000 Hz.

Source: Stach, B. A. (1998). *Clinical audiology: An introduction.* Clifton Park, NY: Singular; and Lloyd, L., & Kaplan, H. (1993). *Audiometric interpretation: A manual of basic audiometry.* Baltimore, MD: University Park Press.

Audiometric Configuration

In addition to the type and degree, the child's hearing loss may also be described according to the overall shape of the threshold curves plotted on the audiogram, or *audiometric configuration* (Table 2-4). The configuration of the hearing loss can provide additional information concerning the amount of access the child has to spoken language. For example, if a child has a gradually falling mild to profound sensorineural hearing loss, he may miss parts of words or sentences, making it difficult for him to understand what he hears, especially in the presence of background noise.

Speech Audiometry

Perhaps the best indicator of a child's access to spoken language lies in the results obtained from speech audiometry. The speech detection threshold is the lowest decibel level at which the child is able to detect speech (not understand what was said). The speech recognition threshold (SRT) is the lowest decibel level at which the child is able to respond correctly to 50% of the two-syllable words presented (e.g., hot dog, baseball, or ice cream). The most comfortable loudness level (MCL) is the decibel level that represents the most comfortable level for the child to listen to connected speech. The MCL is usually established before further speech testing. The uncomfortable loudness level (UCL) represents the threshold of discomfort for the child. The difference in decibels between the child's SRT and UCL is referred to as the dynamic range (UCL − SRT = DR). The dynamic range represents the range between the lower and upper limits of useful hearing (Lloyd & Kaplan, 1993) and is helpful in selecting and fitting hearing aid(s). Many deaf and hard of hearing children, in addition to having higher thresholds of hearing, also have a reduced dynamic range (meaning that the decibel difference between the UCL and SRT is small). If a child has a reduced dynamic range, sound will become uncomfortably loud very quickly. The child may have difficulty wearing a hearing aid unless the range of amplitude can be compressed to keep the amplified speech below the child's UCL.

Word recognition testing (speech discrimination) assesses the child's ability to identify words presented by the audiologist at the child's MCL or 30 to 40 dB above the child's SRT. Word recognition tests designed for use with school-aged children with hearing loss can be open set or closed set. Open set tests do not provide any visual cues to facilitate the child's response (e.g., PB Kindergarten Lists and NU #6 word lists); the child repeats the word that he hears. Closed set tests provide visual cues (e.g., pictures or word lists) from which the child may select a response (e.g., Word Intelligibility by Picture Identification [WIPI] and Northwestern University Children's Perception of Speech [NU-CHIPS]). The choice of word recognition tests will depend upon the age and vocabulary level of the child (Johnson, Benson, & Seaton, 1997). For both open and closed set testing a percentage correct score is obtained.

Speech audiometry test results can provide useful information, but there are a few limitations that one should keep in mind. Because testing is done under optimal listening conditions, it may be an overestimate of the child's functioning in daily listening environments (Ross, 1990). Moreover, the nature of most speech testing is linguistic. If a child has limited English language skills, then speech test results may reflect not only hearing acuity but also the child's limited knowledge of English.

Immittance Testing

An important part of the audiologic test battery is immittance testing. Immittance testing is an objective measure of middle ear function (Flexer, 1999). This testing helps the audiologist determine the type of hearing loss (conductive or sensorineural) evidenced by the child. Immittance audiometry includes tympanometry, ear canal volume, and acoustic reflexes. Interpretation of immittance results indicates the child's middle ear functioning on the day of the test (Flexer, 1999). For example, if the audiogram for a given child is several months old and the child had a middle ear infection (otitis media) on the day of the test that has since resolved, the immittance results may no longer be valid.

Tympanometry measures the compliance or mobility of the tympanic membrane (eardrum) and middle ear system as air pressure is mechanically varied in the ear canal. The compliance/mobility of the tympanic membrane is plotted on a tympanogram. Tympanometry enables the audiologist to differentiate the normally mobile system from the nonmobile system (Hayes & Northern, 1996). Figure 2-4 shows the different types of tympanograms and their interpretation (Northern & Downs, 1991; Stach, 1998).

Tympanogram	Pressure	Mobility	Meaning
Type A	Normal	Normal	Normal middle ear function
Type As	Normal	Low	"s" = stiffness or shallowness
Type Ad	Normal	High	"d" = discontinuity Floppy eardrum; a break or discontinuity in the middle ear bones connecting the eardrum to the cochlea
Type B	Flat	Low	Fluid draining from the middle ear or thickened eardrum; and/or immobile middle ear bones; and/or fluid in the middle ear
Type C	Negative	Normal	High negative pressure (eardrum pulled into the middle ear); eustachian tube malfunction (with or without fluid draining)

Figure 2-4. Interpretation of Tympanograms

Source: Adapted from Northern, J. L., & Downs, M. (1991). *Hearing in children* (4th ed.). Baltimore: Williams & Wilkins; and Stach, B. A. (1998). *Clinical audiology: An introduction.* Clifton Park, NY: Singular.)

Table 2-5. Interpretation of Tympanograms and Equivalent Ear Canal Volume

Tympanogram Type	Physical Volume	Indication
Type A	0.8–1.0	Normal middle ear
Type B	< 0.3	Wax blocking ear canal
Type B	0.8–1.0	Middle ear fluid
Type B	> 2.5	Perforation in the eardrum; or open ear tube
Type C	0.8–1.0	Negative middle ear pressure; eustachian tube not functioning properly

Source: Adapted from Northern, J. L., & Downs, M. (1991). *Hearing in children* (4th ed.). Baltimore: Williams & Wilkins.

Using the same equipment as for tympanometry (immittance meter), it is also possible to measure equivalent ear canal volume. This test measures the volume of air between the immittance probe tip and the tympanic membrane in cubic centimeters. Equivalent ear volume measures enable the audiologist to better interpret tympanometry results. For example, if the child has a flat tympanogram and the ear canal volume is reduced, middle ear fluid may be present. Table 2-5 indicates tympanometry results, equivalent ear canal volumes, and the interpretation of various combinations of tympanogram types and volumes.

Acoustic reflex testing is the measurement of the decibel level at which the stapedius muscle contracts. The stapedius muscle is a small, middle ear muscle that connects the stapes (middle ear bone) to the wall of the middle ear. By measuring the decibel levels at which the muscle contracts and the reflex is measured, the audiologist can obtain additional insight into the type and degree of hearing loss. For example, if the child has a conductive hearing loss caused by fluid in the middle ear, the reflexes will be absent. If the child has a mild sensorineural hearing loss, the reflexes will be present but elevated (Northern & Downs, 1991).

The preceding section has described how various pieces of audiologic data can provide useful information about the potential a child may have to access spoken language through audition. When questions arise about a child's access to sound, the child's audiologist or the school audiologist should be consulted.

For many children who are deaf or hard of hearing, however, vision plays an equal, or greater, role. The following section details some of the vision considerations that have an impact on communication access.

VISION CONSIDERATIONS

A child with a hearing loss may have to depend upon his vision either as a primary source of information (as in the case of the child who is deaf and relying on sign language) or as a supplement to residual hearing (as in the case of the child who

Table 2-6. Summary of Visual Functioning Problems

Visual Functioning	Description of Possible Problems with Visual Functioning:
Visual acuity	The child does not see as clearly as he should; images are not sharp.
Visual field	The area that the child can see (above, below, to the sides, and straight ahead) is limited when holding his/her head and eyes still.
Contrast sensitivity	The child is unable to see the difference between lightness and darkness of objects (e.g., like looking at a faded photograph).
Ocular motor control	The child is unable to see the relative difference between the lightness and darkness of objects; muscular imbalance (e.g., wandering eye).
Visual processing	The child's brain is having difficulty making sense out of what he is seeing.

Source: Rhodes, L. (1995). *Introduction to deaf-blindness workshop.* Paper presented at the Central Missouri Deaf-Blind Task Force.

is hard of hearing and relies on hearing and speechreading). Because vision can be so critical for the deaf or hard of hearing child, it is important that difficulties in visual functioning be identified so that resultant reductions in access can be addressed. Visual access requires appropriate functioning of the visual system, ranging from visual acuity to visual processing. Table 2-6 summarizes some important aspects of visual functioning and some problems that can be found in each aspect (Rhodes, 1995).

A child experiencing vision problems may demonstrate certain behaviors, complaints, or visible symptoms that suggest a vision problem. Table 2-7 summarizes some of the behaviors, complaints, or visible symptoms to look for that might suggest a vision problem in children.

Ensuring that the child's visual system is healthy is extremely important. Remember that even for the deaf or hard of hearing child with normal visual functioning it is exhausting to listen and watch (lips/signs) for extended periods of time. Questions or concerns about a child's visual functioning should be referred to the school nurse, a parent, an occupational therapist, an ophthalmologist, or another appropriate professional.

OPTIMIZING COMMUNICATION ACCESS

This next section addresses measures that can be taken to optimize communication access through the child's hearing and vision. An overview of auditory technologies (hearing aids, tactile aids, cochlear implants, and assistive listening devices) and visual technologies (to address the child's four basic communication needs: face-to-face communication, reception of broadcast media, telephone communication, and an awareness to environmental sounds) will be presented. Implementation of both auditory and visual technologies is discussed in the section on enhancing the environment.

| **Table 2-7.** Behaviors, Complaints, and Visual Symptoms Associated with Visual Problems |||

Behaviors	*Complaints*	*Visual Symptoms*
• Does the child try to brush away a blur, rub eyes all the time?	• Child complains of dizziness, headaches or nausea after close work	• Red rimmed, crusted or swollen eye lids
• Does the child stumble or trip over small objects?	• Child complains of double or blurred vision	• Repeated styes
• Does the child blink more than usual, or is irritable while doing close work?		• Watery or red eyes
• Does the child hold his book close to his eyes?		• Crossed eyes, or a wandering eye
• Does the child cover one eye or tilt his head when looking at something?		
• Does the child have difficulty reading?		
• Does the child who uses sign language miss or misinterpret signs frequently?		
• Does the child who uses Cued Speech miss or misinterpret cues frequently?		
• -Is the child uninterested in distant objects?		
• -Does the child hold his body tense or screw up his face when doing close work?		
• Is the child unable to distinguish colors?		

Source: Adapted from http://www.children-special-needs.org.

Auditory Access and Technology

Many children with hearing loss will use some type of technology to provide them with better access to auditory information. Even a child with a mild hearing loss may need some assistance in very noisy situations. The following section provides information about the types of assistive technologies most commonly used by school-aged children with hearing loss to gain access to sound.

Hearing Aids

A hearing aid amplifies and shapes incoming sounds to make them audible to the child. This amplification device is tuned specifically to the child's hearing loss.

The behind the ear (BTE) or ear-level hearing aid is most commonly used by school-aged children (Northern & Downs, 1991). The BTE aid is coupled to the child's ear via an earmold. The earmold is a custom-made earpiece that directs the sound from the hearing aid to the child's ear (Flexer, 1999). Earmolds should be comfortable and fit properly. Symptoms of a poorly fitted earmold are discomfort to the child or feedback.

Today there are two general categories of hearing aid technology: analog (conventional) and digital (programmable). Conventional hearing aids amplify sound and provide and allow for some manipulation of the amplified signal. Although appropriate for certain types of hearing loss, conventional hearing aids may not provide adequate amplification for children with severe to profound high-frequency hearing losses nor do they compensate for distance and noisy listening situations. Programmable hearing aids are able to be custom fit to the child's individual loss with a program selection that adjusts to difficult listening situations. Programmable/digital aids, however, are significantly more expensive than conventional aids.

Regardless of whether the child is using a conventional or programmable/digital hearing aid, it should be equipped with a strong telecoil or telecoil program. The telecoil is an internal coil of wire that receives electromagnetic energy. Because some telephones and audio loops generate an electromagnetic signal that carries a speech signal, the telecoil provides a convenient way of getting a signal directly into the amplification circuitry of the hearing aid, bypassing the microphone (Berg, 1993). This provides a better, clearer signal to the listener.

The telecoil is activated on conventional hearing aids by the "T" or "M/T" setting on the M-T-O or M-M/T-O switch on the outside of the hearing aid. Most programmable/digital hearing aids have a telecoil program. The telecoil can also be used in conjunction with an assistive listening device.

Another important option for the BTE aid is direct audio input (DAI) capability. Figure 2-5 shows a BTE hearing aid with a DAI boot/audio shoe attachment. The child's hearing aid could be coupled to an assistive listening device by using a DAI boot/audio shoe and the appropriate wire and jack. Both a strong telecoil and DAI options are important for children who use the voice telephone and an assistive listening device (e.g., an frequency-modulated [FM] system). These options are important especially when the child is using his hearing aid/assistive listening device while working on developing/enhancing communication skills.

Another type of BTE hearing aid that is being fit to children with severe to profound sensorineural hearing losses is a frequency transposition hearing aid. This type of hearing aid alters high-frequency sounds by compressing them into the lower-frequency range of usable hearing that is characteristic of children with severe to profound hearing losses (Johnson et al., 1997). Many children using this type of hearing aid have shown significant improvements in their sound and speech reception abilities through extensive training with the device (Johnson & Rees, 1995). Frequency transposition hearing aids have been used as an alternative to a cochlear implant device for some children (Johnson et al., 1997).

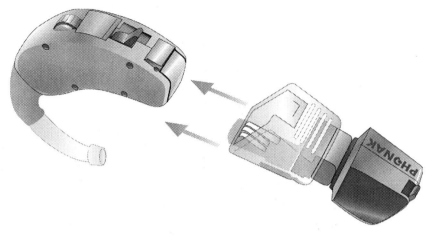

Figure 2-5. BTE Hearing Aid with Direct Audio Input
Source: Courtesy of Phonak.

The success or failure of any appropriately fit hearing aid depends on its consistent use and functioning and a favorable listening environment. Studies have shown that 50% of the hearing aids worn by school-aged children are functioning poorly at any given time (Elfenbein, Bentler, Davis, & Neibuhr, 1988). Hearing aids need to be monitored daily, and a ready supply of batteries should be available. Appendix B provides instructions for checking a BTE hearing aid. Students should be encouraged to be active participants in the monitoring and troubleshooting process with the long-term goal being independence. The functional listening check described in appendix B should be performed after troubleshooting the hearing aid.

Tactile Aids

Tactile aids are vibrotactile devices that receive and convert sound energy to vibrotactile signals to a body-worn processor, which then sends the information through a cord to a stimulator array worn on the skin (typically on the chest or the wrist). Studies have shown that devices that provide speech information tactilely can enhance speechreading and that children with little or no residual hearing may benefit more from a tactile aid than they do from a conventional hearing aid (Weisenberger & Miller, 1987).

The most common vibrotactile aid used is the Tactaid (pictured in Figure 2-6). For some children with multiple disabilities, including hearing loss or those who are deaf-blind, the Tactaid has proven quite useful as a means of connecting the child to his environment. The Tactaid has also been used as a therapy tool for speech development, providing tactile representation of segmental and suprasegmental features as a supplement to auditory input (Johnson et al., 1997).

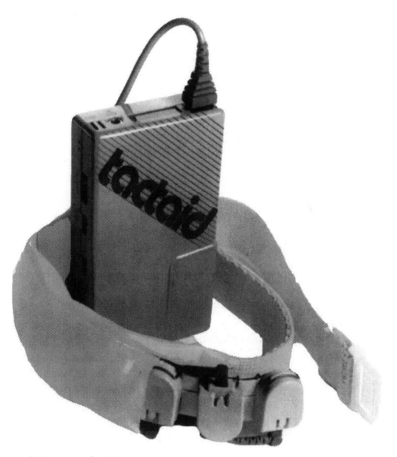

Figure 2-6.   Tactaid 2000
Source: Courtesy of the Audiological Engineering Corp.

Cochlear Implants

Cochlear implants, which represent relatively recent technology, provide the individual with sound, but in a way that differs from a hearing aid. Whereas a hearing aid primarily makes sounds louder, the implant bypasses much of the hearing mechanism of the individual and provides electrical stimulation to the auditory nerve. This device has provided an alternative to individuals with severe to profound hearing loss who do not benefit from amplification. Although results have varied, the technology holds great promise for those who would not have had access to sound in the past.

The cochlear implant pictured in Figure 2-7 is an electronic device comprising a surgically implanted receiver and electrode array and an external transmitter coil, microphone, and speech processor. A microphone attached near the ear picks up sound and changes it to an electrical signal that is sent through a cable to

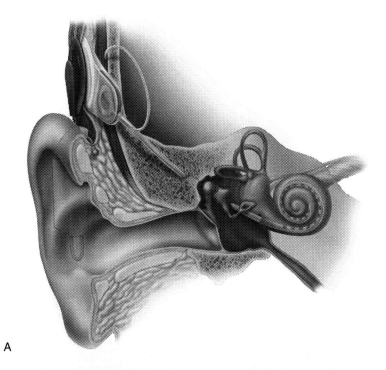

A

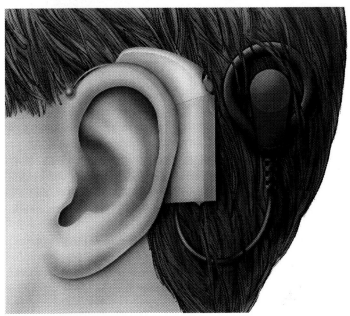

B

Figure 2-7.   Internal (A) and External (B) Components of a Cochlear Implant System

Source: Courtesy of Cochlear, LTD.

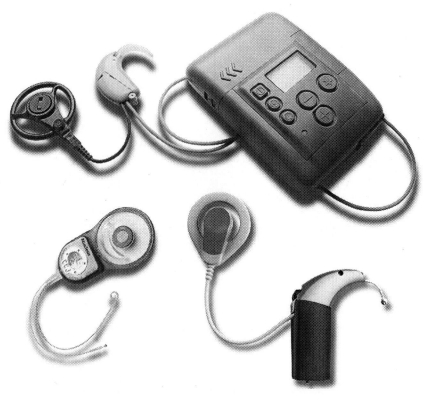

Figure 2-8. Two Types of Cochlelar Implant Speech Processors
Source: Courtesy of Cochlear, Ltd.

an externally worn speech processor. The speech processor digitizes and encodes the signal as a series of electrical pulses. The encoded information, together with the power to operate the implant, is transmitted through the skin by radiofrequency transmission to the implanted receiver-stimulator. The implanted portion is composed of a small button that is embedded in the bone behind the ear (the receiver) and a set of tiny electrodes (the stimulator) that is inserted into the snail-like cochlea. The receiver-stimulator decodes the signal and sends patterns of stimuli to the electrodes within the cochlea to provide stimulation to discrete groups of auditory nerve fibers for higher auditory brain processing (Clark, Cowan, & Dowell, 1997). There are two different speech processors available: one worn as an earlevel device (similar to a BTE hearing aid) and one worn on the body (Johnson et al., 1997). Figure 2-8 shows two different types of cochlear implants and their components.

Once the child is fitted with the external components of the cochlear implant, the speech processor must be programmed or "mapped" by the audiologist. To begin the process, the child's speech processor is connected to the computer.

The audiologist establishes the child's threshold levels (T levels), comfort levels (C levels), and "flags" (turns off) electrodes that might cause problems. The map is determined by setting each of the electrodes to be loud enough for the child to be aware of a sound but not too loud as to cause discomfort. The child's responses are obtained using pediatric hearing evaluation techniques appropriate to the child's age (e.g., behavioral observation audiometry, visual reinforcement audiometry, or play audiometry). During the mapping session, the audiologist will also determine the speech processing strategy to use, the volume setting, the sensitivity setting, program choices (more than one map may be set in a speech processor), and locks and controls (to prohibit children from changing settings inadvertently) (Nussbaum, 2003).

Professionals working with children with cochlear implants need to know how to monitor the implant. Daily monitoring requires that the professionals and the child (depending upon the child's age) know the parts of the implant and how they work. Professionals need to be aware of the child's usual responses while wearing the implant. If a child has consistently responded to speech sounds and then stops, there could be a problem with the device that will require technical troubleshooting. Appendix B ("Troubleshooting Technology") shows a troubleshooting checklist (hardware check) for the Clarion implant. It is apparent that those working with a child who has a cochlear implant should be familiar with the various knobs and settings of the particular device being used. A functional listening check for monitoring the child's performance with the cochlear implant as well as behavioral indicators that might suggest a malfunctioning cochlear implant are also described in appendix B.

Assistive Listening Devices

Whereas hearing aids and cochlear implants can greatly enhance the child's potential for access to spoken language, real-world conditions often reduce the effectiveness of these devices. Conditions such as noise, distance from the speaker and reverberation (echo) will negatively impact the quality of the speech signal and the amount of access the child has to spoken communication. Assistive listening devices are devices that can be used alone or coupled to the child's hearing aid or cochlear implant and function like "binoculars for the ears" (Compton, 2000). Two assistive listening devices that are commonly found in the school setting are personal FM and classroom amplification systems.

Personal FM systems.   The personal FM system relies on FM radiowaves to send a signal from the speaker (using a remote microphone/transmitter) to a receiver coupled to the child's ear in a variety of ways. The microphone/transmitter picks up the desired signal and then transmits it via a radiowave to a receiver worn by the child. The child may use headphones or earbuds, or the receiver could be coupled to the child's personal amplification system or cochlear implant. Figure 2-9 shows a few different ways of coupling the FM system to a personal amplification system. One approach to coupling an FM system to a personal hearing aid is through the use of a teleloop. The teleloop provides speech information in an

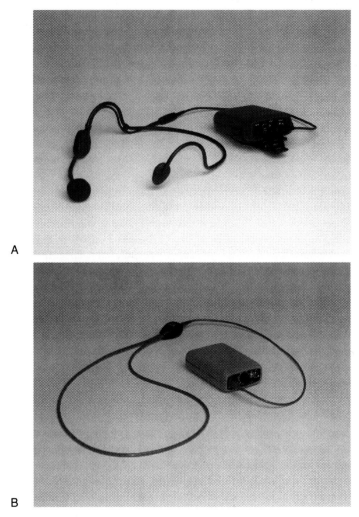

Figure 2-9. FM Receiver Coupling Options. (A) Earbuds; (B) Neckloop.

(*continues*)

electromagnetic field that can be picked up by using the "T" switch on the hearing aid or telecoil program (for digital aids) (Compton, 2000). Although this arrangement enhances the signal to noise ratio, it can be somewhat limiting for classroom use because the child may be unable to hear his own voice or the speech of other students because his hearing aid microphone may not be activated. To avoid this problem, an additional environmental microphone is often recommended in classroom situations.

Various wireless microphone and transmitter options are shown in Figure 2-10. The microphone and transmitter can be housed in the same case and worn around the neck, or the transmitter can be coupled to the microphone (lapel or

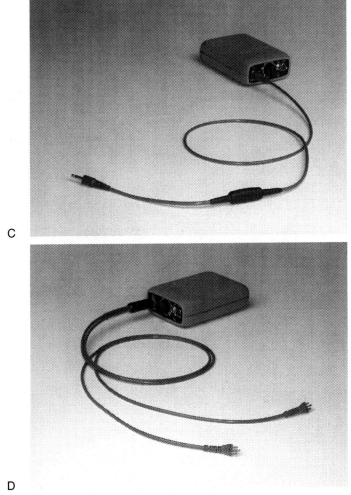

Figure 2-9. (continued)   (C) Direct Audio Input; (D) Cochlear Implant Cable
Source: Courtesy of COMTEK.

head worn) via a cord (Berg, 1993). For group situations, in which children are sitting around a table, a conference table microphone adapter could be coupled to the transmitter. This type of microphone directs the speech from those sitting around the table to the transmitter and then to the receiver(s).

Recently, personal FM systems have been developed that can be worn by the user entirely behind the ear, much like a BTE hearing aid (Figure 2-11). Self-contained FM systems use the same type of microphone/transmitter as the personal FM systems, but the receivers are usually worn in place of the child's personal hearing aid. The internal controls are adjusted to the degree and configuration of the child's hearing loss. Alternatively, the FM signal can be conveyed

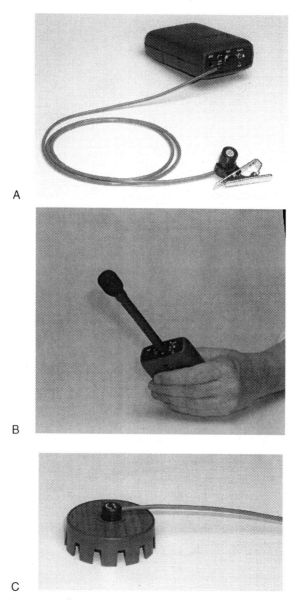

Figure 2-10.   Types of Wireless Microphones with FM Transmitters. (A) Lapel
Microphone; (B) Handheld Microphone; (C) Conference Microphone
Source: Courtesy of COMTEK.

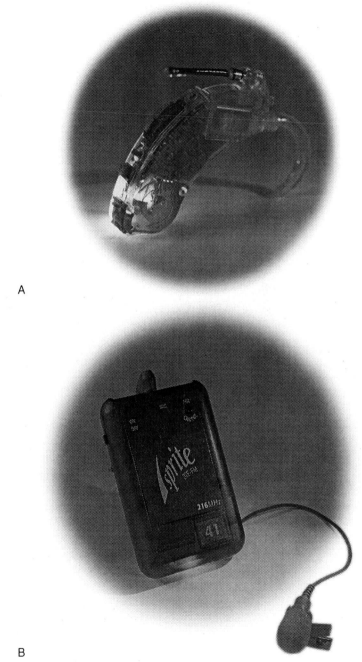

A

B

Figure 2-11. PE800R Sprite Hearing Aid (A) with Built-in FM Receiver (B)
Source: Courtesy of Phonic Ear, Inc.

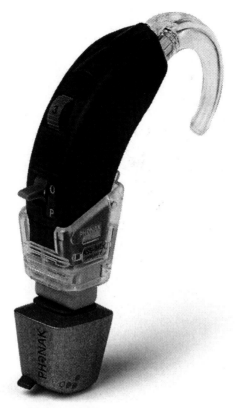

Figure 2-12. BTE with FM Boot (Microlink)
Source: Courtesy of Phonak.

to a personal hearing aid through a DAI boot/audio shoe, which functions as the receiver (Figure 2-12). Some of the new digital hearing aids now incorporate FM technology into the functioning of the hearing aid (Figure 2-13).

It is important to note that if a child is using a personal FM system coupled to his hearing aid, the effectiveness of the system depends on the functioning of the child's hearing aid(s). Troubleshooting of the FM system should always begin by first troubleshooting the child's hearing aid(s) (discussed in appendix B). Once one knows that the hearing aid is functioning properly then the FM system is connected and a listening check is done to be sure the FM signal is present. After listening to the system, one can then perform a functional listening check while the child is using the FM system. A child with a cochlear implant can also use a personal FM system by using a patch cord connecting the speech processor (via an auxiliary jack) to the body-worn receiver. To troubleshoot the self-contained FM system, one can follow the same steps used for troubleshooting the child's hearing aid(s).

Classroom Amplification Systems. Classroom amplification systems are wireless high-fidelity public address systems that are self-contained within a classroom (Crandell, Smaldino, & Flexer, 2005). The teacher uses a wireless FM microphone transmitter (similar to the one used in the personal FM system). The

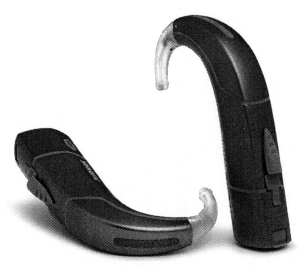

Figure 2-13. BTE Claro (Hearing Aid with FM Technology)
Source: Courtesy of Phonak.

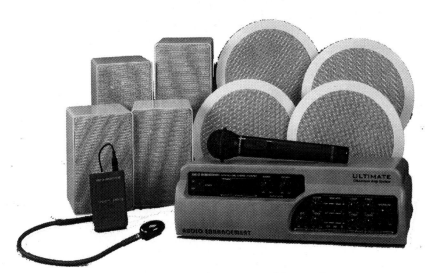

Figure 2-14. Components of a Large Classroom Amplification System
Source: Courtesy of Audio Enhancement.

teacher's speech would then be transmitted by a radio signal, picked up by a receiver/amplifier, and broadcast through a speaker or speakers (one to five floor-, wall-, or ceiling-mounted loudspeakers) for the entire class to hear. The amplified teacher's voice overcomes poor room acoustics (e.g., noise or reverberation) and mild hearing loss to make it easier for students to concentrate on what the teacher is saying regardless of where the child is seated. Figure 2-14 shows the

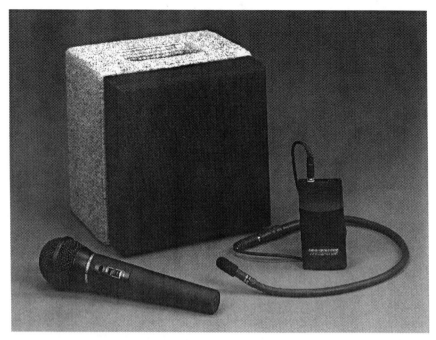

Figure 2-15.   Components of a Portable/Compact Classroom Amplification System
Source: Courtesy of Audio Enhancement.

components of a large classroom amplification system, and Figure 2-15 shows a portable/compact system. These systems improve the listening environment for all of the children in the classroom but may not provide enough amplification for children with more severe hearing losses. There are systems available that allow children to carry their classroom amplification system with them from class to class and set it up on their desks (Figure 2-16). For children with more significant hearing losses or for classrooms composed of children with both typical hearing and hearing loss, a personal FM system or self-contained FM system is a more appropriate choice.

Visual Access and Technology

The use of visual aids and technology is important for all children with hearing loss. Regardless of the degree of hearing loss, the child will benefit from the addition of visual support. This section provides an overview of some of the technologies available to help optimize visual access. These visual technologies will be discussed in the context of meeting four basic communication needs: face-to-face communication (individual and group), reception of broadcast media, telephone communication, and awareness of environmental sounds (Compton, 2000).

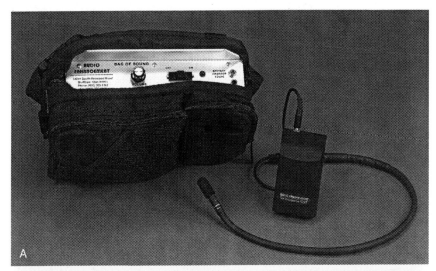

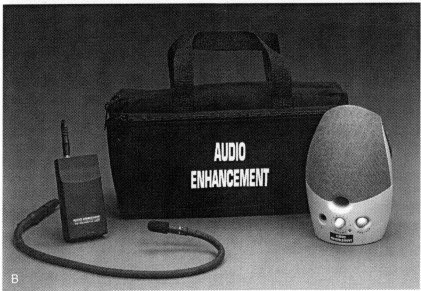

Figure 2-16. Portable (A) and Desktop (B) Classroom Amplification System
Source: Courtesy of Audio Enhancement.

Face-to-Face Communication

Face-to-face communication can occur between two people or in small or large groups. Computer technology can be a useful tool for providing visual access for children with hearing loss in face-to-face communication. In addition to technology designed to enhance auditory access in such situations, there are also technological approaches aimed to enhance visual access, mostly by providing access through text. For example, software that provides chatroom-like capability to networked computers provides a way for children who are deaf or hard of hearing to communicate with each other. Such software helps to facilitate the development of written language skills so that the child will later be able to use the computer to communicate with individuals who may not be skilled in the communication modality used by the child for face-to-face communication, such as sign language.

Other emerging technologies hold future promise for providing children who are deaf or hard of hearing with communication access in mainstream settings. For example, a device has recently been developed that incorporates elements of automatic speech recognition and speech synthesis to enable the user to both receive spoken words in text form and to convert text into synthetic speech. The system, called the iCommunicator (Figure 2-17), is composet of a high-speed laptop computer, a wireless FM transmitter/receiver system, and integrated software for automatic speech recognition and speech synthesis. One situation for which the device holds promise is in the classroom in which a teacher is lecturing. Once the teacher trains the system to recognize her voice (usually requiring about 15 minutes to more than 1 hour) the system can translate spoken speech into text with fairly high degrees of accuracy. An additional feature of the system enables the student with limited speech intelligibility to type in questions or responses and subsequently to use synthetic speech to articulate an utterance. A built-in sign language dictionary that signs isolated words and a text dictionary allowing the user to look up unfamiliar words further enhance the academic utility of this system.

Although promising, such systems do have limitations. The system will only recognize and display the voice of speakers who have "trained" the computer; therefore, the voices of classmates would not be recognized. The teacher would have to repeat what other students say during classroom discussions for it to be displayed on the computer screen. Nontheless, the iCommunicator has the potential to help improve the child's skills in reading, vocabulary, speech, and language.

For face-to-face communication in groups or lectures, computer-assisted real-time translation is a technology that provides access to the spoken message in real time or near real time. The message is typed by a stenocaptioner through the use of a special computer (similar to a court stenographer). The message is then displayed on a computer monitor or LCD screen, and the child with a hearing loss is able to read what is being said. Other systems in use require a transcriber or stenographer to provide a text translation or summary of a spoken discourse [e.g., the C-Print system (Compton, 1992)]. Although these systems provide access, they are expensive, both for the purchase of the initial equipment and for the hiring of a captioner/stenographer.

An inherent aspect of face-to-face communication is the use of skills required to initiate and maintain a dialogue. Many children today, both hearing and deaf, use the Internet and electronic mail (email), both of which can require skills that are involved in any type of dialogue. The use of email can thus serve a useful way

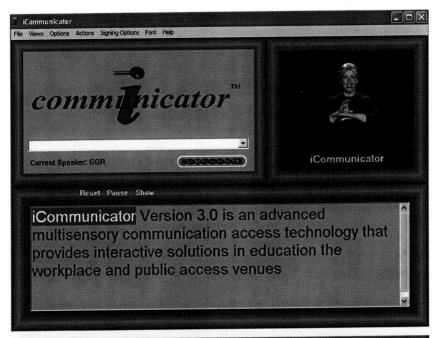

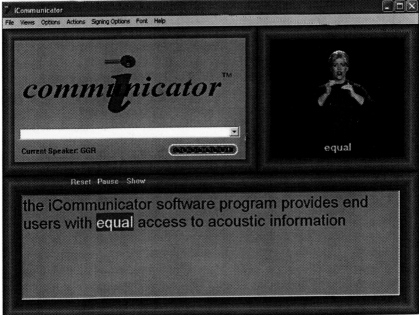

Figure 2-17. The iCommunicator

Source: Courtesy of Interactive Solutions, Inc.

of facilitating communication skill development in children with hearing loss. Children are able to communicate with others regardless of the communication modality. Although promising ways to "even the playing field" for children with limited access to spoken language, successful use of these technologies depends on the child's literacy skills (reading and writing).

Reception of Broadcast Media

Broadcast media consists of information broadcast by television, films and videos, radio, and public announcements (e.g., in an airport or train station). Many broadcast and videotaped programs today are closed captioned, a system that displays subtitles on the viewer's television screen. Most televisions have built-in circuitry to decode captioning of broadcast programming. The viewer must select this feature, typically through a menu that is displayed on the screen. It is important that all classroom materials presented via video, film, or broadcast be captioned to ensure that the child with hearing loss has access to these materials.

Public service announcements are often displayed on an LCD screen in airports and train stations. Many schools are using LCD information displays to inform students of daily scheduled events. For the child with limited access to sound, such accommodations provide an avenue for staying connected to the day-to-day activities within his environment.

Telephone Communication

Children who are unable to understand speech over the telephone may need to have a visual medium for communicating by telephone. A teletypewriter (TTY) or telecommunications device for the deaf (TDD) is a device that permits telephone conversations in print (Figure 2-18). The TTY transmits over regular telephone lines. Each TTY has a keyboard. Typed communication appears either on a soft light-emitting diode 20- or 40-character display panel or on paper (via a paper printer) (Compton, 1991). When a TTY user types a message, the letters or symbols are converted into electrical pulses, which are sent over the telephone line to the receiving TTY, which then must decode these pulses to recreate the message sent. The sender and receiver both see the message on a visual display panel on their respective TTYs. To facilitate good communication via the TTY, the sender and receiver must use a standard TTY etiquette. At the end of each comment, the caller types "GA" (go ahead) to signal that it is the other person's turn to reply. When one caller is ready to end the conversation, he types "SK" (stop keying). If the other person is also ready to end the conversation, she types "SKSK"(goodbye) (Compton, 1989). Many different codes and abbreviations are used as part of the TTY etiquette. Often TTY users will type a descriptor in parentheses to indicate feelings that are typically conveyed by tone of voice (e.g., *grrrr* to reflect anger or *smiling* to show happiness). Some TTYs have printers and answering machine functions and are compatible with PC modems. PC-TTYs use software, modems, or network solutions to allow TTY conversations on the computer. TTY software provides users with a full-screen view of TTY conversations and the ability to retrieve TTY messages from remote locations. Wireless

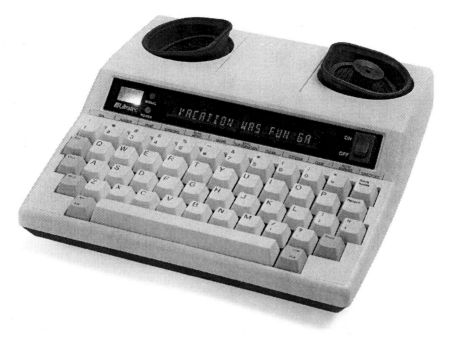

Figure 2-18.   The Supercom 4400 TTY

Source: Courtesy of Ultratec.

TTY/email (two-way) pagers are another option available. These pagers assist with telecommunication access, and most two-way wireless TTY pagers also have email capability.

Telephone conversations are now accessible for all individuals with hearing loss via the telecommunication relay service. The Americans with Disabilities Act mandated that all states provide telephone relay services. If an individual using a TTY wants to call someone who does not have a TTY, the individual would use the relay service. The TTY user contacts the relay service. The relay operator serves as an intermediate between the deaf or hard of hearing TTY user and the hearing nonuser. The relay operator reads the message typed by the TTY caller and dials the person indicated in the message. Once the non-TTY user is contacted the operator voices the message and then types in any spoken response to the TTY user. The conversation proceeds with the relay operator serving as a bridge— print to voice; voice to print—between the two parties. Additionally, the relay service can be used by hearing, non-TTY users to contact a deaf or hard of hearing person who uses a TTY.

Telephone relay services can also be used by individuals with hearing loss who have intelligible speech but little or no speech recognition skills by employing voice carryover (VCO) through the relay service. The person with hearing loss calls the relay operator and indicates that he wants to make a VCO call. The operator would then dial the number and explain VCO. The individual with hearing loss would then speak for himself, and the relay operator would type back what the other person was saying.

Environmental Sound Awareness

Children with normal hearing learn the meaning of various environmental sounds through experience. By hearing sounds such as doorbells, phones, cars, and planes, and associating events with these sounds, the child builds a set of sound-experience relationships that are important for day-to-day functioning. A child who is deaf or hard of hearing cannot be expected to hear environmental sounds such as the telephone, doorbell, smoke alarm, or alarm clock if he is unaided or does not use amplification (Bess, Gravel, & Tharpe, 1996). Awareness of environmental sounds can be accomplished through the use of alerting or signaling devices that provide visual (flashing light), auditory (increase in amplification/change in pitch), or vibrotactile (vibration/sensation) signals. All alerting/signaling devices do three things: (1) detect the sound of the telephone, doorbell, smoke alarm, or other important sounds; (2) either amplify the sound or convert it to another signal; and (3) alert the user (Compton, 2000).

Alerting/signaling systems can generally be grouped in two broad categories: those that are hardwired and those that are wireless. Hardwired systems are physically placed next to or are electronically connected to the signal source. Examples of hardwired systems, as seen in Figure 2-19, are a bed shaker or lamp connected to a clock radio, a lamp connected to a telephone wall jack, and a doorbell wired to a hallway lamp (Compton, 2000).

Wireless alerting systems consist of a transmitter and a receiver. The transmitter picks up the sound via a microphone and sends an FM signal to the receiver, which is connected to a visual, auditory, or vibrotactile alerting device. An example of a wireless system is a battery-powered smoke detector, which not only emits a loud buzz but also sends an FM radio signal to a receiver that vibrates, warning the user of a potentially dangerous situation (Compton, 2000).

Wireless TTY/email (two-way) pagers with a vibration signaling feature as described earlier can also be used to alert the user of environmental signals (e.g., a telephone call or an emergency). Alerting and signaling devices help children with hearing loss gain a greater sense of confidence, independence, and security in all communication environments (home, school, and social settings).

The visual technologies described above can help provide better visual access to communication for the child with hearing loss. See appendix C for a technology resource list.

Enhancing the Communication Environment

Enhancing the communication environment will have a positive affect upon the psychoeducational and psychosocial achievement of children with normal hearing and children with hearing loss (Bess et al., 1996). The communication environment consists of any place in which communication and learning take place. For our purposes we will be referring to the school environment (e.g., classroom/therapy room), but the information that will be provided can be applied to most communication environments (e.g., the home, field trips, or Sunday

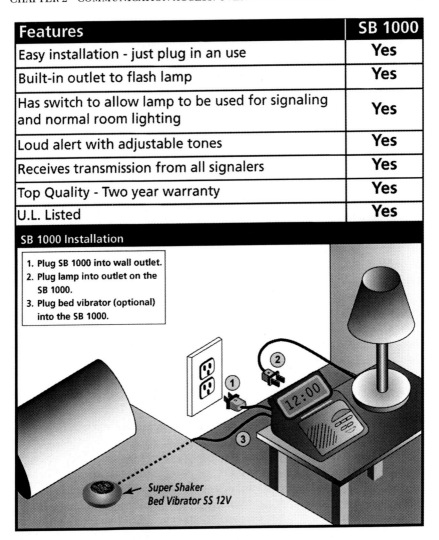

Features	SB 1000
Easy installation - just plug in an use	**Yes**
Built-in outlet to flash lamp	**Yes**
Has switch to allow lamp to be used for signaling and normal room lighting	**Yes**
Loud alert with adjustable tones	**Yes**
Receives transmission from all signalers	**Yes**
Top Quality - Two year warranty	**Yes**
U.L. Listed	**Yes**

SB 1000 Installation

1. Plug SB 1000 into wall outlet.
2. Plug lamp into outlet on the SB 1000.
3. Plug bed vibrator (optional) into the SB 1000.

Super Shaker Bed Vibrator SS 12V

Figure 2-19. Examples of Alerting Devices. Sonic Boom TM Alarm Clock and Super Shaker Bed Vibrator SS12V

Source: Courtesy of Sonic Alert.

school). The process of enhancing the communication environment requires assessing the environment and then making modifications. The following section provides some suggestions for assessing and modifying both the listening and visual communication environment.

The Listening Environment

In schools as in many other communication environments including the home, children are often placed in demanding, degraded, and constantly changing listening situations (Berg, 1993). Background noise, reverberation, and distance will have a negative impact upon the child's ability to listen to and understand spoken communication. Assessing the amount of noise and reverberation in the child's environment is the first step in making modifications to the listening environment.

Background noise is anything that interferes with the child's access to spoken communication and includes other talkers, heating and cooling systems, home and classroom sounds, traffic noise, computer hums, internal biologic noise, televisions, playground and hallway noise, wind, and so forth (Flexer, 1999). To determine the effect of background noise on spoken communication requires an examination of the relationship between the amplitude of the speech and the amplitude of noise in the environment. This comparison is called the *signal to noise (S/N) ratio*. For example, if you have a S/N ratio of 0, it means that the signal and the noise are at the same amplitude level. Children with normal hearing typically require a S/N ratio of +6 dB to understand spoken communication (Flexer, 1999). Children with hearing loss need a +20 dB S/N ratio (Finitzo-Hieber & Tillman, 1978). In an average classroom the S/N ratio is only +4 or +5 dB, and it may be 0 dB, which is less than ideal, even for children with normal hearing (Berg, 1986, 1993).

Sound will reflect repeatedly from the walls, ceilings, and floors of a room with hard surfaces. Repeated reflection (bouncing sound) causes sound prolongation or *reverberation* (Berg, 1993). The reverberant sound results in increased noise levels, thus smearing or masking speech. The longer the reverberation time, the greater this smearing effect (Berg, 1993).

As the distance from the talker to the listener increases, the intensity or loudness of speech decreases. As soon as the child moves further than 6 inches from the speaker's mouth, the speech signal begins to degrade (Flexer, 1999). If the child is involved in group discussion, he may be able to hear the children sitting close to him, but not the children who are seated at a distance.

Aside from acoustically treating the listening environment, the best way to control for background noise, reverberation, and distance is through the use of technology (discussed earlier in this chapter). Appropriately fit hearing aids or cochlear implants coupled to an FM system will significantly enhance the listening environment for the child with a hearing loss. To improve the listening environment for the entire class, a classroom amplification system should be used.

The Visual Environment

As stated earlier, even the child with a minimal hearing loss will need to depend upon his vision for access to communication. Assessing the visual environment requires attention to positioning of the child, visual noise/distractions, lighting, and visual supports (e.g., technology, interpreters, and notetakers).

For communication to be successful for the child with hearing loss he must be positioned appropriately within the communication environment. In the classroom this may require flexibility in seating arrangements, allowing for different seats for different activities (Levitt & McGarr, 1988). If the child needs to speechread or watch signs or cues, it is very important for the child to be positioned in front of the person with whom he is communicating. Speechreading is not possible if the child cannot see the person speaking such as when the teacher is talking while writing on the chalkboard. Hard of hearing children with symmetrical hearing losses should be placed in a central location in the classroom, approximately 3 to 5 feet from the teacher. For optimum use of hearing aids/cochlear implants, the child should be seated in the second row (Brackett & Maxon, 1986). If the teacher is too close, her voice is often directed over the child using hearing aids or a cochlear implant, and the child's head or neck could become strained from looking up at the teacher. When the teacher is reading aloud, she should hold the book below the chin so that the face is visible. If the child is using a sign language interpreter or cued speech transliterater, he should have visual access to both the interpreter or transliterater and the person speaking. Visual access can also be enhanced during group discussions by seating the children in a semicircle so that the child with a hearing loss is able to see the faces of the group members. Although seating arrangements are very important, efforts should be made to limit further isolation of the child with a hearing loss.

Just as background noise interferes with the speech signal, visual noise/visual distractions interfere with the visual reception of speech/signs/cues. If there are a lot of visual distractions in the room (e.g., children moving or lights flashing), it is very difficult for the child with hearing loss to attend.

It is also important to optimize lighting in the room. Overhead and natural lighting provide the best environment for communication. The light should be on the face of the person speaking/signing and not behind this person. The existence of shadows or glare, dimming of lights during the use of audiovisual aids, and the effects of time of day changes or natural lighting need to be monitored (Berry, 1988) to ensure that the child's visual environment is optimal.

Many children with hearing loss receive visual access to spoken communication in the classroom through the use of a sign language/educational interpreter. Educational interpreters act as an intermediate, joining deaf and hard of hearing students with classmates and school personnel who do not sign. However, sign language interpreters represent only one facet of a multifaceted educational enterprise. These students need more than accurate visualization of spoken communication in the classroom. It should not be assumed that because the child is able to see and hear everything in a classroom that the child is learning about all that is covered in class. Education is not solely a matter of transmitting information from the teacher to the student. Some suggest that students learn more from each other through interaction than they do from teachers (Stewart, Schein, & Cartwright, 1998).

Often educational interpreters are considered members of an educational team comprising teachers, communication specialists, and others (Seal, 1998). In many cases the interpreter is the person in the child's school environment who is most familiar with the child's communication strengths and weaknesses. Although one might assume that the interpreter would pass on this information to other members of the team, some interpreters may feel that this is a violation of their profession's ethics. Educational interpreters might argue that sharing this type of information is a breech of confidentiality that will lead the student to distrust interpreters. An alternative presented by Humphrey and Alcorn (1994) suggests that interpreters on educational teams only provide information pertaining to "the interpreting process, the student's language preference, language skills and the appropriateness of interpreting services within a particular educational setting" (p. 307).

As discussed earlier, the educational interpreter serves to equalize the child's language and that of the environment. In most mainstream classrooms the language used by teachers and peers is spoken English. No single sign language or language system is used by all children who are deaf or hard of hearing. The child with hearing loss may communicate best through ASL, an invented sign system (such as Signing Exact English [SEE II]), cued speech, or some variant of ASL such as English-Based Signing, which uses ASL signs in English word order. Communication impediments can emerge if the interpreter is using a form of visual communication that does not match the child's, either because the interpreter is not skilled in the child's form of visual communication or because the school system requires an interpreter to use a particular sign system, such as SEE II. ASL, invented sign systems, and cued speech will be described in detail later in this chapter.

Another important visual support system for the child with a hearing loss is a notetaker. Students who are deaf or hard of hearing often experience difficulty trying to speechread, watch signs/cues, and take notes at the same time. For children in older grades in which notetaking is expected in class, a notetaker can greatly enhance the child's ability to perform effectively. There are additional, technological strategies for ensuring that a child is obtaining important information presented in class that may also prove beneficial (see discussion of technologies for enhancing face-to-face communication earlier in this chapter).

If the child is not reading at grade level, the provision of visual supplements (e.g., notes or pictures) can be beneficial, especially when new concepts are introduced. By demonstrating or using concrete/manipulative learning activities, the teacher or clinician can greatly enhance communication access (Conway, 1990).

The previous sections address a wide range of issues that affect communication access, either auditory or visual. It cannot be overemphasized that without adequately addressing issues of access, the child cannot meet his full potential. Providing communication access is vital to the linguistic, communicative, academic, and psychosocial development of all children, particularly those who are deaf or hard of hearing. The following sections look at issues that affect communication access in various educational settings.

COMMUNICATION ACCESS ISSUES IN VARIOUS EDUCATIONAL SETTINGS

The communication modality used by a child is often related to the educational philosophy employed in the educational setting. Although visual and auditory access play an important role in nearly all educational settings for deaf children, the relative emphasis on audition or vision will differ from program to program. In addition, the nature of the information a child receives through these modalities varies according to different educational philosophies. It is thus relevant to consider current educational philosophies, the communication forms that are employed in programs subscribing to these philosophies, and the relative role and nature of visual and auditory access issues for a student to succeed within various educational settings.

Visual access refers to how the child with hearing loss receives language/communication through vision. The amount of individual access will be influenced by the type of communication modality the child uses, his proficiency with the communication modality, and the proficiency by which those around him use the communication modality. Communication modality reflects the manner in which a language is represented, not taught; however, a specific communication mode may be used as a *medium* for instruction to convey meaning (Paul & Quigley, 1994). The following sections give an overview of the common educational philosophies for children who are deaf or hard of hearing in educational programs and various communication environments. Particular emphasis is given to issues of access that are associated with these educational approaches. The philosophies discussed are total communication, oralism, and bilingual-bicultural (American Sign Language/English as a Second Language).

Total Communication

The total communication (TC) philosophy refers to the use of all forms of communication to teach the English language to children who are deaf and hard of hearing and has been adopted by the majority of school programs in the United States. Forms of communication include listening, speaking, speechreading, signing, gestures, fingerspelling, reading, and writing (Bodner-Johnson, 1996). Speechreading refers to the process of understanding spoken words by watching lip/mouth movements (lipreading), facial expressions, body language, and contextual cues. Fingerspelling refers to hand and finger shapes used to represent each letter of the alphabet to form words, phrases, and sentences. In ASL there are 23 distinct hand shapes that correspond to the letters of the alphabet. The movement of three hand shapes represent two different letters each (e.g., g and q, k and p, and i and j) (Paul, 2000). Figure 2-20 illustrates the manual alphabet.

Because TC is a philosophy of communication rather than a specific methodology, various educational programs have implemented this philosophy differently (Sass-Lehrer, 1999). Many educational programs employ the use of simultaneous communication. Simultaneous communication consists of using signs and speech together to communicate a message. The child uses listening, speechreading, and reading signs and fingerspelling to understand a message, and speaking, signing, and fingerspelling for expression. Simultaneous communication can involve the use of ASL signs in English word order or the use of an invented English-based sign system or manually coded English system that presents a one to one correspondence between each English word and sign (Sass-Lehrer, 1999).

Despite the widespread use of simultaneous communication, a number of concerns have been expressed about the use of simultaneous communication for

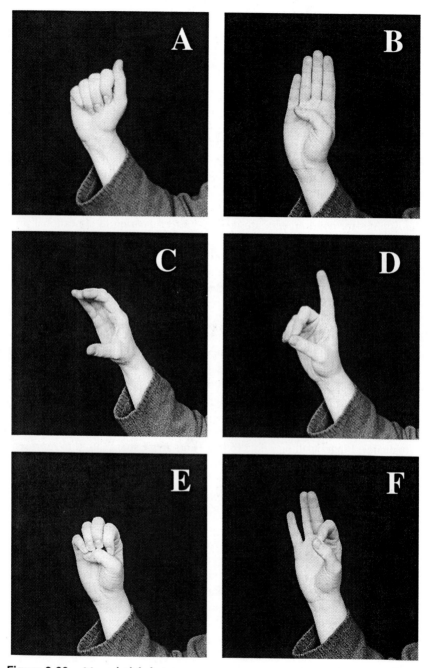

Figure 2-20.   Manual Alphabet

Source: From Paul, P. (2000). *Language and deafness* (3rd ed.). Clifton Park, NY: Singular.

(continues)

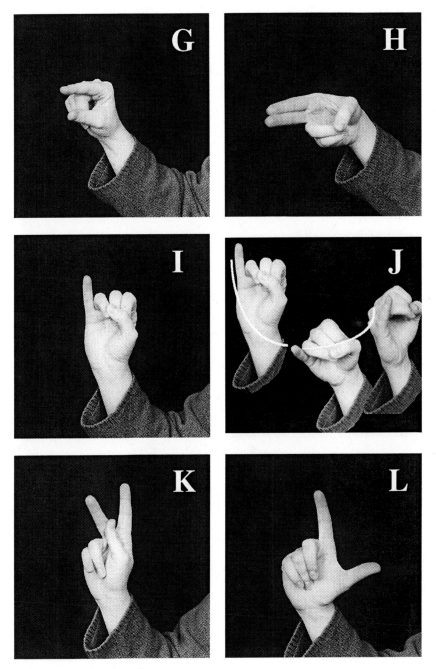

Figure 2-20. (continued)

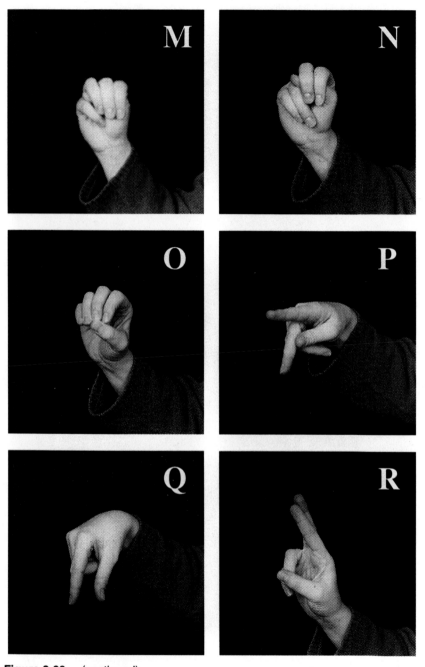

Figure 2-20.   (continued)

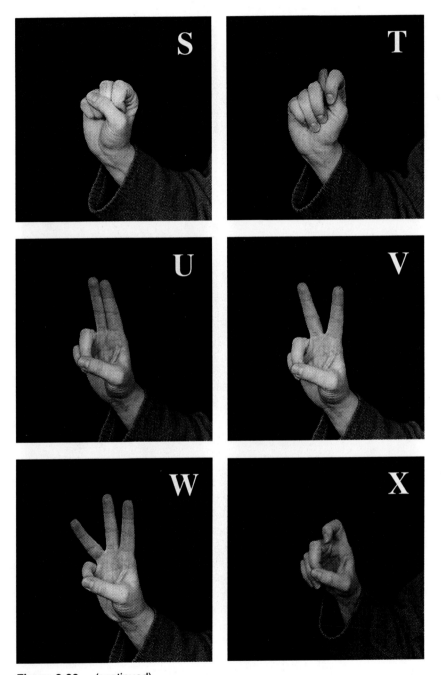

Figure 2-20.   (continued)

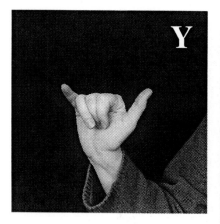

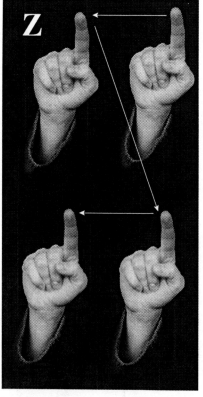

Figure 2-20. (continued)

teaching young children a first language. Because the sign portion of a simultaneously communicated message may be the only portion completely accessible to the child and because this represents neither well-developed English nor well-developed ASL structure, such utterances often fail to provide a good language model to many deaf children (Johnson, Liddell, & Erting, 1989).

The invented sign systems and the manually coded English systems modify or create signs to provide a complete representation of English using English word order and syntax. Invented sign systems use ASL signs as a base and create signs to mark grammatical structures such as pronouns, verb tenses, affixes, and articles (Moores, 1997). The two most widely used invented sign systems, SEE II and Signed English, will be described along with a discussion of English-Based Signing.

Signed Exact English (SEE II)

SEE II categorizes English words in three broad groups: basic (e.g., boy), compound (e.g., cupcake), and complex (e.g., runs). The selection of a sign to represent a word is based on a two out of three rule involving sound, spelling, and meaning. For example, consider the word *run* in the following sentences:

1. John hit a home *run.*
2. The lady has a *run* in her stocking.
3. I love to *run* outdoors.

The same sign for the word *run* is used in all three of the above sentences because two of the three criteria are met: sound and spelling. Many English words with multiple meanings follow the two out of three rule (Gustason, Pfetzing, & Zawolkow, 1975). Other important principles of SEE II as stated by Gustason, Pfetzing, & Zawolkow (1980, pp. xiii–xiv; Stewart & Luetke-Stahlman, 1998) are the following:

1. English should be signed in a manner that is as consistent as possible with how it is spoken or written to constitute a language input for the child that will result in his mastery of English.
2. A sign should be translatable to only one English equivalent.
3. When the first letter is added to a basic sign to create synonyms, the basic sign is retained whenever possible as the most commonly used word; e.g., the basic sign for MAKE is retained whereas the sign is made with C-hands for *create* and P-hands for *produce* (Figure 2-21).
4. When more than one marker is added to a word, middle markers may be dropped if there is no sacrifice of clarity (e.g., the past tense sign is added to *break* to produce *broke,* but *broken* may be signed as *break* plus the past participle or *-en*).
5. When one follows the above principles, respect needs to be shown for characteristics of visual gestural communication.

Gustason and her associates (Gustason et al., 1980; Gustason & Zawolkow, 1993; Stewart & Luetke-Stahlman, 1998) also listed suggestions for the development of new signs; that is, signs for English words that are not contained in the SEE II dictionary. The suggestions are

1. Seek an existing sign. Check other sign language texts. Ask skilled signers in your community, especially deaf native signers.
2. Modify an existing sign with a similar or related meaning. Generally, this means adding the first letter of the word to a basic sign.
3. Consider fingerspelling. This depends, of course, on the age and perceptual abilities of the child, and the length and frequency of use of the word in question.
4. If all else fails and you must invent, try to stay as close as possible to ASL principles.

Signed English

Signed English is an invented system that parallels English. Users of Signed English speak while signing in English word order. It is based on the premise that deaf

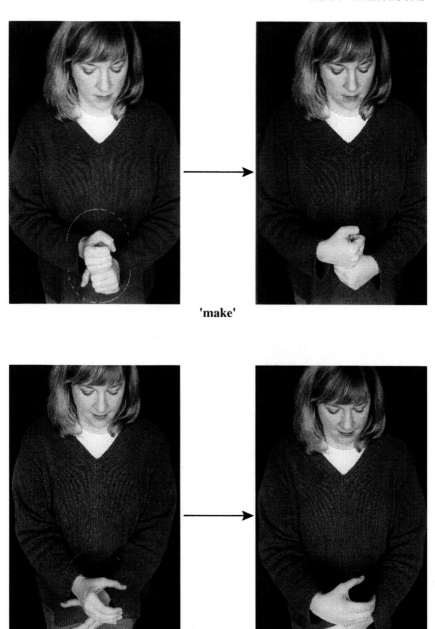

Figure 2-21. Signing Exact English Signs: *make and create*

Source: From Paul, P. (2000). *Language and deafness* (3rd ed.). Clifton Park, NY: Singular.

(*continues*)

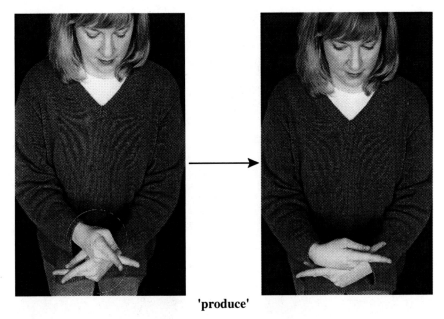

'produce'

Figure 2-21. Signing Exact English Signs: *produce* (continued)

children must depend upon what they see to understand what others say to them (Borenstein, Saulnier, & Hamilton, 1983). Some signs are borrowed from ASL, some are contrived, and others from the SEE systems are presented in the *Comprehensive Signed English Dictionary* (Borenstein et al, 1983).

Signed English has two groups of signs: sign words and sign markers. The Signed English dictionary contains more than 3100 sign words, with the words taken from normal hearing children's spoken language and from vocabulary lists used with young deaf children in homes and classrooms. There are 14 sign markers in Signed English (Figure 2-22). The sign markers represent the most common inflectional and derivational morphemes in the language of deaf children (Paul, 2000).

English-Based Signing

English-Based Signing is different from invented sign systems because it does not follow a clear-cut set of principles but does follow English word order. In the past this type of simultaneous communication has been labeled *pidgin sign English* (Marschark, 1997) and more recently it has been referred to as *sign English* or *conceptually accurate sign English* (Paul, 2000). English-Based Signing entails signing a combination of both English and ASL features executed in an English word order. The language proficiency of the signer will determine the use of the features from either language. If a signer has a high ASL language proficiency

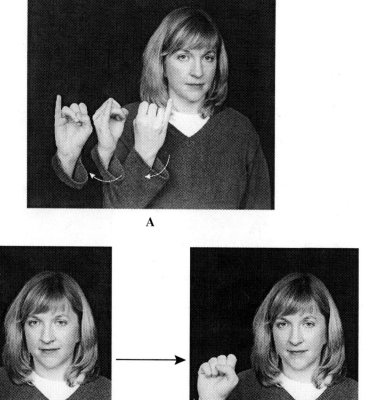

Figure 2-22. Signed English Sign Markers
(A) Verb form:-ing as in playing. (B) Possessive: 's as in *dog's*.

Source: From Paul, P. (2000). *Language and deafness* (3rd ed.). Clifton Park, NY: Singular.

(*continues*)

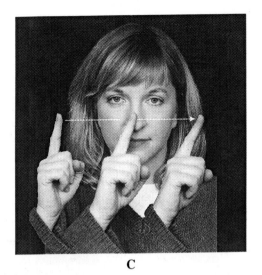

C

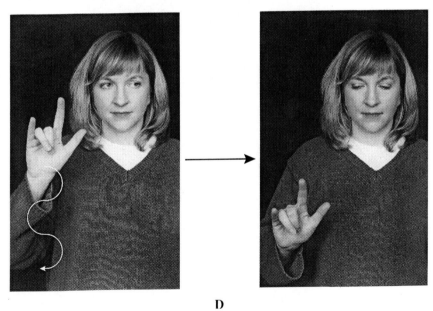

D

Figure 2-22.   Signed English Sign Markers **(continued)**
(C) Irregular plural noun (sign the word twice)—example: *mice.*
(D) Adverb: -ly as in *happily.*

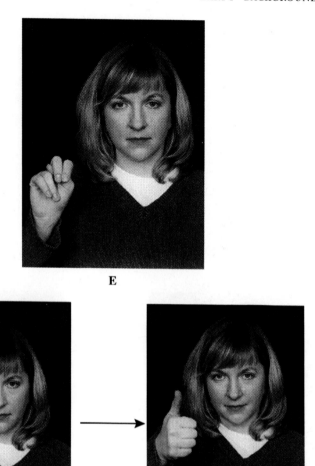

E

F

Figure 2-22. Signed English Sign Markers (continued)
(E) Participle as in *gone*. (F) Comparative -er as in *smarter*.

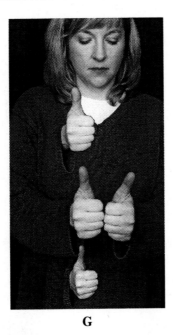

G

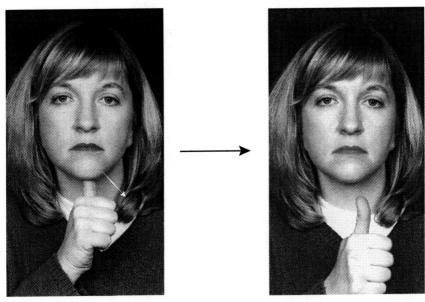

H

Figure 2-22. Signed English Sign Markers **(continued)**
(G) Supportative: -est as in *tallest*. (H) Opposite of: un-, im-, etc., as in *unhappy, impatient*, etc.

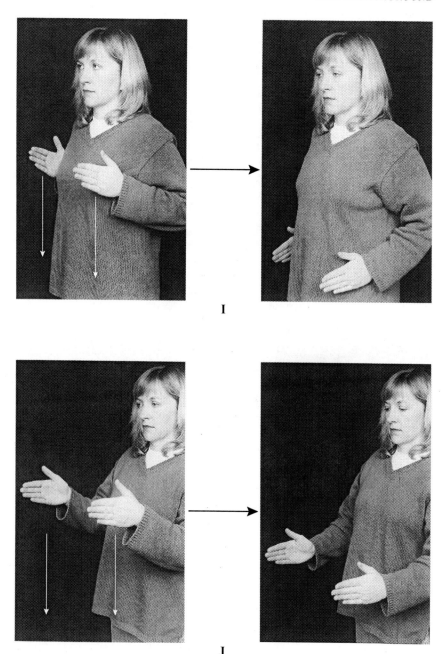

Figure 2-22. Signed English Sign Markers **(continued)**
(I) Agent sign for person as in *teacher*. (J) Agent sign for thing as in
washer.

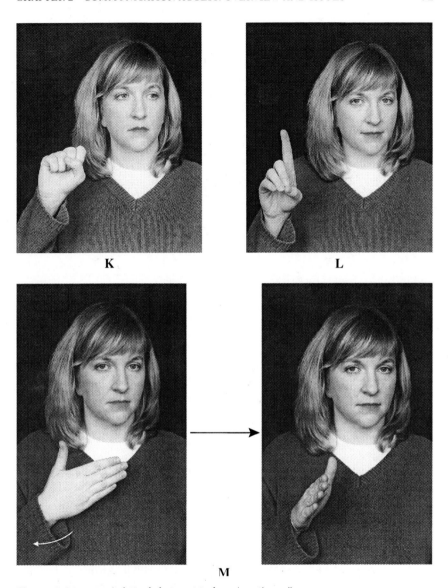

K

L

M

Figure 2-22. Signed English Sign Markers **(continued)**
(K) Regular plural nouns: -s as in *cats*; third person sigular; -s as in *writhes*. (L) Regular past verbs; -ed as in *learned*. (M) Irregular past verb as in *saw*.

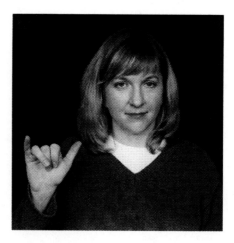

N

Figure 2-22.   Signed English Sign Markers **(continued)**
(N) Adjective: -y as in *cloudy.*

---

and a low English language proficiency, many of the features incorporated in the signing will be taken from ASL. Because of the influence of language proficiency, English-Based Signing may vary from signer to signer (Paul & Quigley, 1994).

English-based signing differs from invented sign systems in the following ways: (1) it was not invented; it evolved; (2) it was not intended to represent or model English; (3) its vocabulary does not necessarily have a relationship to the sound or spelling of English words (Baker & Cokely, 1980); (4) it was not designed to be used in an educational context or to teach English; its purpose was for social communication (Baker & Cokely, 1980); and (5) it can be used with or without voice.

Oral/Aural Educational Philosophies

Oral/aural communication is a communication philosophy that stresses the development of oral communication skills (intelligible speech and the use of speechreading and audition for speech reception) in children who are deaf and hard of hearing so that they can participate fully with a majority of English-speaking individuals (Paul, 2000). Signs or other manual systems are not used with this approach. Although there are a number of variations in how oral educational programs are implemented, all rely to some extent on speech, speechreading, and the use of residual hearing. Some approaches will additionally use touch or taction.

Within oralism there are unisensory and multisensory approaches. Unisensory approaches place the primary emphasis on a single sense, typically audition; however, vision or taction, may also be emphasized primarily (Paul, 2000). Programs stressing a unisensory approach to developing residual hearing or audition include those referred to as auditory, auditory-verbal, aural-oral, aural, acoupedic

(Pollack, 1984), acoustic (Erber, 1982), and auditory global (Calvert & Silverman, 1983); however, the most recent general label used is *auditory-verbal*. One of the primary goals of the unisensory approach is the development of spoken language primarily through the use of amplification, FM systems, or cochlear implants, accompanied by intense listening training (without visual cues). Students are encouraged to learn to listen and learn by listening instead of learning to hear. The use of speechreading is minimized initially but may be developed or motivated later as a result of the intense, earlier focus on audition (Paul, 2000).

The unisensory approach focusing on touch/taction is called the *tactile-kinesthetic approach*, which is based on a motor theory of speech production. This approach has been used with children who are unable to benefit from traditional oral approaches that focus on audition or vision (Calvert, 1986; Calvert & Silverman, 1983). This approach utilizes a tactile device worn by the child to deliver acoustic/speech information via vibratory stimulation to facilitate development of oral communication skills (Weisenberger & Miller, 1987).

Multisensory approaches have been defined as "balanced" approaches because of the equal stress placed on the development of two primary senses, audition and vision (Moores, 1987). Emphasis is still placed on early amplification and auditory management; however, emphasis is also placed on speechreading. For some children with hearing loss the use of audition and speechreading has proven to be more effective in providing them with access to communication than the use of audition alone (Norvelli-Olmstead & Ling, 1984).

Cued Speech

Cued Speech is an example of a multisensory approach to communication. It has long been recognized that speechreading alone as a basis for speech reception is inherently limited because of the similar appearance of many speech sounds (as occurs with the words *be*, *me*, and *pea*). There is visual ambiguity among two-thirds of the speech sounds received.

Invented by Dr. Orin Cornett in 1967, Cued Speech provides a visual accompaniment to speechreading that reduces the ambiguity inherent in speechreading. Cued Speech is a phonemically based hand supplement to speechreading made up of eight hand shapes to represent eight groups of consonant sounds and four hand positions about the face to represent vowel sounds. There are also seven nonmanual signals (NMS) for consonants and four NMS for vowels that represent the mouth movements used to produce English consonants and vowels. Figure 2-23 illustrates the Cued Speech hand shapes and positions and three example of NMS. Combinations of these hand configurations and placements and use of NMS reflect the aspects of pronunciation of words in connected speech that are not readily available through speechreading alone (Williams-Scott & Kipila, 1987). It has been suggested that because Cued Speech is sufficient for representing phonology, students who use Cued Speech should be expected to develop phonologic and, consequently, phonemic awareness that is critical for developing literacy (Paul, 2000).

Unlike the other approaches included under the philosophy of oralism, many children who use Cued Speech also use sign language (either ASL, English-Based

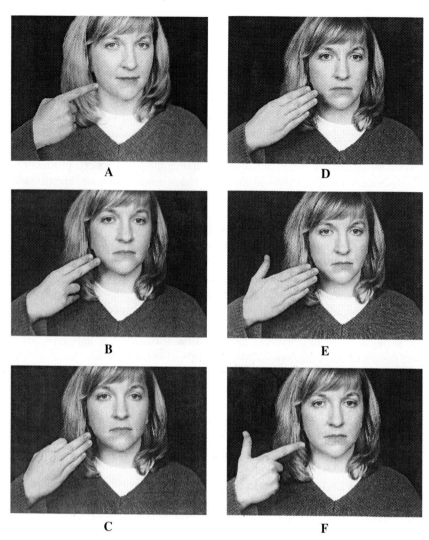

Figure 2-23. Cued Speech Hand Shapes and Positions
Hand shapes: consonants. (A) d, p, zh. (B) k, v, tH, z. (C) n, s, r. (D) b, n, wh. (E) t, m, f. (F) l, sh, w.

Source: From Paul, P. (2000). *Language and deafness* (3rd ed.). Clifton Park, NY: Singular.

(*continues*)

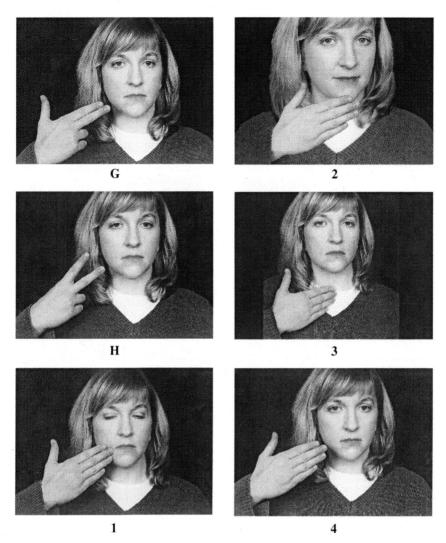

Figure 2-23. Cued Speech Hand Shapes and Positions **(continued)**
Hand shapes: consonants. (G) g, j, th. (H) ng, y, ch. Locations for
"vowels" (point of contact). (1) Corner of mouth. (2) Tip of chin.
(3) Center of neck. (4) Noncontact movement: begins 4 inches to side
of chin.

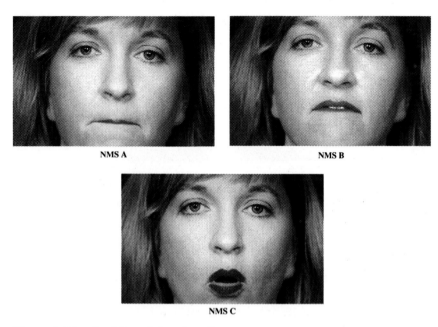

NMS A   NMS B

NMS C

Figure 2-23. Cued Speech **(continued)**
Three examples of nonmanual signals of cued speech/language

Signing, or one of the invented systems) for communication. Obviously, the child cannot sign and cue at the same time. Cued Speech is often used in the classroom (via a Cued Speech transliterater) when spoken English is the language of instruction, whereas sign language is used for other aspects of communication. Many children who use Cued Speech for receptive communication will use sign language for expressive communication. LaSasso and Metzger (1998) have suggested that Cued Speech be used in bilingual-bicultural (ASL/English) programs to represent English visually, thus providing visual access to both languages.

Cued Speech is used to provide the child with speech reception but is not commonly used for speech intelligibility training. In Cued Speech the phonemes of English are divided into visually contrastive sets (Woodward & Barber, 1960) but not according to placement or manner of production of the phonemes. The speech-language clinician may be able to use Cued Speech to help the child determine the correct pronunciation of a word and that may in turn directly impact the child's ability to correctly pronounce the word. Alternatively, hand systems such as Visual Phonics (International Communication Learning Institute) may provide a more phonetically appropriate hand system for supplementing speech teaching. Visual Phonics consists of 46 hand cues and corresponding written symbols. The hand cues are in some way suggestive of how the sounds are produced. The cues help the child to conceptualize the production of the sound and then to see how it relates to its printed correlate.

Bilingual-Bicultural Philosophy (American Sign Language/English as a Second Language)

The bilingual-bicultural philosophy of educating children who are deaf and hard of hearing is based on the use of ASL as the primary language of instruction in the classroom with English taught as a second language primarily through print (Gallimore & Woodruff, 1996; Mahshie, 1995). Bilingualism involves the ability to use two different languages successfully with some individuals being stronger in one language and some in the other language (Maxwell, 1990). A child who is deaf or hard of hearing is considered bilingual if he is able to communicate effectively in both ASL and English. Biculturalism implies an understanding of the mores, customs, practices, and expectations of members of a cultural group and the ability to adapt to their expectations. A child who is deaf or hard of hearing is considered bicultural if he is capable of functioning within the deaf community and the majority culture (Gallimore & Woodruff, 1996).

In a significant publication that questioned current educational practices with children who are deaf and hard of hearing, Johnson et al. (1989) suggested that ASL is the language choice of adults who are deaf and that it offers access to school curricula and other world knowledge. They pointed out that ASL is a visual-gestural language complete with phonology, morphology, syntax, and semantics. There is evidence that when children learn two languages, they do not do so independently and that aspects of learning one language facilitate the other (Cummins, 1984). Proponents of bilingual-bicultural programs further suggest that by providing children with a visual language to which they have access, the child will develop an important first language during the critical period for language development. This in turn will facilitate development of a second language, English, in these children.

ASL entails using manual and nonmanual features instead of speech. The manual features refer to the shapes, positions, and movements of the hands, whereas the nonmanual features refer to facial expressions (movements of the cheeks, lips, tongue, eyes, and eyebrows) and movement of the shoulders and body (e.g., body shifts). Signers express language using manual and nonmanual features simultaneously (Paul, 2000). ASL uses emphasis through nonmanual features or size or intensity of signs to differentiate among concepts. The use of ASL by the child depends on the his motor and visual skills and not the degree of his hearing loss.

ASL is a complete language although very different from English. Because ASL and English are separate languages, they cannot be used simultaneously. There is no direct correlation between each sign and the spoken word. Like other sign languages, ASL does not have a written form; ASL users do not read or write their messages in ASL. Information is expressed and received via the child's primary language, ASL, which is analogous to speech for the child whose primary language is a spoken language (Paul, 2000).

Some linguists suggest that once a child acquires a strong visually based language through ASL, a second language, such as English, can be developed through reference to the first language (Johnson et al., 1989; Strong & Prinz, 1997). Others have suggested that ASL and English are acquired concurrently but should be presented separately (Quigley & Kretschmer, 1982). Bilingual-bicultural programs do promote spoken language development (auditory and speech) but recognize that the languages of ASL and English are distinct and do not support the use of signs and speech simultaneously. Bilingual-bicultural programs that use ASL as the primary language employ deaf adults who are native users of the language as well as hearing adults who are proficient in both ASL and English. Bilingual-bicultural programs emphasize deaf studies to promote the child's understanding of deaf culture and communities and to facilitate the child's development of a positive self-image. Currently a limited number of programs use the bilingual approach.

Summary

Communication access is fundamental to educational and human growth. The opportunity and ability to communicate are so basic that people with normal hearing rarely think about their absence. Professionals working with children with hearing loss therefore have the responsibility of providing for communication assessment, access, and development. This chapter provided an overview of the issues that the clinician needs to consider when determining and optimizing the child's ability to access communication through both hearing and vision.

References

Baker, C., & Cokely, D. (1980) American Sign Language: A teacher's resource text on grammar and culture. Silver Spring, MD: T. J. Publishers.

Berg, F. S. (1986). Classroom acoustics and signal transmission. In F. S. Berg, J. C. Blair, S. H. Viehweg, & A. Wilson-Vlotman (Eds.), Educational audiology for the hard of hearing child. New York: Grune & Stratton.

Berg, F. S. (1993). Acoustics and sound systems in schools. Clifton Park, NY: Singular.

Berry, V. S. (1988). Classroom intervention strategies and resource materials for the auditorily handicapped child. In R. J. Roeser & M. P. Downs (Eds.), Auditory disorders in school children. New York: Thieme Medical.

Bess, F. H., Gravel, J. S., & Tharpe, A. M. (Eds.). (1996). Amplification for children with auditory deficits. Nashville, TN: Bil Wilkerson Center Press.

Bess, F. H., Dodd-Murphy, J., & Parker, R. A. (1998). Children with minimal sensorineural hearing loss: Prevalence, educational performance, and functional status. Ear & Hearing, 19, 339–354.

Bodner-Johnson, B. (1996). Total communication: A professional point of view. In S. Schwartz (Ed.), Choices in deafness: A parent's guide to communication options (2nd ed., pp. 207–217). Bethesda, MD: Woodbine.

Borenstein, H., Saulnier, K., & Hamilton, L. (1983). The comprehensive signed English dictionary. Washington, DC: Gallaudet College Press.

Brackett, D., & Maxon, A. B. (1986). Service delivery alternatives for the mainstreamed hearing impaired child. Language, Speech and Hearing Services in the Schools, 17, 115–125.

Calvert, D. (1986). Speech in perspective. In D. Luterman (Ed.), Deafness in perspective (pp. 167–191). San Diego, CA: College-Hill Press.

Calvert, D., & Silverman, S. (1983). Speech and deafness. Washington, DC: Alexander Graham Bell Association for the Deaf.

Clark, G. M., Cowan, R. S. C., & Dowell, R. C. (1997). Cochlear implantation for infants and children. Clifton Park, NY: Singular.

Compton, C. L. (1991). *Doorways to independence*. Washington, DC: Gallaudet University.

Compton, C. L. (1992). Assistive listening devices: Videotext displays. *American Academy of Audiology*, 19–20.

Compton, C. L. (2000). Assistive technology for the enhancement of receptive communicator. In J. Alpiner & C. McCarthy (Eds.). *Rehabilitative audiology: Children and Adults* (3rd ed.). Baltimore: Lippincott Williams & Wilkins.

Conway, D. (1990). Semantic relationships in the word meanings of hearing impaired children. *Volta Review, 92*, 339–349.

Crandell, C., Smaldino, J., & Flexer, C. (1995). *Sound-field amplification: Applications to speech perception and classroom acoustics*. Clifton Park, NY: Singular.

Culbertson, J. L., & Gilbert, L. E. (1986). Children with unilateral sensorineural hearing loss: Cognitive, academic, and social development. *Ear & Hearing, 7*, 38–42.

Cummins, J. (1984). *Bilingualism and special education: Issues in assessment and pedagogy*. Clevedon, Avon, England: Multilingual Matters.

Elfenbein, J., Bentler, R., Davis, J., & Niebuhr, D. (1988). Status of school children's hearing aids relative to monitoring practices. *Ear & Hearing, 9*, 212–215.

Erber, N. (1982). *Auditory training*. Washington, DC: Alexander Graham Bell Association for the Deaf.

Finitzo-Hieber, T., & Tillman, T. (1978). Room acoustics effects on monosyllabic word discrimination ability for normal and hearing-impaired children. *Journal of Speech and Hearing Research, 21*, 440–458.

Flexer, C. (1999). *Facilitating hearing and listening in young children*. Clifton Park, NY: Singular.

Gallimore, L., & Woodruff, S. (1996). The bilingual-bicultural (Bi-Bi) approach: A professional point of view. In S. Schwartz (Ed.), *Choices in deafness: A parent's guide to communication options* (pp. 47–59). Bethesda, MD: Woodbine.

Gustason, G., Pfetzing, D., & Zawolkow, E. (1975). *Signing exact English* (rev. ed.). Los Alamitos, CA: Modern Signs Press.

Gustason, G., Pfetzing, D., & Zawolkow, E. (1980). *Signing exact English*. Los Alimitos, CA: Modern Signs Press.

Hayes, D., & Northern, J. L. (1996). *Infants and hearing*. Clifton Park, NY: Singular.

Humphrey, J. H., & Alcorn, B. J. (1994). *So you want to be an interpreter: An introduction to sign language interpreting*. Salem, OR: Sign Enhancers.

Johnson, C. D., Benson, P. V., & Seaton, J. B. (1997). *Educational audiology handbook*. Clifton Park, NY: Singular.

Johnson, C. D., & Rees, K. (1995). Amplification options for infants and toddlers. *Seminars in Hearing, 16*, 140–150.

Johnson, R. E., Liddell, S., & Erting, C. (1989) *Unlocking the curriculum: Principles for achieving access in deaf education* (Gallaudet Research Institute Working/Occasional Paper Series 89-3). Washington, DC: Gallaudet Research Institute.

Joint Committee on Infant Hearing. (2002). Joint Committee on Infant Hearing 2000 position Statement. *American Journal of Audiology, 9*, 9–29.

LaSasso, C., & Metzger, M. (1998). An alternate route for preparing deaf children for bibi programs: The home language as L1 and cued speech for conveying traditionally-spoken languages. *Journal of Deaf Studies and Deaf Education, 3*, 265–289.

Levitt, H., & McGarr, D. (1988). Speech and language development in hearing-impaired children. In. F. H. Bess (Ed.), *Hearing impairment in children* (pp. 45–60). Parkton, MD: York Press.

Lloyd, L., & Kaplan, H. (1993). *Audiometric interpretation: A manual of basic audiometry*. Baltimore: University Park Press.

Mahshie, S. (1995). *Educating deaf children bilingually*. Washington, DC: Gallaudet University Press.

Marschark, M. (1997). *Raising and educating a deaf child: A comprehensive guide to the choices, controversies, and decisions faced by parents and educators*. New York: Oxford University Press.

Maxwell, M. (1990). Simultaneous communication: The state of the art and proposals for change. *Sign Language Studies, 69*, 333–390.

Moores, D. (1997). *Educating the deaf: Psychology, principles, and practices* (4th ed.). Boston: Houghton Mifflin.

National Institutes of Health (1993). *Early identification of hearing impairment in infants and young children.* (NIH Consensus Statement, Vol. 11, No. 1, pp. 1-24). Washington, DC: Author.

Northern, J. L., & Downs, M. (1991). *Hearing in children* (4th ed.). Baltimore: Williams & Wilkins.

Norvelli-Olmstead, T., & Ling, D. (1984). Speech production and speech discrimination by hearing-impaired children. *Volta Review, 86,* 72–82.

Nussbaum, D. (2003). Cochlear implants: Navigating a forest of information. . . . One tree at a time. Washington, DC: Gallaudet University's Laurent Clerc National Deaf Education Center.

Paul, P. (2000). *Language and deafness* (3rd ed.). Clifton Park, NY: Singular.

Paul, P. V., & Quigley, S. P. (1994). *Language and deafness* (2nd ed.). Clifton Park, NY: Singular.

Pollack, D. (1984). An acoupedic program. In D. Ling (Ed.), *Early intervention for hearing-impaired children: Oral options* (pp. 181–253). San Diego, CA: College-Hill Press.

Quigley, S., & Kretschmer, R. E. (1982). *The education of deaf children: Issues, theory, and practice.* Austin, TX: Pro-Ed.

Rhodes, L. (1995). *Introduction to deaf-blindness workshop.* Paper presented at the Central Missouri Deaf-Blind Task Force.

Ross, M. (1990). *Hearing impaired children in the mainstream.* Monkton, MD: York Press.

Sass-Lehrer, M. (1999). Techniques for infants and toddlers with hearing loss. In S. Raver (Ed.), *Intervention strategies for infants and toddlers with special needs: A team approach* (2nd ed.). Upper Saddle River, NJ: Prentice-Hall.

Seal, B. C. (1998). *Best practices in educational interpreting.* Needham Heights, MA: Allyn & Bacon.

Stach, B. A. (1997). *Comprehensive dictionary of audiology.* Baltimore: Williams & Wilkins.

Stach, B. A. (1998). *Clinical audiology: An introduction.* Clifton Park, NY: Singular.

Stewart, D., & Luetke-Stahlman, B. (1998). *The signing family: What every parent should know about sign communication.* Washington, DC: Gallaudet University Press.

Stewart, D. A., Schein, J. D., & Cartwright, B. E. (1998). *Sign language interpreting: Exploring its art and science.* Boston: Allyn & Bacon.

Strong, M., & Prinz, P. (1997). The study of the relationship between American Sign Language and English literacy. *Journal of Deaf Studies,* 2(1), 37–46.

Williams-Scott, B., & Kipila, E. (1987). Cued Speech: A professional point of view. In S. Schwartz (Ed.), *Choices in deafness: A parent's guide.* Kensington, MD: Woodbine House.

Weisenberger, J. M., & Miller, J. D. (1987). The role of tactile aids in providing information about acoustic stimuli. *Journal of the Acoustical Society of America, 82,* 906–916.

Woodward, M. F., & Barber, C. G. (1960). Phoneme perception in lipreading. *Journal of Speech and Hearing Research, 3,* 212–220.

Yoshinago-Itano, C. (1999). Benefits of early intervention for infants with hearing loss. *Otolaryngologic Clinics of North America, 32,* 1089–1102.

Issues in Assessment and Intervention

Introduction

This chapter describes a number of overarching issues important to assessing the communication skills of children who are deaf or hard of hearing and that affect the development and implementation of an intervention plan for these children. The issues presented here apply to children of all ages. Later chapters will focus on particular aspects of assessment that apply to children in particular age ranges.

THE SCOPE OF ASSESSMENT AND INTERVENTION WITH CHILDREN WITH HEARING LOSS

The Scope of assessment and intervention (Table 3-1) seems to lend itself to a developmental framework. The framework includes prelanguage communication, early language, later language, and, finally, adolescent language. It should be kept in mind that these levels or stages do not necessarily represent specific ages; children with hearing loss often present skills and difficulties that cross a number of different stages. For example, a 9-year-old with a progressive hearing loss may present skills that are typical of average children in the later language stages, whereas a congenitally deaf 6-year-old may have some skills that are characteristic of children in the early language stage, yet lack some skills that are characteristic of typical children in the prelanguage stage. The developmental aspect of the Scope is a guide and a possible determiner of current level and future goal directions. The Scope is also divided into expressive and receptive skills with the

Table 3-1 Scope of Areas That Need to Be Considered in Examining the Communication of Deaf and Hard of Hearing Children at Different Stages of Language Development

	Receptive	*Expressive*
Prelanguage	• Pragmatic skills (e.g., intentionality) • Eye contact and turn-taking • Audiovisual (AV) awareness and discrimination • Preliteracy skills	• Pragmatic skills (e.g., intentionality) • Eye contact and turntaking • Vocalization • Preliteracy skills • Visual-gestural
Early Language 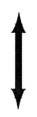	• AV skills • Content • Form • Use • Visual-gestural (if appropriate) • Reading	• Spoken • Voice/prosody • Articulation • Linguistic content, form and use • Visual-gestural (if appropriate) • Use of space • Sign production • Linguistic content, form and use • Written • Mechanics • Linguistic content, form and use • Narrative structure
Later Language 	• Language • Context • Conversational • "School language" • Continued development of content, form and use (including figurative language, vocabulary development, and syntax)	• Context • Conversational • "School" language • Spoken • Speech refinement • Voice • Articulation
Adolescent	• AV reception continued • Sign language and cultural identity • Reading refinement	• Spoken language refinement • Reality check • Interaction with the hearing world

knowledge that these skills may be woven together or worked on independently as appropriate for a given child.

Prelanguage

As shown in Table 3-1, there are a number of expressive and receptive skills along a developmental continuum to be addressed. Among the earliest skills developed in the prelanguage stage are a variety of pragmatic abilities. These include eye contact, turn-taking (e.g., nonlinguistic, visual, and gestural), intent, and response. It should be noted that the level of eye contact appropriate for a deaf or hard of hearing child might actually be greater than that expected of hearing children. Because of the deaf or hard of hearing child's reliance on vision for access to spoken or signed languages, consistent attention and eye contact is an important prerequisite for communication to occur. For the young child showing limited eye contact, activities will probably need to be incorporated into therapy that will build on the child's ability to establish and maintain eye contact for increasing lengths of time.

Turn-taking is an important precursor of communicative behavior. It is thus important to determine whether or not a child can take turns visually in a game with a caregiver (i.e., peek-a-boo), or if the child will pass a ball or other object back and forth with the caregiver or another child. In addition to 1:1 turn-taking (linguistic or nonlinguistic), another feature of turn-taking that is critical, and perhaps less naturally developed in youngsters with hearing loss is the ability to take turns in group situations. The ability to track the group and determine the speaker at any given time is an important communication skill for the child when communicating in school with hearing and deaf peers. Eye contact and turn-taking will facilitate the child's ability to successfully navigate a circle time activity in preschool as well as family conversation around the dinner table.

Lund and Duchan (1993) state that children perform nonlinguistic behaviors not merely to express themselves but to accomplish something. These communicative efforts performed by the child to achieve an end are *intentions*. It is important for the clinician to ascertain the child's sophistication and efficiency in intentionally getting her needs, wants, and preferences met without language. For example, does the child tend to have a tantrum or act out behaviorally until an adult is able to guess what she wants? Does the child point or guide the adult to what she wants, or does she use a random or patterned set of gestures or vocalizations to indicate her needs? These represent different levels of communicative ability and indicate a different starting place for intervention.

As with any child being seen for a speech-language evaluation, it is important to elicit a sound/word repertoire. The clinician determines spontaneous sounds made as well as stimulability for developmentally appropriate sounds. Additional factors that may need to be assessed include the ability to vocalize spontaneously as well as on demand, the presence of sufficient breath support and proper speech breathing, and vocal quality (i.e., pitch, resonance, and loudness).

Two additional areas to be addressed that are specific to children with hearing loss are auditory and visual awareness and discrimination skills to support

Table 3-2 Erber's Stages of Auditory Development	
A. Detection	Detection is the basic process of determining whether a sound is present or absent.
B. Discrimination	Discrimination is the ability to perceive the differences between speech and nonspeech sounds.
C. Identification	Identification is the ability to attach a label to a stimulus and may include the ability to repeat or replicate.
D. Comprehension	Comprehension is the ability to demonstrate understanding and often includes an appropriate response.

From Erber, N. P. (1982). *Auditory training.* Washington, DC: Alexander Graham Bell Association for the Deaf.

listening and speechreading. According to Kaplan, Bally, and Garretson (1987), speechreading includes not only the interpretation of lip and articulator movements but also facial expression, body language, gestures, accessible auditory information, and clues from the context/situation and from language redundancy. Young children at the prelanguage level are expected to be developing awareness/detection skills and discrimination abilities. The clinician is responsible for determining the baseline skill level in these areas and setting an achievable goal for the child to work toward. To orient the clinician to the model of listening and speechreading represented in this book, a brief description of the hierarchy used by Erber (1982) is given in Table 3-2. This hierarchy represents a developmental framework for acquisition of auditory skills that is used by any aural rehabilitation specialist who works with deaf children and adults. These developmentally more advanced levels will be referred to in the section on Early Language.

Finally, it is important to assess and promote preliteracy skills in children at this developmental level. Examples of these skill areas include the following:

- Interest in various forms of print (this may include exposure to fingerspelling for children learning sign language)
- The ability to manipulate books appropriately (directionally and eventually page by page)
- The ability to visually scan from left to right

The existence of a hearing loss may inadvertently limit the child's access to print (e.g., home exposure or story time at the library). This places the child with hearing loss at risk for disinterest and a lack of facility/confidence with print that may continue throughout her life.

These are some of the important skills to be assessed and developed in children with hearing loss who are exhibiting skills at the prelanguage level. The next sections describe some of the knowledge and skills evident during the early language period of development.

Early Language

As the child's language grows it is important to look at not only her access to language but also her ability to understand it, use it, and act on it. The parameters to be addressed are the same as those for hearing children and include language content, form, and use exhibited by the child. Content covers the domain of semantics and includes vocabulary knowledge, word classes, intentions, nonliteral language, and humor (Lund & Duchan, 1993). Form refers to the phonologic, morphologic, and syntactic structures used by the child. The area of pragmatics is contained in the child's use of language. For children who use a visual gestural system, it is essential to determine the child's proficiency with sign language as well as her ability to receive, comprehend, and use spoken language. Children using spoken and signed languages need to have their facility in both languages assessed to gain an accurate picture of language proficiency.

Receptively, it is important to continue to monitor and build the child's visual and auditory skills. As stated previously awareness, discrimination, identification, and comprehension skills for listening and speechreading should be cultivated. Although ideally children at the early language stages of development will exhibit some identification and comprehension skills, it is not unusual for deaf children to have only limited abilities at these higher, more demanding levels of speech reception.

The child will need to be challenged to optimize her potential for accessing spoken language via listening and speechreading. As the child begins to acquire spoken and signed language, these language skills can be integrated into listening and speechreading practice. This is referred to in Kaplan et al. (1987) as *synthetic level therapy*. In addition, a certain amount of analytic training will benefit the child. *Analytic training* includes more concentration on awareness, discrimination, and identification of smaller units of speech via listening and speechreading. For example, the clinician and child may work on reception of specific vowel and consonant sounds. This would include what each sound looks like on the lips as well as what it sounds like to the child. Spoken language expression at the early language stages should be assessed not only for language as outlined earlier but also for speech production including articulation skills, resonance, voice (quality and pitch), and prosody.

The determination of a child's reading comprehension abilities may be the most accurate way of examining the child's ability to comprehend English. When using receptive reading comprehension as a basis for judging receptive English language abilities, it is essential to rule out the existence and subsequent interference of reading problems. Identifying decoding problems may indicate the need for greater attention to phoneme/grapheme (sound/letter) correlations in therapy with the child. Expressive language assessment in written language can be accomplished via an analysis of an elicited or spontaneous language sample (e.g., having the child write about a recent trip or weekend activities). The emphasis of these types of assessments should be on vocabulary and syntax, because it is in this period that the child is expected to demonstrate significant development in both of these areas. Consultation or collaboration with the classroom teacher is essential during these assessments to help determine which deficits are language-based skills and which are academically oriented.

If assessment of sign language is deemed appropriate, the parameters to be assessed are the same as those for spoken language. Articulation of signs is referred to as *sign production skills*. This includes the correct production of a sign in terms of hand shape, palm orientation, location, and movement. Also important is the child's appropriate use of sign space and her ability to fingerspell accurately and appropriately. Because English language rules are different from those of American Sign Language (ASL), linguistic content, form, and use should also be evaluated in terms of the sign language or system used by the child. A Sign Language expert or an individual proficient in assessing ASL should be integrated into the assessment process. This may require contracting with an evaluator from a local school for the deaf or another facility with individuals trained in this type of assessment.

Easterbrooks and Baker (2002) suggest several sources for evaluating students' ASL skills. The first is a Checklist of Emerging ASL Skills (McIntire, 1994; Valli & Lucas, 1995; Wix & Supalla, n.d.). To use this checklist, the evaluator identifies a language skill to assess and then observes the student in both natural conversation and prompted activities to determine if it is currently in the student's repertoire. A second checklist, the ASL Development Checklist, was developed by Evans, Zimmer, and Murray (1994). This checklist provides a series of indicators to judge whether a deaf student has components of ASL in her communication system.

It is again important to keep in mind that the focus should be on ASL and not the student's English ability. The student should be evaluated by three different evaluators using the checklist. The evaluators must be skilled in ASL and be familiar with the students being evaluated. For each indicator on the checklist, the evaluator will judge the student's ASL skills relative to other students they know who have the same degree of hearing loss and are of the same age.

Later Language

Expressively and receptively, it is important to evaluate and address difficulties a later language learner might exhibit in various aspects of language that encompass spoken language, visual gestural communication, written language, and contextual language. As stated earlier, written English may be a more representative means of assessing English language knowledge of a deaf or hard of hearing child, particularly when there are significant speech production problems. If the child with a hearing loss does not speak or has limited facility for spoken language, the written word will clearly yield a more complete basis for examining the child's English language knowledge and use.

As the deaf or hard of hearing child develops and becomes a more proficient language user and achieves academically, it is important to continue to ensure she reaches her full linguistic, academic, and communicative potential. All of the areas previously assessed should continue to be evaluated at developmentally appropriate levels and the appropriate intervention provided. In addition, it is important to assess the child's language skills in terms of conversational language and "school" language. These are skills that the hearing language learner develops during her school years and that will impact a deaf or hard of hearing child's academic and social success. Conversational language facility reflects the child's ability to communicate with peers. For example, does the child evidence the ability to take the listener's perspective, providing sufficient yet not redundant information when sharing experiences? Does the child navigate colloquialisms, idioms, and nonliteral language forms? Has she developed adequate vocabulary to support academic and social needs? Can she use and understand a variety of age appropriate forms of humor?

"School" language refers to the child's ability to navigate and use the language of the classroom. For example, does the child understand the directions given in school? Is she able to understand the language forms and questions used by the teacher or those that appear in typical academic texts? Can she define words?

Text becomes more and more important for achievement as a child develops as a student. Reading comprehension and written language may be assessed as described in the preceding section. In addition, the narrative structure used by the child in writing will yield important information regarding the sophistication of the child's English language skills (e.g., the use of cohesion, sophisticated syntax, or sequencing of ideas). A strong language base in English or strategies for using ASL to support English language learning must be in place by this time. The speech-language therapist is an integral team player in this process.

Adolescent Language

As the language user reaches adolescence, continued assessment and intervention are as important as at the earlier stages. The difficulty at this time is that the child may become less willing to participate in the therapeutic process. The continued development and improvement of the skills contained in the Scope (see Table 3-1) support and ensure academic success beyond the secondary level or success in the work world. In addition, linguistic proficiency and communicative sophistication become inextricably woven into the child's formation of identity.

The Scope presented in this text should be viewed as a fluid concept. Each child will move through the various skills and stages at different rates. Some may be precocious and others delayed. In addition, each child may be at different stages for different skills. It should also be noted that some skill areas may not progress as rapidly as others, or they may plateau. If this happens, decisions should be made with the family and/or the child to determine future intervention for that area. Options at that point may include abandoning work in that area, modifying the goals to reflect a more attainable functional level of achievement or perhaps alternative strategies for attaining the goal. For example, a high school student who has been unable to achieve any intelligible speech may choose to abandon articulation goals. On the other hand, the student may choose to alter the goal and attempt to develop simply accurate mouth movements that may aid in face-to-face interactions.

THE PURPOSE OF ASSESSMENT

Communication assessment is an ongoing process with the aim of achieving a number of different goals. Among the major purposes for assessment are the following:

1. Screening and referral
2. Eligibility and placement
3. Instructional planning
4. Monitoring progress (Kratcoski, 1998)

Determining the appropriate procedures to use in evaluating a deaf or hard of hearing child is often complicated by the need to meet school district and state requirements for assessment on one hand and the need to obtain information that can lead to effective and efficient communication intervention on the other. Assessment is further complicated by the limitations of the academic year—one cannot spend so much time on assessment and evaluation that intervention is delayed. This presents a dilemma to the clinician who must balance the need for assessment aimed at various purposes with the need to initiate intervention in a timely manner.

The following section will describe a few general concepts concerning the evaluation of communication skills of deaf and hard of hearing children. Although the general orientation to assessing a deaf child is similar to that one might consider in assessing a hearing child, there are a number of special considerations that need to be kept in mind.

THE BROAD CONTEXT FOR EVALUATION

It is often tempting to consider the deaf or hard of hearing child simply in terms of hearing or speech. It is of utmost importance, however, to consider the child from the broader perspective of her ability to communicate. The child's communicative competence represents the best indicator of how well the child is able to interact with and learn from her environment. Communicative competence is the knowledge required of an individual to communicate appropriately within a given speech community, as well as the skills required to make use of that knowledge (Singh & Kent, 2000). Communicative competence can be viewed as the overlap among the child's speech and language system, knowledge, and cognition. It thus becomes important to consider not only factors such as speech and auditory ability but also the child's overall ability to communicate with others. In other words, all the factors that are normally considered in evaluating a hearing child's communicative competence apply equally to the child with a hearing loss.

The selection of specific tests will depend on an initial prioritization of the factors described in the section discussing the Scope of assessment and intervention given earlier in this chapter. An informal screening often provides adequate information to enable the clinician to develop a list of essential areas in need of further assessment. These may include, but are not limited to, the following:

- Oral mechanism
- Receptive skills
- General language functioning
- Phonology and articulation
- Morphology and syntax
- Semantics (vocabulary)
- Classroom achievement of performance
- Learner characteristics
- Intelligence
- Personality characteristics
- Environmental or home characteristics
- Classroom environment
- Additional disabilities

MULTIPLE LANGUAGE INFLUENCES

During the past few years, much attention has been given to the issue of multiple language use in young school children. Growing numbers of children in U.S. public schools come from homes in which English is the second language (Goldstein, 2000). Advocates for deaf children suggest viewing and teaching English as a second language to children with hearing loss (Johnson, Liddell, & Erting, 1989; Mahshie, 1995). Thus, a major goal for education of deaf or hard of hearing children may be for some of them to become bilingual in ASL and English. The form of the second language, English, may be either written or spoken, depending on the needs of each individual child. For some deaf children, English may become a third or possibly fourth language. For example, a deaf child from Mexico may have spoken and signed languages in Spanish and then be exposed to English and ASL when she enrolls in the public schools in the United States.

Cummins (1984) hypothesized two levels of language competence needed to be fluent and competent in either a first or second language. The first level he defines as basic interpersonal communication skills (BICS). This is a level defined mostly by conversational interaction for which the speaker can rely on the context and a more predictable topic. The second level is defined as cognitive academic language proficiency (CALP). This level is needed for critical thinking, problem solving, inferencing, and other higher-order thinking skills. These two levels described by Cummins appear to be closely aligned with the language knowledge needed to succeed in schools: everyday discourse (interpersonal conversation) and instructional discourse (the language of the school) (Wallach & Miller, 1988).

Conversational language is informal and contextual and involves more frequent turn-taking and shared assumptions, whereas school language (both face to face and written) is formal and decontextualized and involves considerable background knowledge and comprehension of assumptions thought to be shared by the culture at large. The amount of knowledge imparted through instructional discourse is considerable during the school years and probably involves language proficiency at a "deeper" level (CALP) than that involved with interpersonal skills.

The authors have found the above concepts useful to keep in mind when assessing deaf and hard of hearing children. First, the knowledge that a specific child may indeed have several language influences in her life is important when trying to get an overview of what language the child knows. For example, she may use speech for individual words, while using sign language for the combination of words. Both modes must be addressed to ensure full knowledge of the language competence of the child. In addition, a child may be able to comprehend and use speech well for conversational interaction with family and peers; however, this does not assure that the child can comprehend or use speech well enough to participate in the classroom situation or learn new information in a timely manner. For example, the child may use speech to verbally interact with family and peers but have considerable difficulty with the language of the school. Making a differentiation between interpersonal language and school language is an important aspect of assessing the child's abilities and will probably be accomplished through intensive on-going evaluation and intervention.

PSYCHOSOCIAL CONSIDERATIONS

It is recognized that the vast majority of deaf and hard of hearing children are born into families with hearing parents. As a result, most deaf children exist in a family and social milieu in which they experience being different from those around them. Although little research has been done to examine the cultural issues involved in families in which a deaf child is born of hearing parents, there are perhaps some analogies that can be drawn from transracial adoptions, a situation in which adoptive parents and children are "different" in both physical and cultural ways. Patton (2000) suggests that

> "While the parents of some (transracial) adoptees are conscientious about exposing their children to their cultural origin, others see these concerns as irrelevant. Whether raised with such awareness or not, international and African-American adoptees report a disjuncture between the ways they experience themselves and the. . .treatment to which they are subjected at school. Indeed, such experiences are often the catalyst for their cultural explorations as adults." (p. 13)

These children can be considered members of a *nonfamilial* culture, a concept described by and borrowed from Pohan and Bailey (1997). The authors describe the experience in the following way in relationship to gay and lesbian youth with straight parents:

> "What makes this void so devastating is that while students of different ethnicities, races, and religions can go home for emotional support from family, students who are gay and lesbian often have no place to go for the much needed support." (pp. 12–15)

Although the limited studies tend to focus on transracial adoptions or gay and lesbian youth with straight parents, the concept appears equally applicable to the child with hearing loss who feels at odds with all those around her. Marschark (1997) discusses how deaf children with hearing parents have "atypical" experiences that can adversely affect their social, linguistic, and even intellectual development. This experience may have significant effects on the child's identity development and ability to reconcile their identity within the world around them.

Marschark (1997) also discusses the medical and cultural perspectives of deafness and their impact on the child, particularly when the family embraces the deficit over the difference paradigm. A medical perspective is one that focuses on the pathology of hearing loss and a desire to fix the "broken" ear. A cultural perspective focuses on hearing loss/deafness as a difference not a disability. For a hearing parent of a deaf child who adheres to a medical/pathologic perspective of his or her child, the child is viewed as deficient, or in some way "broken." Hearing parents who adopt a more cultural perspective on hearing loss may be able to overcome some of the negative impact of the nonfamilial experience of their child.

Longres (1995) and Troiden (1989) suggest that the sociologic environment in which an individual exists and the interactions she is afforded is important to the identity development process and subsequent difficulties because of the child's "differentness." Individuals, particularly those without familial support, need opportunities to see and interact with others like themselves to normalize their experience and view it in terms of a difference rather than disability. For children in mainstream educational settings the environment does not readily provide the types of experiences/interactions necessary to facilitate efficient and healthy identity development.

Strategies for Enhancing the Deaf or Hard of Hearing Child's Self-Perception

There are strategies and techniques that can be incorporated to diminish the alienation or disenfranchisement of the mainstreamed student with hearing loss. All of the techniques will require effort on the part of the specialists, teachers, and advocates working with the child as well as her parents. The audiologist or speech-language pathologist may be the individual who needs to accept the responsibility to educate the school community and strive for the implementation of the strategies and techniques designed to foster a healthy self-concept for the deaf or hard of hearing child.

Child-Focused Strategies

The techniques are two-pronged, focusing on both the child and the environment in which she exists. The identity of the child as a deaf, hard of hearing, or hearing impaired-individual is a necessary element. (Most people in the deaf and hard of hearing community prefer the terms *deaf and hard of hearing* rather than *hearing-impaired*, because the latter term is viewed as focusing on the individual's limits or deficits.) If the child is taught to or expected to identify as a hearing person, it is highly likely that she will identify as a "broken" hearing person.

Instead, it is suggested that she be able to develop a healthy identity as a deaf or hard of hearing individual. This process is achieved by assisting the child in developing an awareness of her strengths and areas for improvement in the context of being a whole person. This moves the paradigm away from concentrating on the child's ears and mouth to who she is as a learner, communicator, and individual. There will still be subsequent attention to the specifics of increasing her awareness of her communication strengths and weaknesses. This, however, is only done after and as part of the understanding that she has developed of herself as a whole person. Based on the child's recognized strengths and areas for improvement resulting from an ongoing, holistic evaluation of the child, the speech-language pathologist (SLP) would foster the development of skills and abilities for communicating in a variety of settings with a variety of communication partners. This would serve to make therapy individualized and specific but also rewarding, allowing for the child's strengths to be featured in the context of addressing goal areas. Finally, it would be important to provide opportunities to use these skills in a variety of settings to increase confidence and comfort.

Environment-Focused Strategies

As mentioned earlier, there will also be an initiative to address the environment in which the child exists. This will include her home, her community, and, specific to the audiologist or speech-language clinician serving as advocate and educator, the school community. The school climate will play a large role in determining the success or failure of the child's healthy identity formation. A school climate of pity and pathology concerning the child's hearing loss will infiltrate and affect the child's own perspective. If, on the other hand, it embraces the diversity of hearing loss and provides opportunities for the child to normalize her experience and display her strengths, the impact can be far more positive. The school climate is often dictated by the teachers, staff, and administrators. Therefore, it is integral to this process for the audiologist or speech-language therapist to begin with the school staff. Education regarding the importance of developing a supportive and nurturing climate will be the first step. When the school staff understands and fosters this idea, additional strategies and techniques can be woven into the fabric of that particular school's climate. This will necessitate increasing the knowledge base of teachers, administrators, specialists, and staff through in-service training. Asking deaf adults from the community to come and speak during in-services will provide those in the school with familiarity about deaf and hard of hearing people and give the adults in the school the opportunity to experience communication challenges. This will educate them about the options, considerations, conventions, and etiquette for communication with individuals who have hearing losses. When appropriate, interpreters should be brought in to facilitate communication between the hearing school staff and the deaf individuals from the community. It will also be important to invite a variety of deaf and hard of hearing people to visit. This will allow for the diversity of the deaf and hard of hearing community to be realized. School personnel can benefit from understanding that deaf and hard of hearing people communicate in a variety of ways and that they mirror the diversity of the hearing community in terms of race, ethnicity, religion, sexual orientation, and socioeconomic and educational levels.

A helpful next step is to work toward the inclusion of hearing loss/deafness in the school's multicultural education framework. Multiculturalism is an important part of every school's curriculum and is an appropriate and advantageous strategy for educating the school community about hearing loss and the achievements and diversity within the deaf community. The audiologist and speech-language clinician as well as deaf individuals from the community will need to provide information about hearing loss and deaf culture. This also becomes the opportunity to begin including students in the process. Children in all classes can learn about deaf and hard of hearing people and their culture. Although class(es) with deaf or hard of hearing student(s) may need additional education, the entire school could be included.

Use of Interpreters.   Educational interpreters as well as interpreters hired for meetings and presentations are integral components of the process. These individuals often serve as the link between the deaf and hearing worlds. It is important that everyone in the school understand the role and the qualifications of the interpreters. A national Registry of Interpreters for the Deaf (RID) exists and can be helpful in understanding interpretation for the deaf and in locating interpreters. The organization's web site, www.rid.org, includes helpful information such as certification levels and types as well as the code of ethics. Interpreting for the deaf, as opposed to interpretation into spoken foreign languages, is a highly developed, sophisticated, and, to greater and lesser degrees depending on location, regulated discipline. Interpreters who are nationally certified are bound by the code of ethics and required to maintain certification through continuing education. Nationally registered interpreters can hold CI (Certificate of Interpretation), CT (Certificate of Transliteration), or CI/CT endorsements. These indicate what type of interpretation they are able to provide. CI indicates that the interpreter can use ASL. CT indicates that the interpreter translates using a more English-based manual system. CI/CT interpreters can use either ASL or an English-based system. It is important to realize, however, that different states have different criteria for interpreters and specifically educational interpreters. Some states use the RID certification levels whereas others have their own systems and levels. Other states or jurisdictions may have no formal system for rating and hiring educational interpreters.

Similarly, transliterators for individuals using Cued Speech should be as qualified as possible. Generally, individuals are certified through TECUnit Inc, a national certifying body. More information regarding Cued Speech and transliteration can be found at www.cuedspeech.com or www.cuedspeech.org. Tansliterators function much like interpreters and should be considered and worked with in a similar manner.

There are conventions for working with interpreters, and both deaf and hearing consumers working with them need to familiarize themselves with these conventions. It is important to discuss with the interpreter what a specific individual's needs are related to communicating with deaf individuals. Some hearing people can understand some sign combined with voice and only need interpreters to expressively communicate for them. Some deaf people choose to voice for themselves and others do not. It is important to work out the expectations and needs among the communication partners and the interpreter. The interpreter is the conduit of information and should not be addressed directly during communication interactions. Often people unfamiliar with the interpreting process will say "Tell her . . ." (indicating the deaf person). This can be avoided by viewing the interpreter as a channel for information; one should maintain eye contact with the deaf person with whom one is interacting. It is helpful to have the interpreter positioned near to the hearing person so that the deaf or hard of hearing person can maintain as much eye contact with the hearing person while still being able to follow the interpreter.

Educational interpreters are sometimes hired by school systems as an interpreter/tutor. This is not an ideal situation because it requires the interpreter to step out of her role as interpreter and provides direct support to the student. This can sometimes complicate the relationship and lead to difficulties among the student, the interpreter, and the teacher or therapist. It is most beneficial if the SLP, educational audiologist, teacher of the deaf, or reading specialist provide the additional support the student needs. Educational interpreters should also be among the most well trained and highly qualified interpreters. Unfortunately, because of budget constraints, this is often not the case. Anecdotally, there is evidence that educational interpreters are sometimes hired without any formal certification or skill level. The educational interpreter is the only means for some students to access the information in the classroom and if the interpreter is not highly skilled, the child and her education will suffer.

Interpreters and transliterators also assist in creating a more accessible and interactive learning environment for the deaf or hard of hearing child. The deaf child is more able to participate if she has the interpreter voicing what she is comfortable signing but unable or uncomfortable voicing. This allows the student to express herself and show evidence of her knowledge in an optimal manner.

Rules for Communication.   Another consideration is the communication within the classroom. There should be clear communication rules within the classroom, specifically for larger group interactions. The interpreter is only able to sign for one voice at a time. Thus, clear communication rules need to be established and maintained so that the deaf child has equal access to what is being said in the classroom.

These "communication rules" are about respect as much as they are about access. The promotion of communication access through shared responsibility will foster a climate of respect. Shared responsibility is the idea that all communication partners have a commitment and duty to the communication process. It is not simply the deaf child's responsibility to make sure that communication is effective. Recognition that an interpreter is present for both parties helps to promote shared responsibility. Also in one-on-one interactions the child with a hearing loss and the hearing child or adult should be able to employ communication strategies to establish, maintain, and or repair communication. The speech-language clinician or educational audiologist can teach these skills. All members of the community benefit when a climate of respect and shared responsibility infiltrates a school environment. The particular benefit to the child with a hearing loss is that the environment becomes safe, comfortable, and nurturing.

Establishing Goals That Are Positive to a Child's Self-Image

Once an appropriately nurturing environment has been established, the school community will be prepared to meet the academic, communicative, and psychosocial needs of a child with a hearing loss. In this school the deaf or hard of hearing student will be able to fully participate in all academic, social, and extracurricular activities. Current trends in education support the idea that children who are involved and invested in the education process are successful and develop strong self-images (Haberman, 1991).

The child with a hearing loss will flourish in an environment such as the one described but will also need additional support. This additional support will address identifying the child's strengths as well as identifying the communication and learning needs she may have. The identification of the child's strengths is important in the process of identifying and addressing areas for improvement. Not only will the strengths create a balance for the child, but they can also become strategies and techniques for overcoming or working through weaknesses. Identification of the areas for improvement will provide the goals for the student's Individualized Education Plan (IEP).

The goals developed from assessment and negotiation with the child and her family may be addressed and achieved quickly or over extended periods of time. When they are achieved quickly they can then be moved to the skill or strength areas. Sometimes, however, skills are slower in development and eventual mastery. In fact, some skills may at some point be identified as unachievable. When this happens, decisions need to be made regarding discontinuing work on the goal or modifying the expectation for achievement. For example, a child with a hearing loss may develop intelligible speech, and many sounds may be produced correctly except for the sibilant sounds (i.e., s and /s/, and so on). When this happens, it may become necessary to accept a particular distorted production as the best possible. This new target will then become the standard by which the child's speech production is judged. In other cases goals may be discontinued and replaced with others. An example of this is the older child who does not develop speech that is intelligible at any level. One strategy used in this situation is to encourage the child to turn off her voice and simply work on improving accurate mouth movements to represent words. This has anecdotally been observed to be a more effective communication tool than voicing attempts that in no way represent the target word.

In addition to the modification of goals that may take an extended period to be achieved or changed is the idea of the child's perception of the continued focus on a particular outcome. A child will be aware that similar goals are being addressed for months or years. It is necessary to keep the child motivated to persevere in the attention to these goals. However, it is also important to ensure that the child has an accurate understanding of her skill level. To achieve both of these, the child should be praised and reinforced for the attempt but not misled regarding the accuracy of that attempt. Anecdotal reports from deaf adults indicate that some speech-language clinicians praised the speech demonstrated, but then when the deaf adult used that speech in public the hearing person did not understand. This impression has been supported by recent research (Mahshie, Moseley, & Robins, 2002).

The lack of a clear perception of her own intelligibility often results in a negative experience for the deaf person and mistrust of the SLP. Honesty and reinforcement of the effort put forth by the deaf or hard of hearing child is more useful in the long term.

Positive Role Models

The child with an accurate self-concept will then be ready to encounter the world equipped for the many experiences offered. Unfortunately, for many children with hearing loss these encounters do not include deaf or hard of hearing peers or adults. As mentioned earlier, interaction with peers and adult role models is essential to normalizing differences and development of a positive self-image. Children with hearing loss can benefit from efforts to increase access to deaf and hard of hearing peers and adult role models. Being able to interact with other children who share the similar obstacles and feelings will help the children process what they are experiencing. The adults allow the children to see what they can become and get a perspective that their own parents cannot offer.

Strategies for Enhancing Self-Esteem

Finally, it is necessary to provide a variety of self-esteem building activities that allow the child to be successful within and outside of the school community. All the opportunities presented to children with normal hearing should be provided to deaf and hard of hearing children. Additionally, experiences that are specific to deaf and hard of hearing children are important. Experiences that allow the child to use her communication skills in successful ways will also lead to greater confidence and self-esteem. Interpreters are again important and the staff interpreter or one provided by the destination of the field trip will be essential to the child's ability to maximize the experience.

Summary

There are certainly obstacles and barriers in the overall development of children with hearing loss. It is, however, possible through the effort of advocates and educators to minimize the negative impact and overcome many of them. Children with hearing loss are successful and well adjusted when they attend programs that have implemented attitudes, techniques, and strategies similar to those discussed in this chapter. The psychosocial development of children with hearing loss is the foundation upon which academic, communicative, and personal successes are based. It is negligent to ignore this aspect of students' lives. In addition, everyone in the academic community benefits from the approach advocated in this text.

ASSESSMENT—OBTAINING INFORMATION

Communication assessment involves obtaining all available information concerning a child's ability to communicate. It is recognized that many school districts have a prescribed set of standardized tests that are required for eligibility, development of IEPs, and academic placement. Such tests can provide some useful information. However, use of these tests alone is often inadequate for determining starting points for therapy and the appropriate modalities for teaching certain skills. The following discusses some of the issues and additional considerations for obtaining information for assessing communication.

Interview

In assessing the communication abilities of deaf and hard of hearing children, it is often difficult to get a complete picture of strengths and weaknesses through testing alone. In most cases, individuals in the child's environment are able to provide details about how the child communicates needs, how variable the child's spoken language may be, how adaptable the child is as a communicator, and in what circumstances the child is best able to communicate. It is essential to have a clear understanding of the child's communicative functioning in a variety of settings and contexts. It is not unusual for a parent to describe a child's communicative abilities in a way that differs from the perception of teachers, clinicians, and others in the child's school environment. It is thus important to sort out what seem to be differing reports of communication ability to determine where the child's range of abilities might lie. It is possible that the child is more comfortable or more effective in communicating in some situations than in others. Alternatively, the parent or teacher's familiarity and communication style will play an important role in determining how "'effective'" the child is perceived as a communicator.

It is additionally important to know about any family-based factors that might impact the child's progress in therapy. Among the factors that might influence how therapy is structured for a child are the language used in the home, the availability of opportunities to use spoken language, sign language or manual systems such as cues at home, siblings and the communicative "'competition'" in the home, the acceptance of a child's deafness by immediate and extended family, and family problems that might affect the emotional well-being of the child. The interview also provides an opportunity to explore factors that might suggest the existence of disabilities (beyond deafness) that could impact communication ability.

Standardized Tests

A variety of terms have been used to describe tests that comprise the majority of those available instruments for measuring a child's speech, language, and hearing abilities. Although terms such as standardized tests, formal tests, and norm-referenced tests have all been applied to such instruments, the present authors feel that these are not equivalent terms and some distinction among these categories of instruments is needed. A *standardized test* is one that has a prescribed set of procedures for administration. If there are associated norms that have resulted from administering this test to large numbers of children representative of a particular population, then the test may also be considered *norm-referenced*. However, not all standardized tests are norm referenced—only those for which normative data have been obtained and provided to the user. Although the term *formal tests* might apply to all standardized tests, norm-referenced or not, the term does not contribute additionally to the current discussion and so will be used minimally in this text.

Norm-Referenced Tests

A few norm-referenced tests have been developed for use with deaf children. These tests are unique in that they provide normative data for comparing the performance of deaf and hard of hearing children to that of other deaf and hard of hearing children. Often, these measures provide a useful means of demonstrating that the progress being made by a child is either adequate or inadequate and can thus contribute to decisions about the appropriateness of academic placement and services.

There are also a number of reasons for administering certain tests that have been normed not on children that are deaf or hard of hearing but rather on hearing children. A primary reason is that the tests that have been developed and normed on deaf children are limited both in number and scope. There are areas of speech and language for which adequate tests have not been developed and normed for deaf children. Additionally, because the goal is often to facilitate the deaf or hard of hearing child's attainment of language levels comparable to that of her peers, some comparison of a child's performance to that of her hearing peers is desirable. A partial list of norm-referenced language tests used with deaf children is given in Figure 3-1.

An additional reason for using tests normed on hearing children is the concern in deaf education that expectations are often low and that children often rise to (or are limited to) our level of expectation. If the expectation for a deaf child is that she reach levels comparable to those of her hearing peers, there is an inherent limitation to comparing communication performance of deaf children only to that of other deaf children. Comparing the test performance of a deaf child to that of her hearing peers implies the expectation that the child has the potential of performing comparably to her hearing peers, at least in some aspects of communication.

Assessment of Children's Language Comprehension (ACLC):
Areas of language assessed: receptive language, syntax
Standardization: hearing children
Age range: 3 to 6½ years
Available through: Consulting Psychologists Press, Inc.*
577 College Ave.
Palo Alto, CA 94306

Boehm Test of Basic Concepts:
Areas of language assessed: semantics
Standardization: hearing children
Age range: preschool, elementary
Available through: The Psychological Corporation
555 Academic Ct.
San Antonio, TX 78204

Carolina Picture Vocabulary Test:
Areas of language assessed: receptive signed vocabulary
Standardization: children with hearing loss
Age range: 2½ to 16 years
Available through: Pro-Ed
8700 Shoal Creek Blvd.
Austin, TX 78757

Clinical Evaluation of Language Fundamentals (CELF):
Areas of language assessed: language processing and production
Standardization: hearing children
Age range: grades K through 12
Available through: The Psychological Corporation
555 Academic Ct.
San Antonio, TX 78204

Expressive One-Word Picture Vocabulary Test (EOWPVT):
Areas of language assessed: expressive vocabulary
Standardization: hearing children
Age range: 2 to 12 years
Expressive One-Word Picture Vocabulary Test - Upper Extension
Age range: 12 to 16 years
Available through: Academic Therapy Publications
20 Commercial Blvd.
Novato, CAr 94949

Figure 3-1. Selected Published Language Tests

(continues)

Gouchner Idiom Screening Test (GIST):
   Areas of language assessed: comprehension of idioms
   Standardization: children with hearing loss
   Age range: high school, college
   Available through: Interstate Printers & Publishers, Inc.*
   Danville, IL 61832

Grammatical Analysis of Elicited Language (GAEL):
   Pre-sentence level
   Simple sentence level
   Complex sentence level
   Areas of language assessed: syntax
   Standardization: hearing children and children with hearing loss
   Age range: pre-school through early elementary
   Available through: Central Institute for the Deaf
   818 S. Euclid Street
   St. Louis, MO 63110

Peabody Picture Vocabulary Test (PPVT):
   Areas of language assessed: receptive vocabulary
   Standardization: hearing children, youth, and a selected sample of adults
   Age range: 2½ to 18 years
   Available through: American Guidance Service
   4201 Woodland Rd.
   Circle Pines, MN 55014

Preschool Language Scale (PLS):
   Areas of language assessed: auditory comprehension and verbal ability
   Standardization: hearing Head Start children
   Age range: 1 to 7 years
   Available through: The Psychological Corporation
   555 Academic Ct.
   San Antonio, TX 78204

Receptive One-Word Picture Vocabulary Test (ROWPVT):
   Areas of language assessed: receptive vocabulary
   Standardization: hearing children
   Age range: 2 to 12 years
   Available through: Academic Therapy Publications
   20 Commercial Blvd.
   Novato, CA 94949

Figure 3-1.   (continued)

(continues)

Rhode Island Test of Language Structure (RITLS):
Areas of language assessed: syntax
Standardization: hearing children and children with hearing loss
Age range: children with hearing loss 3 to 20 years; hearing children 3
    to 6 years
Available through: University Park Press*
300 N. Charles St.
Baltimore, MD 21201

Test of Adolescent Language (TOAL):
Areas of language assessed: comprehension and production of spoken
    and written grammar and vocabulary
Standardization: hearing children
Age range: 11 to 18 years
Available through: Pro-Ed
8700 Shoal Creek Blvd.
Austin, TX 78757

Test of Expressive Language Ability (TEXLA):
Areas of language assessed: expressive
Standardization: hearing children and children with hearing loss
Age range: early elementary
Available through: G. B. Services*
100 Waterton Rd.
Westin, ON, Canada M5P 2R3

Test of Language Competence (TLC):
Areas of language assessed: figurative language
Standardization: hearing children
Age range: 9 to 19 years
Available through: The Psychological Corporation
555 Academic Ct.
San Antonio, TX 78204

Test of Language Development:
Primary (TOLD-P)
Intermediate (TOLD-I)
Areas of language assessed: syntax and semantics; production and
    comprehension
Standardization: hearing children
Age range: primary 4 to 9 years; intermediate 8½ to 13 years
Available through: Pro-Ed
8700 Shoal Creek Blvd.
Austin, TX 78757

Figure 3-1. (continued)

(continues)

Test of Problem Solving (TOPS):
 Areas of language assessed: thinking and reasoning; e.g., explaining
  inferences, determining causes, negative why questions, determining
  solutions, avoiding problems
 Standardization: hearing children
 Age range: 6 to 12 years (may be used above 12 years)
 Available through: Linguisystems, Inc.
 3100 4th Ave.
 East Moline, IL 61244-9700

Test of Receptive Language Ability (TERLA):
 Areas of language assessed: receptive
 Standardization: hearing children and children with hearing loss
 Age range: early elementary
 Available through: G.B. Services*
 100 Waterton Rd.
 Westin, ON, Canada M5P 2R3

Test of Syntactic Abilities (TSA):
 Areas of language assessed: comprehension of written syntax
 Standardization: children with hearing loss
 Age range: high school, college
 Available through: Dormac, Inc.*
 P.O. Box 752
 Beaverton, OR 97005

Test of Written Language (TOWL):
 Areas of language assessed: written language
 Standardization: hearing children
 Age range: 7 to 19 years
 Available through: Pro-Ed
 8700 Shoal Creek Blvd.
 Austin, TX 78757

Figure 3-1. (continued)
*Address provided is for the last known publisher.

Although it is obvious how such information might be valuable, there are
clearly impediments to interpreting the performance of children who are deaf
or hard of hearing on many norm-referenced tests developed for hearing children. It is often necessary to alter the administration of these tests in significant
ways. The most typical alteration relates to the way that a question or task is
presented. For example, the Peabody Picture Vocabulary Test (Dunn & Dunn,
2000) was normed on a hearing population by asking the child to point to one of
four pictures depicting a particular vocabulary or lexical item. For a child who
is deaf, presentation of the stimuli via speech would be an obvious problem.
Clinicians often administer this test to their deaf or hard of hearing children by

signing the desired items, but there are obvious problems in interpreting results obtained in this way. A sign may contain iconic information that will provide cues to the child that may lead to a correct response while the child may have little lexical knowledge of the item presented. There is some value, however, in obtaining such information, but it is important that the results be qualified in terms of the modifications in administration. The results can provide a "'qualified'" description of how the child is performing compared with her hearing peers and also provide useful information concerning the linguistic knowledge already acquired by the child that can be used in establishing goals for therapy.

Criterion-Referenced Tests

Another category of tests should be mentioned: criterion-referenced tests. Haynes and Pindzola (1998) described such tests as follows:

> Rather than indicating a person's relative standing in skill development, criterion referenced tests measure a person's development of particular skills in terms of absolute levels of mastery. . . .Items on criterion-referenced tests are often linked directly to specific instructional objectives and therefore facilitate the writing of objectives. Test items sample sequential skills, enabling a teacher not only to know the specific point at which to begin instruction but also to plan those instructional aspects that follow directly in the curricular sequence.

As Haynes and Pindzola point out, the focus of criterion-referenced tests is clearly different from that of norm-referenced tests. Whereas norm-referenced tests focus on group similarity, criterion-reference tests emphasize individual performance. Although such instruments would be of obvious value, there are very few criterion-referenced tests available that are specifically designed for deaf children.

Informal Assessment

In many cases the specialist must rely on information that is obtained through informal assessment procedures. Informal procedures are typically self-devised tasks and activities designed to establish a child's knowledge and use of a particular skill. The clinician might examine a child's knowledge of prepositions, for example, by using toys and objects to determine whether the child can either describe (in sign or English) a prepositional relationship or understand such a relationship. Informal assessment procedures may also involve less structured observations aimed to characterize the ways that a child communicates or that capture some of the patterns a child exhibits. In many cases, such informal procedures become incorporated into therapy, thus yielding what is more appropriately called diagnostic therapy. Such observations enable the clinician to assess how the child interacts in a classroom with teachers and peers or with parents or other caregivers.

Informal tests, by definition, do not employ standardized procedures for administration, but this does not mean that informal procedures are casual or without specific purpose. Indeed, the aim of informal procedures is typically to assess a particular skill or set of skills. Although in some cases the purpose may be very general (e.g., the child's overall interaction with her peers), in other situations informal procedures will enable the clinician to obtain very specific information about particular knowledge or skills (e.g., does the child understand and use prepositions such as in, on, and under?).

A particular informal procedure must thus be defined both in terms of the particular attribute being assessed and the procedure to be used to obtain that information. In considering the aspect of communication to be assessed, it is important that the clinician be knowledgeable of the appropriate developmental sequence for a particular skill to be able to adequately characterize the child's performance.

There are, of course, many different procedures one could use to evaluate a particular skill. The clinician-developed procedures can be based on those employed in standardized tests or based on many procedures that have been employed in research to describe a particular linguistic ability. For example, analyzing a language sample for specific categories of child intentions, such as *regulatory, personal*. (Halliday, 1975) (see chapter 5). It is also important to realize that informal procedures are also subject to the need for validity and reliability that applies to more formalized tests (Haynes & Pindzola, 1998).

The Need for Ongoing Assessment

It is important to get initial information about a child's communicative strengths and weaknesses to establish appropriate starting points for intervention. However, assessment is not a single event but rather a process. In some cases, therapy may have as its focus further evaluation of a particular aspect of communication. In other cases, therapy will require periodic assessment to determine progress toward or mastery of a particular goal. In both cases, assessment is not limited to a single event in time but is rather integrated into treatment. This will be elaborated on further later in this chapter.

Issues Related to Assessing Communication Access

Communication access is an essential prerequisite for communication and, as such, needs to be evaluated. Chapter 2 discusses relevant ways to evaluate the child's hearing, vision, and environment to assure the child is getting maximum sensory information.

Overview of Issues Involved in Assessing Speech

Assessing speech is, of course, a necessary starting point for intervention. The information about a child's knowledge and skills related to spoken language allows the professional to determine both what the child can do and what limitations might appropriately be the focus of therapy. There are a number of general considerations that one might have in assessing a deaf child's speech that must be kept in mind to accurately interpret test results.

The Child's System—Phonological Considerations

As the deaf or hard of hearing child develops a spoken language system, it tends to be systematic. Although there often are errors in the articulatory patterns used, these errors tend to be used consistently to represent a particular phonologic contrast (e.g., using stops for fricatives). It is thus important that the child's entire phonologic system be examined and characterized, so that the implications of changing a particular pattern can be seen.

Phonetic versus Phonologic

At first glance the assessment of speech of a deaf child seems relatively straightforward and obvious. To establish a child's sound repertoire (i.e., the speech sounds the child has or does not have), the clinician will sample speech and conduct an inventory of various segmental and suprasegmental speech characteristics. Those present are considered acquired whereas those absent are in need of remediation.

This view, however, is problematic. The process of acquiring aspects of speech is not simply binary—either present or absent. Steps are involved in acquiring a speech skill, and the clinician must evaluate the particular stage of acquisition of various speech skills. For example, suppose that a deaf child does not present evidence of producing a vowel, such as /i/. One of the first questions that needs to be asked is whether or not the child has the sensory prerequisites to be able to either develop the necessary internal representation of the segment so that there is a clear target of what is being attempted or so that she has some way of monitoring the result of her production attempt. Second, the child must acquire the oral motor skills needed to produce the segment, in a variety of contexts and utterance positions. Finally the child must be able to show that she is able to produce the pattern appropriately for a particular word or utterance (such as using the vowel /i/ in conjunction with a picture of a baby eating a cookie). This latter aspect involves true phonologic usage of the skill.

In examining the articulatory errors of a deaf or hard of hearing child, it should be recognized that the source of an error is not always easy to determine. For example, in using a standard three-position articulation test such as the Goldman-Fristoe (Goldman & Fristoe, 2000) or Fisher-Logemann (Fisher & Logemann, 1971), one might find that the child does not articulate the /f/ segment in any contexts. In considering where to begin therapy, however, this information alone may not be adequate. An additional consideration relates to the source of difficulty the child is experiencing in producing the target words correctly. Does the child have the oral motor skills needed to articulate the /f/ segment? Is the ability to produce the segment adequately stable so that she can articulate it in a variety of phonetic and sentence contexts? Does the child have an adequate understanding of the words that require this oral motor pattern (i.e., does she understand that the /f/ pattern applies to particular words on the page)?

There are a limited number of test instruments that can be used to assess a child's motor production abilities. Probably the most recognized is that developed by Ling (2002) as an imitative task to determine which sounds a child can produce independent of meaning. The Phonetic Level Evaluation (Ling, 2002) provides a structured and ordered set of imitation tasks that enable the clinician to systematically sample the child's ability to produce certain articulatory patterns in varied contexts.

The Phonetic Level Evaluation is typically used to determine a few segments on which the clinician should focus motor production work. It is not designed to be given in its entirety but rather to be administered until a number of teaching goals are able to be established. The child's ability to use acquired articulatory skills in words can be assessed through the use of standard articulation tests or through analysis of a spontaneous speech sample. For example, the Fisher-Logemann (1971) or the Goldman-Fristoe (2000) test provides a reasonable sampling of the child's ability to produce various speech segments in initial, medial, and final word positions. Alternatively, Ling (2002) has made suggestions for eliciting and analyzing a spontaneous speech sample to obtain a picture of a child's phonologic usage of various articulatory patterns.

Suprasegmentals

The speech of deaf and hard of hearing children is often characterized by both segmental and suprasegmental speech errors (Osberger & McGarr, 1982). The suprasegmental attributes that are typically difficult for a deaf or hard of hearing child to acquire include adequate control of fundamental frequency, intensity, and duration. Consequently, a deaf child is likely to exhibit one or more of the following speech characteristics: average fundamental frequency that is too high or too low, pitch breaks, inappropriate vocal intensity, and the production of utterances that have inappropriate pauses. Additionally, the speech of deaf individuals is often longer in duration than the speech of hearing individuals, with the result being utterances with fewer syllables per exhalation.

The impact of such suprasegmental characteristics on speech intelligibility is not always easy to assess. Although some studies suggest that the suprasegmentals have only limited impact on speech intelligibility (Maassen & Povel, 1985), it is likely that many of the suprasegmental errors exhibited by deaf individuals are the result of inadequate control of basic systems underlying speech (such as respiration or phonation) and accordingly would have a negative impact on the ability to produce intelligible speech. There is little dispute, however, that such speech errors have a limiting effect on the naturalness of speech produced by a deaf child and so require some attention in therapy.

Although assessing suprasegmental aspects of speech is important, few test instruments provide information about suprasegmentals. One exception is The Fundamental Speech Skills Test (FSST) (Levitt, Youdelman, & Head, 1990). This test was developed to permit standardized sampling and evaluation of the "fundamental" speech skills of deaf individuals. The test is divided into four sections designed to assess general production skills (such as breath control, and voice quality) pitch control (variability and overall pitch level), suprasegmental production (stress and intonation patterns), and spontaneous speech (evaluation of all skills during less structured activities). Whereas norms are provided for children and adolescents to age 20, the test can also be used as a criterion-referenced test (Mahshie & Allen, 1996).

The National Technical Institute for the Deaf (NTID) Voice and Speech Examination (Subtelney, Orlando, & Whitehead, 1981) permits evaluation of a number of different speech attributes by a trained listener. Based on a reading of the Rainbow Passage (Fairbanks, 1960), the listener assigns a 1 (severe problem) to 5 (no problem) rating to describe the client's ability to control pitch, loudness, breath stream, prosody, rhythm, nasal resonance, and overall intelligibility. Although norms for deaf speakers are not provided, results from the NTID Voice and Speech Examination can be used to establish goals for nonsegmental aspects of speech, as well as other fundamental aspects of speech production such as breath stream support and control.

Intelligibility

A child's ability to effectively use speech for communication requires that the child not only have the cognitive and linguistic prerequisites to encode thoughts into linguistic form, but that the child also have adequate intelligibility so that she can be understood by others. Intelligibility is defined as extent to which an individual's speech can be understood. The concept of intelligibility is not to be confused with naturalness, which is the extent to which an individual's speech is considered comparable in quality and content to that of a hearing individual.

Intelligibility measures can play an important role in therapy. First, such measures provide an overall index of how the child's speech might function for communication. Those with relatively intelligible speech obviously have an important prerequisite for being able to use speech for face-to-face communication (although intelligible speech alone is not sufficient for such communicative interactions to be successful). If speech is minimally intelligible, then there is an obvious limitation to using speech in such interactions. This in turn will suggest that the child learn to employ nonspeech strategies (such as gesturing or writing) to communicate effectively whereas a communication partner must rely on speech.

An additional reason for evaluating intelligibility is to provide the deaf or hard of hearing client with a measure of her own speech that provides a measure of potential use for communication. It is not uncommon during the therapy process to encourage the client with statements about success with achieving a particular speech task. Indeed recent research suggests that deaf individuals often perceive their speech as being more or less intelligible than objective measures might suggest (Mahshie et al., 2002).

Measuring intelligibility, however, can be involved. Factors such as the measure used, the nature of the stimulus materials, and the familiarity of the judge with the speech of the individual can all affect the overall rating of intelligibility. One convenient approach developed at NTID (Subtelney et al., 1981) is a five-point scale that rates an individual as being completely intelligible

1. Speech cannot be understood.

2. Speech is very difficult to understand; only isolated words or phrases are intelligible.

3. Speech is difficult to understand; however, the gist of the conversation can be understood. (Intelligibility may improve after a listening period.)

4. Speech is intelligible, with the exception of a few words or phrases.

5. Speech is completely intelligible.

Figure 3-2. The National Technical Institute for the Deaf (NTID) five-point Intelligibility Scale

Source: Adapted from Subtelney, J., Orlando, N., & Whitehead, R. (1981). *Speech and voice characteristic of the deaf.* Washington, DC: Alexander Graham Bell Association for the Deaf.

(rating of 5) to being completely unintelligible (rating of 1). The complete scale and descriptors of each scale rating are given in Figure 3-2. Whereas some questions have been raised about the limitations of this rating system (Samar & Metz, 1988) the use of such a scale provides a fairly reliable and easy way of describing the general level of intelligibility exhibited by an individual.

Summary

A sampling of available instruments that can be used to assess a range of speech skills in deaf and hard of hearing children is given in Table 3-3. It is important to recognize the importance of evaluating a range of speech skills, both segmental and suprasegmental, as well as the level of acquisition of a particular skill into spoken language. It is also essential that a deaf or hard of hearing child's speech intelligibility be evaluated often and that this assessment be communicated effectively to the child and to the parents of that child to promote a realistic picture of a child's overall ability in spoken English.

Issues Involved in Assessing Language

Many of the variables discussed in the preceding section apply to the assessment of language with deaf and hard of hearing children. For example, SLPs need to consider the reason for testing (justifying the need for services or identifying strengths and weaknesses) to help determine which test or method to use for evaluation. In addition, the lack of availability of tools designed for deaf and hard of hearing children makes it necessary to adapt tests that were created for other populations.

Some additional aspects of testing should be kept in mind when the clinician attempts to get a complete picture of the deaf or hard of hearing child's language. The child's use of different modes of communication is important to consider.

Table 3-3	Representative Tests That Can Be Used to Evaluate Speech Skills of Deaf and Hard of Hearing Children

Test	Information
Andrew's Voice Evaluation (1988)	• Parameters of voice including intensity, pitch, quality, environmental factors
Fisher-Logemann Test of Articulation Competence (1971)	• Production of consonants and vowels at the word and sentence level
Fundamental Speech Skills Test (1990)	• Breath control, voice quality, pitch control, suprasegmental production and overall intelligibility • Developed specifically for deaf and hard of hearing populations
Goldman-Fristoe Test of Articulation (GFTA) (1972)	• Production of consonants in words and short passages; for use with the KLPA to determine phonologic patterns
Khan-Lewis Phonological Analysis (KLPA) (1986)	• For the use with the GFTA to determine phonologic patterns and their degree of severity
Ling Phonetic Level Speech Evaluation (2002)	• Production of suprasegmentals and segmentals of speech • Developed specifically for deaf and hard of hearing populations
Ling Phonologic Level Speech Evaluation (1976)	• Use of suprasegmentals and segmentals at the phonologic level • Developed specifically for deaf and hard of hearing populations
National Technical Institute for the Deaf Voice and Speech Examination (1981)	• Parameters of voice including intensity, pitch, quality, prosody, rate, breath support, and overall intelligibility • Developed for specifically deaf and hard of hearing populations

From Mahshie, J., & Allen, A. (1996). Speech and voice skills. In M. J. Moseley & S. J. Bally (Eds.), *Communication therapy: An integrated approach to aural rehabilitation.* Washington, DC: Gallaudet University Press.

For the signing child, some information needs to be obtained about what the child knows about language that is expressed through the mode of signing. The typical formats that are used for English may not suffice to get the best information with this child. For example, one often-used way of determining sentence structure development for young children is through figuring mean length of utterance (MLU). Unlike English, which has a linear morphologic structure, ASL may involve one movement which represents several morphemes simultaneously. For example, *dark blue* is represented by one long movement. Applying an MLU to a signing child may, thus, not represent her knowledge of the structure of English.

Specific movement involved in signing may be very similar for different words, making the assessment of vocabulary a challenge. For example, the words *control* and *manage* have a similar movement and depend on the context for differentiation. In trying to do a thorough analysis of the child's vocabulary, the clinician needs to consider this similarity. In addition, question formation in sign language involves facial expression, which may not be familiar to the SLP, but differentiates the type of question being asked (e.g., raised eyebrows indicate yes/no questions).

Other differences exist in the use of sign language that may not be familiar to the SLP but represent knowledge of language content, form, and use. Sign language teachers, parents, and other fluent signers may be helpful in assisting the SLP in understanding the language development of the child who is primarily using sign. Videotaping an evaluation session and letting a skilled signer view it may be a valuable way to get this additional input. A creative and flexible approach to evaluation of the child who primarily uses sign is necessary to identify her knowledge of language.

The same concepts as discussed earlier are also true for children who have more than one oral language, for example, Spanish and English. The SLP needs to know what the child knows in both languages to plan a comprehensive program aimed to increase basic language use. Because most SLPs will probably be trying to encourage English skills, they may be able to "build" on the knowledge that the child has in another language to teach English comprehension and use. For all children, the interaction of the various areas of language is another important variable when the child is evaluated. Many of the language tests available will assess only one aspect of language: e.g., the Test of Syntactic Abilities (Quigley, Steinkamp, Power, & Jones, 1978) looks at syntax only, the Peabody Picture Vocabulary Test (Dunn & Dunn, 2000) looks only at vocabulary, an aspect of semantics. All areas of language (syntax, morphology, phonology, semantics, and pragmatics) need to be examined regularly, as well as cognitive and social areas that impact communication. Current theoretical approaches to language acquisition emphasize the interactional nature of these variables (Haynes & Shulman, 1998). For example, Yoshinaga-Itano & Stredler-Brown (1992) hypothesized that for those children skilled in asking questions to obtain information, aspects of pragmatics will affect growth in vocabulary.

Yoshinaga-Itano (1997) made recommendations for a comprehensive assessment of deaf and hard of hearing children that examines the interaction of several areas of language. (See appendix G.) A focus on the three areas discussed in appendix G—pragmatics, semantics, and syntax—will provide a broad picture of the child's language abilities. In addition, a comprehensive assessment such as she describes can also yield information about the child's social and cognitive abilities.

Children's language changes constantly as they learn new concepts and appropriate ways to express themselves. Ongoing diagnostic therapy will continue to help the SLP constantly update the child's language knowledge.

GENERAL CONSIDERATIONS FOR INTERVENTION

Planning an intervention program for deaf and hard of hearing children in the mainstream involves consideration of a number of variables before the intervention process actually begins. In addition, these variables may be regularly monitored and adjusted as needed during the course of the intervention program.

Communication Access and Child's Mode of Communication

First and foremost, the deaf or hard of hearing child must have access to communication on an ongoing basis. The SLP may be the one to assure that the child's hearing aid, cochlear implant, or FM system, is functioning at the beginning of the session/day in school. In addition, monitoring the learning environment to assure that it is conducive to the deaf child (e.g., quiet room, proper lighting, and placement in the room) can be done on a daily basis. (See chapter 2 for an in-depth discussion of these factors.) An environment that is supportive of access is of obvious importance.

Many educators and linguists recommend that if a deaf or hard of hearing child uses sign language as her primary mode of communication, new information, including teaching speech and/or written English, may be better understood and learned by the child if she is instructed in sign language (Johnson et al., 1989). For example, a clinician can help a child develop written narrative skills by first telling the story in ASL to the child and then repeating or writing the story in English (M. Nichols, personal communication, 1996). The rationale is to allow the child to first understand the underlying concepts of what is being discussed/taught and then adjusting the form of the story to fit a second language/mode. (See the section on Multiple Language Influences in this chapter.) If the SLP does not sign, there may be some creative opportunities to use this concept at least part of the time. For example, the use of other children/teachers/parents who *do* sign may be integrated into a part of the therapy sessions.

Therapy Setting

There has recently been a move toward a model of collaboration with the classroom teacher (McCartney, 1999). The focus of this model is on maximizing the deaf or hard of hearing child's language/learning in her natural context during the school years—the classroom. This approach generally assumes that the classroom teacher (CRT) and SLP will plan together how to achieve goals for a specific child within the context of the classroom (Nelson, 1998). The participation of the SLP may take different forms, depending on the needs of the child. One example might be the SLP working with a child or group of children to supplement their comprehension and participation in the current lesson. This may involve sitting in a special place in the room and assuring that the child is following the lesson given by the teacher (e.g., through expansion or repetition of directions).

Another form of participation in the classroom may be planning a special lesson for the entire class, which has special goals for the child/children on the SLP's caseload. For example, the SLP may be involved in a vocabulary review in a biology class, with special visual techniques that will help the hard of hearing child to define, analyze, and practice new vocabulary. The SLP could make a chart on the board of all words the children know (plant, sun, etc.) and new words (chlorophyll, etc.). The children can participate verbally, they can copy the words, the words can be put in different colors, the children can make short sentences, both verbally and in writing, and they can discuss relationships between *plants* and *chlorophyll*, etc. These types of activities will highlight the new vocabulary and help the deaf or hard of hearing child to practice the new vocabulary.

The use of a collaborative model depends on a mutual understanding between the CRT and the SLP as well as the support of the school administration. However, a collaborative approach to achieving specific communication goals must be considered in the contexts of the child's specific needs. Factors such as the acoustics of the classroom and the psychosocial needs of the child may either support or exclude this approach as being in the best interest of the deaf and hard of hearing child. It may be the responsibility of the SLP to help advocate for whatever model is most helpful and appropriate for the deaf and hard of hearing child. Additional discussion of a collaborative model is provided in chapter 8 on adolescent language.

The familiar alternative to collaboration is a pull-out model including consultation with the CRT. The SLP may work with the child or a group of children outside the classroom setting (e.g., in an unused classroom or therapy room). Often this takes the form of individual therapy for the child to facilitate academic and social development. Hopefully, there will be constant discussion with the CRT regarding the content of the school curriculum and a "matching" of goals for the classroom and the speech-language therapy setting.

The pull-out model is also frequently used with small groups and may be particularly challenging when the clinician is working with deaf and hard of hearing children. Assuring communication access to all group members may be difficult if the children all have different communication needs, e.g., signing, Cued Speech, or oral/aural. Whether these children can be grouped together may depend on the support services available to the clinician (e.g., an interpreter or a teacher's aid) and the clinician's comfort level in working with a heterogeneous group. In addition, deaf and hard of hearing children have varying needs that may or may not be consistent with their age. The specific goals for each child of the same chronologic age may be so different (see the discussion of the fluidity of the scope of therapy, discussed earlier in this chapter), that this will affect the placement of children within small groups or the efficacy of group work in general.

In many cases, however, it may be appropriate to use a combination of these models to help create the optimal setting for a particular child. For example, the child may benefit from having the SLP teach the class with a focus on her new vocabulary but may still need additional work in that area that can be done more efficiently in a pull-out setting. Preteaching of new vocabulary (in individual therapy) based on consultation with the CRT is also a useful technique for supporting the classroom performance of children with hearing loss. This allows the child to anticipate and have familiarity with the language she will experience in class the following day or week. The authors are familiar with a number of SLPs who utilize both classroom and pull-out approaches to address/ the clinical goals of deaf and hard of hearing children on their case load. For example, the clinician may go into the classroom every third time he sees the child, while working on skills that will be needed for classroom success during the other two pull-out sessions.

Another possible consideration in deciding upon the therapy setting, is *who* may be involved in therapy in addition to the child. Peer tutors may be an effective way to provide a benefit to both the younger and the older child. Older deaf or hard of hearing children may gain insight and esteem by working with young children in areas for which they exhibit a relative strength. Parents may be involved in the therapy setting itself, particularly with younger children. Many intervention programs for young children at the preschool level provide for extensive involvement from parents. The parents may serve as tutors for any child in the classroom, may serve as aides for the teacher in the classroom, or be otherwise present to observe and participate in the same class as their child. In addition, parents may be involved with home activities, journals, etc. to help their child with specific activities.

Teachers (e.g., classroom, art, physical education, and music), principals, counselors, and other school personnel may be utilized in pull-out therapy sessions, as well as in the classroom. The use of other individuals provides excellent opportunities for communicating with a wider array of individuals, e.g., practicing receptive and expressive skills and generalizing new skills. In addition, when therapy is planned in tandem with classroom content, other individuals may have excellent information to offer that may be utilized in the therapy session. The more closely therapy can shadow the focus of classroom work the greater the benefit received by the child.

Integrated Therapy Model

The authors have consistently discussed a holistic view of the child in which the child is viewed in their psychosocial and linguistic and physical contexts. Following this holistic and broad view of working with the child, an integrated therapy model is proposed to permit a horizontal approach to the therapy process. A horizontal approach is one in which many goals may be approached simultaneously through a carefully chosen activity that incorporates several goals at the same time (Fey, 1986). Two examples of integrated therapy are shown in Table 3-4. Both of these activities incorporate several of the areas that are important for the child.

Within the framework of an integrated therapy model, the clinician may move back and forth on a continuum from an adult-centered approach (one in which the structure is planned and there is little deviation from that structure during therapy time) to a child-centered approach in which the child takes

Table 3-4	Examples of Goals and Activities Involved in Integrated Therapy
Topic	Colors: brown, red, yellow, blue, green, purple, white, black, and gold
Materials	"Brown Bear, Brown Bear, What Do You See?" by Bill Martin/Eric Carle, construction paper cards of target colors, mirror
Goals to be addressed	• Speech: production of the word; accurate lip movements, production of the initial sound and/or the correct vowel sound • Listening: discrimination or identification of color words • Speechreading: discrimination or identification of color words • Language: expressive and receptive knowledge and use of the color words/signs • Cognition: matching colors • Literacy: exposure to the book, text, and color words
Topic	Baking potatoes and serving to friends
Materials	Microwave oven or conventional oven, potato
Goals to be addressed	• Semantics: fast/slow 　—(microwave vs. conventional oven) • Syntax: past tense, e.g., baked, washed 　—(potatoes, dishes) • Pragmatics: asking questions 　—taking turns • Cognitive: sequencing the activity: 　—"What do we do first?" 　—"What do we do next?" • Speechreading 　—environmental strategies: 　　Good lighting 　　Turn toward the speaker 　—anticipatory strategies: 　　"Do you want butter or sour cream?" 　—repair strategies: use as needed 　—identification of specific words: 　　e.g., potato, fast

the lead or "sets the tone" of the session and the clinician follows the child's lead while using that time to reach therapy goals. "Incidental learning" can easily occur when the child brings a specific interest to the therapy session. For example, the child may wish to tell the clinician about the art project she just completed in school. The discussion of this activity may prompt a variety of possibilities for reaching goals for the child: sequencing, new vocabulary, pragmatics (such as turn-taking or taking the listener's perspective), writing, and so forth. An approach that attempts to integrate and connect goals through a particular activity frequently provides both a meaningful and efficient means of addressing multiple therapy goals. It is important for the SLP to take advantage of "teachable moments" that arise.

One of the components of planning carefully in an integrated model is to introduce new learning experiences for the child within the framework of something she already knows. It has been well documented in the literature that individuals learn new information more easily when it is presented at a level just above their level of comfort. The clinician thus is challenged to develop approaches that put some demands on the child, but not to overwhelm the child with tasks for which prerequisite skills are not present. This concept has been described in the literature as the *minimum distance principle* or the *zone of proximal development* (Haynes & Shulman, 1998; Nelson, 1998). For example, if one of the focal points of the lesson is to teach new vocabulary, working on articulation with those particular new words may make the task too complex for the child. The vocabulary can be learned first, perhaps for several sessions, and then articulation work can be planned with those words. For example, in the activity about colors in Table 3-4, speech on the color words that the child *does* know can be emphasized in one session and the articulation of new color words can be emphasized later.

Goal Development and Obtaining Data

The development of appropriate goals depends very much on development of a clear picture of the child's strengths and weaknesses. Goal development with deaf and hard of hearing children should proceed as with any child in therapy. It is suggested that the areas outlined in Table 3-1 be considered and that areas of concern be identified and constitute the long term objectives for that child (for example, improved understanding of figurative language, or development of ability to use idioms during conversation and writing activities). Long- and short-term IEP goals would address all of the areas mentioned in Table 3-1 that are relevant to a particular child. Within each of those areas, a hierarchy of short-term goals would be specified, depending on each child's starting point and the outcome desired. As with any child, the short-term goals will change as the child progresses. Often in public schools data banks of IEP goals exist and are used in IEP development. Unfortunately, the goals are generally not applicable to children with hearing loss. However, once modified or created, a clinician can develop her own bank of measurable goals that address more specifically the areas outlined in Table 3-1. Because each child may have needs that are atypical of her chronologic age, it is valuable to constantly and regularly evaluate the child's progress through consistent observation, interviewing of involved individuals (including the child herself), and evaluation. In addition, facility in one domain (e.g., receptive skills) does not necessarily equate to the same level of skill in another domain (e.g., expressive). Additionally, one might find that a skill attained in one modality or language may not be evident in another. For example, sign skills, spoken English skills, and written English skills may be at developmentally different levels and require differing levels of support.

Obtaining Data through Diagnostic Therapy

The process of ongoing evaluation and goal adjustment allows the clinician to provide *diagnostic therapy*. Traditionally, SLPs have provided diagnostic assessments first and then planned a therapy program based on the results of that evaluation. There is little documentation in the literature about what methods work "best" for deaf and hard of hearing children. Thus, the need to constantly adjust and reconsider the child's needs and therapy priorities becomes paramount in working with these children. SLPs working with deaf and hard of hearing children regularly report that they consider what they do to be diagnostic therapy (R. Reinstein, personal communication, 2001).

The process of adequate and accurate data collection is important for two reasons: 1) to allow the SLP to do diagnostic therapy and 2) to provide ongoing information about the efficacy of programming for deaf and hard of hearing children. Each of these areas will be discussed in the following paragraph.

Keeping data for several children at once is a constant challenge for the SLP. Traditionally, IEPs and behavioral objectives have required that a percentage increase in improvement be documented. This usually involves keeping "score" of how many correct responses occur in a given time. SLPs typically do this by writing (e.g., tick mark or check) whenever a specific response is deemed correct. This can be done in a variety of ways when many children are involved. For example, SLPs can record responses for only one child per therapy session, one area of therapy (e.g., vocabulary) at one time, once a week in a certain area for different children, or other ways that lend themselves to the particular situation.

More recently, there has been a move toward a more ethnographic or "field notes" method for showing progress in a given child. Written observations provide one means of doing this, e.g., by keeping an ongoing account of how and what the child is doing on a particular day. Written observation can be done through the use of portfolios (Kratcoski, 1998). Examples of written items in a portfolio that may help with ongoing evaluation are the initial referral forms, language samples, story retell samples, observation notes, work samples, teacher interviews, parent interviews, student interviews, and testing data (Kratcoski, 1998). For children with hearing loss who use sign language as a mode of communication, videotaping may also be helpful and can be included in the portfolio. A portfolio provides a means of documenting what the child is doing and a means for evaluating the child's progress and serves as an excellent resource for the child as she moves from grade to grade and classroom to classroom.

Data to Establish Efficacy of Treatment

The nature of deaf education and therapy for children has moved from one end of the continuum to the other during the past 20 to 30 years: from an emphasis on oral/aural education to an emphasis on bilingual-bicultural (emphasis on ASL and written English) education and many other options in between. Clinicians, educators, and parents may have strong views on one or the other of these issues and there is constant discussion among professionals about the direction of communication and education for deaf and hard of hearing children. Documentation of what works for a particular child with a particular set of communication issues is important in ultimately determining the efficacy of various models of working with deaf and hard of hearing children. Individual documentation in conjunction with a focus on sharing this information with other professionals in the field of deafness may help provide the ability to determine "best practices" in the field of deaf education.

Collaboration with Families

The involvement of families in the intervention process with deaf and hard of hearing children is necessary and important. The family includes the parents or other involved adults, siblings, and *the student herself.* The family perspective on the intervention process, e.g., what kind of communication mode parents choose for their young child, parents' perception of the child's progress, and their communication with the SLP, can all contribute to a positive and profitable intervention experience. Keeping parents aware of what is happening day by day in the intervention process allows them to become involved with the child at home. For example, many clinicians report use of a dialogue journal with parents to describe briefly what is accomplished each time the child sees the SLP or send home a "calendar" on the first day of each week with intended outcomes for the week. Regular phone calls or personal conferences contribute to the parents' knowledge, as well as providing additional information for the SLP. Some of this information may take the form of an interview that goes into a portfolio for later comparative purposes (see earlier discussion of portfolios).

The deaf or hard of hearing child can often give the SLP insights into programming that help make planning and intervention more effective. Older children can be included in the planning and goal-setting process (Wilson & Scott, 1996). Middle and high school students may be able to identify very specific communication needs that can help guide the intervention process. For example, a child may want to work on idioms because she does not understand some of what she reads in the news or sees on TV, or the child may want to learn about communication strategies to use when they go with their friends to McDonald's to order a hamburger.

Very young children may also be able to have a positive impact on the therapy process when they are asked for input. For example, one of the authors worked for many weeks with a young, third grade child, who appeared to have very little motivation for learning. The clinician worked hard to determine new therapy techniques and tried "everything" to interest this child—books, games, toys, and technology—and in desperation asked the girl "what do you like to do?" The girl responded by indicating she loved recess and jumping rope and could not do it well because of motor problems. Lessons built around the theme of jumping rope and related areas (e.g., interacting with other kids, vocabulary built around what you can do at recess, and sequencing the process of making rope as well as jumping rope) were combined with speechreading, sequencing concepts, use of narrative structure, and so forth and were well received as well as effective.

Another consideration for intervention and working with parents is the issue of prognosis for the child's communication skills. SLPs may find themselves in the position of having to reconcile parental goals with their own (SLP) clinical judgment. Building rapport with the family is essential to reconciling differing expectations about the focus and likely outcomes of therapy (Mahshie & Allen, 1996). It is important to establish a clear picture of the child's needs, skills, and interests. Sometimes the SLP is needed to mediate between an adolescent and a parent; for example, the high school junior who communicates via sign language and exhibits limited speech skills and poor voice quality may wish to focus therapy on receptive skills or SAT preparation and no longer use the limited therapy time for articulation practice. The parent may still be very focused on expressive speech production goals. Helping the parent understand the prognosis for improvement in different areas sometimes yields consensus among the constituents (child, parent, and SLP). Often it is important to be clear and specific about what the prognosis is and what areas afford the greatest likelihood of improvement and subsequent support to academic success.

Summary

This chapter has focused on broad considerations for assessment and intervention with deaf and hard of hearing children. Included are discussions on the Scope of assessment, purposes of assessment, the context for evaluation, multiple language influences, obtaining information in the assessment process, the need for ongoing assessment, and issues in assessing speech and language. In addition, the Scope of language planning was discussed, as well as the therapy setting, an integrated therapy model, goal development, diagnostic therapy, data collection, and collaboration with teachers and family.

References

Cummins, J. (1984). *Bilingualism and special education: Issues in assessment and pedagogy.* Clevedon, Avon, England: Multilingual Matters.

Dunn, L. M., & Dunn, L. M. (2000). *Peabody picture vocabulary test—III.* Circle Pines, MN: American Guidance Services.

Easterbrooks, S. R., & Baker. S. (2002). *Language learning in children who are deaf and hard of hearing: Multiple pathways.* Boston: Allyn & Bacon.

Erber, N. P. (1982). *Auditory training.* Washington, DC: Alexander Graham Bell Association for the Deaf.

Evans, C. Zimmer, K., & Murray, D. (1994). Discovery with words and signs; a resource guide for developing a bilingual and bicultural preschool program for deaf and hard of hearing children. Winnipeg, Manitoba, Canada: Sign Talk Development Project.

Fairbanks, G. (1960). *Voice and articulation drillbook* (2nd ed.). New York: Harper and Row.

Fey, M. E. (1986). *Language intervention with young children.* San Diego, CA: College-Hill Press.

Fisher, H. B., & Logemann, J. A. (1971). *The Fisher-Logemann test of articulation competence.* Iowa City, IA: Houghton Mifflin.

Goldman, R., & Fristoe, M. (2000). *Goldman-Fristoe Test of Articulation* (2nd ed.) (GFTA-2). Circle Pines, MN: American Guidance Service.

Goldstein, B. (2000). *Cultural and linguistic diversity resource guide for speech-language pathologists.* Clifton Park, NY: Singular.

Haberman, M. (1991). The pedagogy of poverty versus good teaching. *Phi Delta Kappan, 73*(4), 290–294.

Halliday, M. A. K. (1975). *Learning how to mean: Explorations in the development of language.* London, England: Edward Arnold.

Haynes, W., & Pindzola, R. (1998). *Diagnosis and evaluation in speech pathology* (5th ed.). Needham Heights, Ma: Allyn & Bacon.

Haynes, W. O., & Shulman, B. B. (1998). *Communication development foundations, processes, and clinical applications.* Baltimore: Williams & Wilkins.

Johnson, R. E., Liddell, S. K., & Erting, C. J. (1989). *Unlocking the curriculum: Principles for achieving access in deaf education.* (Gallaudet Research Institute Working Paper 89-3). Washington, DC: Gallaudet University.

Kaplan, H., Bally, S. J., & Garretson, C. (1987). *Speechreading: A way to improve understanding* (2nd ed.). Washington, DC: Gallaudet University Press.

Kratcoski, A. M. (1998). Guidelines for using portfolios in assessment and evaluation. *Language, Speech, and Hearing Services in Schools, 29*(1),3–9.

Levitt, H., Youdelman, K., & Head, J. (1990). *Fundamental speech skills test.* Englewood, CO: Resource Point.

Ling, D. (2002). *Speech and the hearing-impaired child: Theory and practice* (2nd ed.). Washington, DC: Alexander Graham Bell Association for the Deaf.

Longres, J. (1995). *Human behavior in the social environment* (2nd ed.). Itasca, IL: Peacock.

Lund, N. J., & Duchan, J. F. (1993). *Assessing children's language in naturalistic contexts* (3rd ed.). Englewood Cliffs, NJ: Prentice-Hall.

Maassen, B., & Povel, D. J. (1985). The effect of segmental and suprasegmental corrections on the intelligibility of deaf speech. *The Journal of the Acoustical Society of America, 78*(3), 877–886.

Mahshie, J., & Allen, A. (1996). Speech and voice skills. In M. J. Moseley & S. J. Bally (Eds.), *Communication therapy: An integrated approach to aural rehabilitation.* Washington, DC: Gallaudet University Press.

Mahshie, J., Moseley, M.J., & Robins, A. (2002). *Self-assessment of speech intelligibility by deaf and hard of hearing individuals.* Paper presented at the meeting of the American Speech and Hearing Association, Atlanta, GA.

Mahshie, S. N. (1995). *Educating deaf children bilingually.* Washington, DC: Gallaudet University, Pre-College Programs.

Marschark, M. (1997). *Raising and educating a deaf child.* Oxford, England: Oxford University Press.

McCartney, E. (1999). *Speech/language therapists and teachers working together: A systems approach to collaboration.* London, England: Whuur.

McIntyre, M. (1994). *The acquisition of American Sign Language by deaf children.* Burtonsville, MD: Linstock Press.

Nelson, N. W. (1998). *Childhood language disorders in context—Infancy through Adolescence.* Boston: Allyn & Bacon.

Osberger M. J., & McGarr, N. (1982). Speech production characteristics of the hearing impaired. *Speech Language, 8,* 221–283.

Patton, S. (2000). *Birth marks: Transracial adoption in contemporary america.* New York: New York University Press.

Pohan, C., & Bailey, N. (1997, Fall). Opening the closet: Multiculturalism that is fully inclusive. *Multicultural Education,* pp.12–15.

Quigley, P., Steinkamp, M. W., Power, D. J., & Jones, B. W. (1978). *Test of syntactic abilities: Guide to administration and interpretation.* Beaverton, OR: DORMAC.

Samar, V., & Metz, D. E. (1988). Criterion validity of speech intelligibility rating-scale procedures for the hearing-impaired population. *Journal of Speech and Hearing Research,31,* 307–316.

Singh, S., & Kent, R. D. (2000). Illustrated dictionary of speech-language pathology. Clifton Park, NY: Singular.

Subtelney, J., Orlando, N., & Whitehead, R. (1981). *Speech and voice characteristic of the deaf.* Washington, DC: Alexander Graham Bell Association for the Deaf.

Troiden, R. (1989). The formation of homosexual identities. In G. Herdt (Ed.), *Gay and lesbian youth.* New York: Harrington Park Press.

Valli, C., & Lucas, C. (1995). *Linguistics of American Sign Language* (2nd ed.). Washington, DC: Gallaudet University Press.

Wallach, G. P., & Miller, L. (1988). *Language intervention and academic success.* Boston: College-Hill Press.

Wilson, M. P., & Scott, S. (1996). An Integrated therapy model. In M. J. Moseley & S. J. Bally (Eds.), *Communication therapy: An integrated approach to aural rehabilitation.* Washington, DC: Gallaudet University Press.

Wix, T., & Supalla, S. (n.d.). *American Sign Language acquisition assessment.* Tucson, AZ: Arizona Schools for the Deaf and Blind.

Yoshinaga-Itano, C. (1997). The challenge of assessing language in children with hearing loss. *Language, Speech and Hearing Services in Schools, 28,* 362–373.

Yoshinaga-Itano, C., & Stredler-Brown, A. (1992). Learning to communicate: Babies with hearing impairments make their needs known. *The Volta Review, 94,* 107–129.

Assessment
and Intervention

Graney (1998) proposed that children can be placed into general intervention groupings depending on how much access they have to spoken English. She further suggested that the child's access can be determined as children move from pre-kindergarten into the elementary years. These groupings will thus suggest the type and amount of intervention provided for an individual child. The authors of this book have expanded on Graney's groupings and included case studies that represent the following five general types of children:

1. The child with a cochlear implant. This child is likely to emphase speech and auditory skills and may have varying degrees of access to spoken English and to language.
2. The child who will develop spoken English and language skills that, on the surface, appear similar to those of hearing children. With hearing aids, the auditory skills of these children are sufficient to allow them quite a bit of access to spoken English and thus, to the English language.
3. The child who has a severe to profound loss and becomes a speaker. These children will depend on speechreading, visual cues, and tactile information to learn speech and language. These skills need to be explicitly taught and the children will acquire them to varying degrees.
4. The child who learns sign language as a first language. These children may develop some spoken English, which must be taught, and will acquire it to varying degrees.

5. The child who learns sign language at a later age and has limited access to spoken English. These children may have little or no spoken English and may have limited language skills. They will develop language and functional speech to varying degrees.

These groupings have been clinically useful to the authors; however there are always children who do not fit into these categories. For example, there may be children who learn sign language as a first language, have good language skills but have limited access to spoken English, and have very little, if any, usable speech. As has been emphasized repeatedly in this book, each child must be considered individually when planning assessment and intervention.

The following four chapters will focus on the intervention process. Each chapter will discuss one of the four areas defined in the Scope: prelinguistic, early language, later language, and adolescent language. Case studies will be used to demonstrate the application of these areas and the overlapping nature of the skills within individual children. Five children, each representing one of the above groupings, will be discussed from the development of prelinguistic skills through adolescent language. The purpose of the case studies is to demonstrate the needs of different deaf and hard of hearing children at various stages of development and to show the scattered nature of the skills demonstrated by many of these children. It is hoped the presentation of these case studies will help the reader clarify the nature of the intervention process for various deaf and hard of hearing children in the school setting.

Prelanguage Communication: Assessment and Intervention

Introduction

Young hearing children learn prelanguage skills from the day they are born. These skills are thought to help them learn to manipulate their environment and, thus, learn to express wants, needs, and interests before they have a mode of communication to use. In addition, during this early period of time, they are learning to interact with objects and people in their environment. Most hearing children will develop these skills before they have their first words, although these skills will continue to be developed and refined throughout the early stages of language development.

The deaf or hard of hearing child may not have the input needed to develop these skills and, thus, may be behind in the prerequisites for verbal (speech or sign) communication from the beginning of life. Children with hearing loss, even those who have some verbal communication, may be missing some of these early skills, which will make communication more difficult for them. Thus, it is important, *at every age*, to evaluate these early skills and, if appropriate, incorporate them into the therapy program as needed.

Before beginning any test protocol or intervention activity, the child must have the needed access to language being used for the evaluation. For example, if the child wears hearing aids or a cochlear implant, the speech-language pathologist will determine if it is working properly during the evaluation, make sure room noise is at a minimum, and so forth. These areas of access were discussed in depth in chapter 2.

In this chapter, the prelanguage skills discussed in the Scope (chapter 3) are discussed in depth. In addition, assessment and intervention ideas are discussed, and case histories demonstrate the inclusion of these areas in the intervention program.

RECEPTIVE AND EXPRESSIVE PRAGMATIC SKILLS

As defined in the Scope, these skills include eye contact, facial expression, turn-taking, and the comprehension and use of intentions. Each area will be discussed in the following.

Eye Contact

The child who is deaf or hard of hearing must maintain eye contact with the communication partner, regardless of the mode of communication being used. Very few published evaluation tools examine this area in a structured manner. Informal dynamic assessment will yield considerable information about the child's understanding and use of eye contact. To get a representative sample of how the child is using eye contact, the clinician should examine the child's eye contact with several communication partners (for example, the clinician, a parent, teacher, or a sibling or peer). These people are likely to be involved with the child at this age, and the results of evaluation may show some differences in the child's responses to people of different ages and roles.

As a prerequisite to maintaining eye contact with other individuals, there are a few questions that the clinician may consider to better understand variations in eye contact that might occur:

- Does the child have good visual acuity? Private and public preschools as well as elementary and secondary schools will probably have a nursing consultant or staff who will do a visual screening for the young child.
- If the child wears glasses, are they being used?
- What types of attentional strategies are effective in getting the child to look at the speaker's face (e.g., tapping the child on his shoulder or part of his body, tapping the floor so he can feel the vibration, switching the lights in the room on and off to get his attention, calling his name, bending down to put the speaker at eye level with the child, or pointing to an object) (Mohay, 1997)?
- Does the child look at the speaker's face when he initiates communication?
- If the child has intermittent eye contact, the speech-language pathologist may want to check his ability to track an object (e.g., following a moving object (toy or food) from side to side or up and down).

The observations may be documented by using a self-made checklist or using a time-sampling methodology (Goetz, Haring, & Anderson, 1983). A time-sampled checklist for eye contact would involve observing the child for 20 seconds, recording for 20 seconds (e.g., writing down the object of his eye gaze), and then repeating this process for a period of time (e.g., 10 minutes). This procedure would document the consistency and object of eye contact over time and provide baseline information about what is of interest to the child and how long she can maintain eye contact.

In addition, a simple checklist that uses tic marks to indicate a response to the questions raised above would provide a way to document and later track changes in the child's behaviors. This procedure is reasonably easy to set up and can be used during a specific context in therapy, for example, a period of play.

If it is the judgment of the clinician that maintaining eye contact is a problem, activities aimed to improve eye contact can be incorporated into the therapy plan at any level of the child's expertise. Cueing or pointing to the speaker's own eyes after getting the child's attention may sometimes be all that is needed to help the child focus on the speaker's face. Discussing the importance of looking at the speaker may be useful with school-aged children. Pictures may be used to show profiles of speakers' facing each other and may also serve as a cue for reminding the child to attend.

For the child who cannot maintain eye gaze, gradually increasing the number of seconds the child can focus or track may be a profitable goal. This goal can easily accompany speechreading, speech and auditory training, or any other area of intervention.

Facial Expression

There is some indication that young deaf and hard of hearing children may not be skilled in using facial expression as an adjunct to understanding a message (Nussbaum & Waddy-Smith, 2001). Very young hearing infants are known to respond to familiar faces (mother) during the first few months of life (see a summary of research in Haynes & Shulman, 1998). These children learn to identify smiles and expressions of anger very early. Clearly, nonverbal facial behaviors may help the deaf or hard of hearing child to understand the message that is being communicated. Experienced clinicians report that they often include work on comprehending facial expressions within their therapy plans at the prelanguage level and sometimes with children already using language (e.g., Nussbaum & Waddy-Smith, 2001).

Ongoing assessment of the child's ability to recognize and identify facial expressions is beneficial. By noting the contexts in which the child does or does not react appropriately to specific facial expressions such as happiness, sadness, anger, surprise, sleepiness, and any others appropriate in a particular child's environment, it is possible to expand the child's use and identification of appropriate facial expressions.

Therapy activities may involve matching line drawings of specific facial expressions, matching line drawings to magazine pictures or photographs, and matching line drawings or photographs to the speech-language pathologist's actual facial expression. These activities will assure that the child recognizes the expressions in different contexts and with different people. Pictures may be shown to the child when the child uses certain facial expressions to emphasize what he is doing. For example, if the child is surprised to see a new toy in therapy and expresses that facially, the speech-language pathologist may show him the similar picture or have him look in a mirror. If the child is sad on occasion, the speech-language pathologist may use the pictures or mirror to initiate communication with the child. These steps in recognition usually precede the child's comprehension of the expressions of others. Again, when the child consistently acts appropriately to the expression of the clinician (or others engaging in the therapy process), comprehension may be assumed. Situations may be set up in therapy to try to determine whether the child is comprehending; for example, the clinician may role-play sadness ("the doll lost her shoe") and observe the response of the child to see if it is appropriate to that context. These activities may also be used for speechreading (the affective words), auditory training, new vocabulary, and other areas included in intervention.

Turn-Taking

Infants are exposed to turn-taking with their caretakers from the time they are born (Snow, 1977). For example, the mother will stroke the baby while the baby is active and then be quiet herself while the baby actively feeds. These behaviors and others that are similar are thought to be the beginning of the participatory act of communication, in which each partner takes a turn. As the child gets older, the turn-taking becomes more complex, and the child learns new activities that precipitate a turn, e.g., pointing or gesturing to something, which the caretaker then names or comments upon or taking a turn with a toy and then letting the communication partner take a turn also. Turn-taking activities may be limited or changed with the deaf child, and he may not learn the importance of the ability to take turns in a communicative interaction.

To assess a child's turn-taking skills, informal observation with recording again appears to be one of the most effective ways of determining if the prelanguage child is aware of this aspect of communication. The child may be observed in a preschool classroom setting, with adults and peers, in a play setting during therapy, or at meals or snack time. The older child who is still functioning within the prelanguage level may interrupt consistently with actions that are inappropriate for the context or may be unresponsive to initiations from adults or peers. Questions to be asked may include the following:

- Does the child demonstrate back-and-forth interactions with the communication partner?
- In what contexts do these interactions occur?
- What behaviors are observed during the child's turn? For example, does he make sounds or take action that is coordinated with the partner?

If it is deemed by the speech-language pathologist that turn-taking should be a goal for therapy, it can be incorporated into the other goals for the child. For example, games may be used that involve the child and clinician taking a turn (finding pictures hidden in the room or building blocks where each person takes a turn stacking a block). Nonverbal signaling may be used to help the child know when it is his turn to respond (for example, putting a block or object in front of the child or pointing to the child).

Intentions

The hearing child at around 6 months will begin to intentionally communicate through the use of gestures (Haynes & Shulman, 1998). Deaf children are also observed to use these same types of gestures at an early age (McAnally, Rose, & Quigley, 1994). These gestures are not to be confused with the use of sign language, but rather indicate the process young children go through when they learn they can influence their environment but do not yet have a structured means (i.e., oral or signed language) to do so.

The different types of gestures children use at this level have been categorized in various ways, but generally fall into the four categories discussed by Zinober and Martlew (1985). They are the following:

1. Expressive gestures, with which the child demonstrates emotional types of gestures: examples include clapping hands and waving hello or goodbye.
2. Instrumental gestures, with which the child tries to regulate or control the actions of the adult: for example, holding his arms up to be picked up and pulling a sleeve to get the adult to move to some specific place.
3. Enactive gestures, with which the child demonstrates some action that symbolically represents actions of people: for example, holding his hand to his ear to pretend it is a telephone or pretending to sleep. Volterra and Erting (1994) discuss additional types of behaviors evidenced by young children that would fall into this realm. These types of actions will also demonstrate the child's beginning of symbolic play, which is thought to be helpful in the development of language (Westby, 1988).
4. Deictic gestures, with which the child points to an object or shows objects to other people with the perceived intent of finding out more about it: for example, playing and pointing to various objects that the partner will name. Pointing may also serve an instrumental function if it is intended to control the behavior of the adult, for example pointing to the refrigerator with the perceived intent of getting something to drink or eat.

Deaf and hard of hearing children have been shown to use the same types of gestures as hearing children but tend to expand on them and use them longer than most hearing children (McAnally et al., 1994). They have been observed to combine gestures to represent ideas, for example, showing who gives what to whom through gesture, rather than words (Goldin-Meadow, 1975).

There are some published instruments that evaluate gestures in young children. For example, the Rossetti Infant-Toddler Language Scale (Rossetti, 1990). This type of test for young children may give the speech-language pathologist diagnostic information about the child's strengths and weaknesses that can easily be translated to therapy goals. Gestures may also be assessed through informal checksheets as described earlier in this chapter or through time-sampling procedures (e.g., marking specific behaviors at preset intervals, e.g., every 30 seconds). Comprehension of gestures made by the adult may also be evaluated (e.g., patting the chair when the speech-language pathologist wants the child to sit down or pointing to a toy that she wants the child to retrieve).

For many children in the public schools, the major goal will be to move beyond gestures to a spoken or signed system of language. Unless the child has extremely limited or no speech skills, the speech-language pathologist may be hesitant to teach gestures. It is, however, useful to evaluate the child's use of gestures because they indicate how the child is able to manipulate and interact with his environment. The gestures that the child uses provide a starting place for therapy; they point to ways the child can interact with his environment, even if he does not have the linguistic means to do so. Knowing what the child knows provides a starting point for working on a linguistic means of expression for this concept. For example, a child may wave "hi" and "bye-bye" and may then be taught to use these words through the mode that is appropriate. If the child demonstrates understanding of regulatory behaviors, such as raising the hands to be picked up or pointing to the refrigerator for milk, then the child can work into vocabulary such as *up* or *milk*.

In working with the child to develop a communication system, it is important to give him practice in all the various intentions that he will need to know to effectively communicate (Power & Hollingshead, 1982).

RECEPTIVE AUDITORY/VISUAL SKILLS

This section examines the importance of auditory and visual receptive skills in the prelanguage child. To ensure access to language, both of these areas must be assessed before the clinician initiates intervention.

Auditory Skill Assessment

It is obviously important to examine the extent to which a child can receive auditory information from his environment. The audiologic information will indicate what types of sounds the child is aware of and what sounds can be discriminated or identified. (See discussion of audiologic information in chapter 2.)

For children needing to learn awareness of sound, many voice-activated toys are available, such as stuffed animals and "dancing" flowers. Tapes are available that produce environmental sounds; actual environmental sounds, such as a door closing, may also be used. These tapes can be used to assist the child in detecting various kinds of sounds that vary in acoustic attributes.

Many other activities are found in published sources that provide a means of helping the child through the early stages of auditory learning. [See "Auditory Learning Resources" in Appendix B, as well as selected sections of the Ski*Hi Model (Clark & Watkins, 1985)].

Visual Skills

In addition to eye contact and facial expression, it is important for the child to be able to focus on the mouth and, therefore, make use of visual speech sounds for speechreading.

Comprehension of speechreading may be assessed by introducing familiar words and assessing whether the child can point to an object or picture. Early speechreading is integrally interwoven with language ability; thus, it is difficult to determine whether the child's speechreading abilities are related to inability to identify visual information or lack of knowledge of the language. Observation over time may help to clarify the differences. For example, if it becomes clear that the child uses the English word for a certain object in concept, then that vocabulary item may be used to evaluate speechreading ability.

RECEPTIVE AND EXPRESSIVE VISUAL GESTURAL SKILLS

The term *visual-gestural system* refers to a signed language or system. As discussed earlier in the book, some children in the public school system may come from homes in which American Sign Language (ASL) is used, either as a first language or as a means of communicating in a more limited way within the family. Visual-gestural communication must thus be taken into account when the clinician evaluates the prelanguage child, because gestures (as discussed earlier) must be distinguished from "baby signs." The young child first learning sign language will probably not be able to form an accurate adult model, but rather will have aspects of a particular sign that may need to be identified to understand what concepts and vocabulary the child is using. As noted earlier, establishing the child's knowledge of sign language is important to obtain a comprehensive picture of the child's overall language functioning.

As discussed earlier in this book, there are several alternatives to assessing early signs if the speech-language pathologist is not familiar or comfortable with the language (see chapter 3.) If expressive sign language is desired, the child will need someone who is skilled in the language to help learn to produce the signs. If possible, the speech-language pathologist should collaborate with a sign language specialist to know what vocabulary and combinations of utterances are appearing in the child using sign language. If English through voice is also a goal for this child, the production and comprehension of English words can be encouraged through the use of already known concepts in sign language. This area will be discussed more fully in the chapters on early and later language.

VOCALIZATION

For the prelanguage child, it is likely that informal evaluation of vocalizations will be the most helpful in determining the child's ability in this area. Observation with recording of a phonetic inventory is the most likely way to achieve this goal. A sample of sounds made by the child may be recorded and transcribed in different contexts. Lund and Duchan (1983) recommended doing a sample in more than one context to give the child numerous opportunities to produce different sounds. It may be helpful for the clinician to obtain samples from several of the different situations experienced by the child (e.g., classroom, therapy room, mealtime or snack time, and special subject areas such as art, music, or playground).

Recording can be accomplished on-line or by audio or video taping for later transcription.

Some of the questions the clinician should ask are the following:

- What vowel sounds is the child making spontaneously?
- What consonant sounds is the child making spontaneously?
- What stage or stages of speech development appears to be used by the child? (e.g., cooing, babbling, or jargon)
- Does the child use any phonetically consistent sounds (e.g., using /i/ every time a particular light goes on)? These phonetically consistent sounds may not yet be words, the same form used in different appropriate contexts, but are used in a consistent manner.
- Is the child stimulable for any vowel sounds?
- Is the child stimulable for any consonant sounds?
- Are there consistent categories of sounds produced by the child (e.g., low front vowel, stop consonants, or others).
- Is the child using syllabic structure, even if not babbling?
- Is the child able to vocalize on demand?
- Does the child attempt to imitate the adult when requested to do so?
- Is the child able to sustain vocalization and use appropriate vocal intensity and pitch?

One of the more commonly used published tests for examining these early vocalizations is the Ling Phonetic Level Inventory, which was designed for children with hearing loss (Ling, 2002). This test looks at both suprasegmental and segmental production. According to a survey by Abraham, Stoker, and Allen (1988), the Ling test is the test most commonly used by speech-language pathologists to evaluate children at the preschool level, although at the prelanguage level, the child may not have enough speech control to use this tool.

In most cases, the kinds of vocalizations that are being facilitated at this stage of spoken language development are quite basic. This may include tasks such as vocalizing on demand, altering the duration of vocalization, and beginning to initiate a range of different vowel or consonant vowel utterances (Ling, 2002). Of course, the specific focus of intervention aimed to improve vocalization will depend on the child's skill level. Awareness and response to sound were discussed earlier under auditory skills, as well as in chapter 2, and may precede or accompany actual production work. Sound production may be worked on through any means that brings about the correct production of the sound and helps the child to be able to automatize its production, that is, produce it easily and without having to think about how the sound is produced (Ling, 2002).

To facilitate production, it may be necessary to rely on a range of sensory modalities—visual, tactile, and auditory. For example, the child may be getting some information from his hearing aids or an assistive listening device, may also watch the clinician's mouth during production, and may also obtain feedback through tactile stimulation. An example of this latter modality is the feeling of a stream of airflow on the fingers during production of the fricative /s/.

There are various ways in which the clinician can facilitate production of a sound. For example, a published program called Visual Phonics (International Communication Learning Institute (ICLI), 1982) will show cues around the mouth that mimic the manner of production of various sounds. For example, /p/ is demonstrated with the fingers in front of the mouth touching each other and then "popping" open—to represent the stop-release aspect of this segment. Articulation of /s/ is shown by drawing the "s" in the air with your forefinger, moving outward from the mouth—to demonstrate the continuant property of this sound.

Other, ad hoc types of hand cues may alternatively be used. For example, tapping under the chin or at the back of the throat for /k/ or /g/ production to demonstrate place and manner of production. Tapping the upper lip can, likewise, cue the production of /t/ and /k/. Ling (2002) provides a number of useful suggestions for various types of intervention activities that may prove useful in facilitating production of specific speech segments.

There are numerous computer programs that provide the deaf or hard of hearing child with visual feedback about her own productions. For example, the IBM Speechviewer provides a visual display of various aspects of phonation (fundamental frequency, intensity, and duration). Additional features of the system provide the child with feedback about vowel accuracy and limited feedback about the accuracy of isolated words. For a deaf or hard of hearing child, the feedback provided by computer-based speech practice systems such as the Speechviewer can provide useful visual correlates that can facilitate self-monitoring.

A major reason for promoting vocalization in the child at this stage is to help him understand that he can produce and control speech sounds. Equally important, however, is to quickly facilitate the child's use of these sounds to communicate meaning. For example, if the child learns to produce the neutral vowel /^/, it may easily be transferred to a meaningful situation, perhaps indicating *up* with a gesture or any other intention that appears appropriate for the child. Any specific speech work, as just described, will fit well with the integrated aspects of intervention, for example: working on maintaining eye contact for a period of time, then having the child practice the production of /p/-containing syllables, incorporating /p/-containing syllables in speechreading activities, reading a story that contains production models of /p/-containing syllables and words (for example, *Hop on Pop* by Dr. Seuss, 1963), or modeling vocabulary words that have the same sound.

Portions of the skill areas covered in this chapter may be evaluated through published instruments that involve parent reports as well as observations by the clinician. Most of the published tests are not standardized on children with hearing loss but still provide useful information that is pertinent to planning at the prelanguage level. Examples of such inventories are the Transdisciplinary Play-Based Analysis (Linder, 1997), the Rossetti Infant-Toddler Language Scale (Rossetti, 1990), the Battelle Developmental Inventory Screening Test (Newborg, Stock, Whek, Guidubaldi, & Svinicki, 1984), and Birth to Three: Screening Test of Learning and Language Development (Ammer & Bangs, 2000). Examples of parent-reported inventories specifically developed for deaf or hard of hearing children are the Meaningful Auditory Integration Scale (MAIS) (Robbins & Osberger, 1990) and the Meaningful Use of Speech Scale (MUSS) (Robbins & Osberger, 1991) (See appendix A).

PRELITERACY SKILLS

Considerable attention has been given recently to promoting literacy in deaf children. This focus has resulted from the longstanding recognition that reading difficulties among deaf learners are common. The majority of deaf students graduating from high school are reading between the third and fourth grade level. As a result of the prevalence of reading problems among deaf children (CADS, 1991) educators have begun to discuss some of the early areas that appear to be important for the later development of literacy.

Young children must first be exposed to a literate environment at a very early age. A literate environment is considered to be one that includes print as an important part of the visual context in which the child functions, for example, homes that include print in many different forms: books (both child and adult), magazines, newspapers, telephone messages, grocery lists, calendars or any other form of print that is consistently present and available to both the young children and the adults in the family.

In addition, young children must learn how to manipulate a book to understand and use the reading process. For example, they must learn how to distinguish print from nonprint and learn how to interact with the book: right side up and page turning from left to right. In addition, they begin very early to recognize some printed symbols, e.g., *stop* signs, a TV character's name, and their own name on a name tag at preschool (Wallach & Miller, 1988).

Hearing parents read to young hearing infants from the day they are born or before. These parents may let babies play with books when they are very young: e.g., holding the book, turning it upside down, and so forth. This exposure to print and the value of reading are thus available to the infant as he grows and explores his world. In addition, deaf parents sign books to their young children from a very early age (Moseley & Schick, 1999) and have books available for their child to manipulate. There is some speculation that hearing parents with deaf or hard of hearing children may do less reading to their children, because the child may not be able to understand the words. Thus, it may be that the manipulation of books is not a major goal in these homes.

The speech-language pathologist working with the prelanguage child may help the parents by discussing behaviors the parents can encourage that may ultimately help their child in the reading process, for example, exposure to various kinds of print as discussed above, letting the child manipulate books, and reading to him. The reading process may be different with the deaf and hard of hearing child. As well as informing the parents about ideas to use at home, the clinician may use reading as part of the therapy plan to help encourage language development as well as set the stage for learning to read when the child is in school.

Adults, whether parent or clinician, can seat the child so that the child can see his face. Adult and child may sit opposite each other with the adult pointing to pictures, naming or discussing them while assuring the child is watching the adult's face. Deaf parents will point to a picture, sign the name of it and then point again (Moseley Schick, 1999). Ezell, Justice, Mattingly, and Parsons (2000) examined a group of preschool children in Head Start and determined that print awareness can be encouraged in young children by "tracking" the words with a finger (left to right; top to bottom) and by occasionally calling attention to the names and sounds of letters. Ratner, Parker, and Gardner (1993) pointed out that different types of books encourage different aspects of reading. For example, some children's books play with sounds and call attention to the rhymes and rhythm of sound (e.g., *Hop on Pop* by Dr. Seuss, 1963, and other such books). Rhyming is one of the aspects of later reading that appears important for decoding new words (LaSasso & Metzger, 1998).

Ratner et al. (1993) also discuss the importance of reading books that are repetitive and help the child to comprehend and predict what is coming next in the book. Examples include books such as *Brown Bear, Brown Bear* (Martin & Carle, 1970), in which repetition occurs with new vocabulary. (An example from the book is "Brown Bear, Brown Bear, what do you see? I see a yellow duck looking at me. Yellow duck, yellow duck, what do you see? I see a blue horse looking at me," and so on. The child turns the page to see the new animal each time, and many children learn to "read" the pictures by learning and predicting which animal comes next within a similar text.) Ratner et al. (1993) includes a list of books in her article that address the above concepts (see appendix A).

Schleper (1996) developed a program entitled *The Shared Reading Program* for deaf children at the Clerc Center on Gallaudet's campus.

> The Shared Reading Project is built on the premise that hearing people can learn to read storybooks to deaf and hard of hearing children by observing how deaf adults do it. The Project is an accommodation that gives parents and caregivers visually based communication and booksharing strategies they can use to share books with their young deaf and hard of hearing children. The Shared Reading Project is based on 15 booksharing principles derived from research about how deaf adults read books to young deaf children. Deaf tutors serve as models and coaches to help hearing parents learn the skills needed to share books with their young deaf and hard of hearing children. The ultimate goal of the project is to help deaf and hard of hearing children become better readers in school and improve their academic achievement. (Delk & Weidekamp, 2001)

Many of these principles may be useful to nonsigners as well as to the parent who is learning to sign with their child and may also be useful to the speech-language pathologist who is incorporating the reading process into intervention activities. (See appendix A for a resource list for use in joint bookreading with language-disordered preschoolers.)

CASE STUDIES

The remainder of this chapter examines five different children introduced earlier. Each child is described at the prelanguage level, and assessment-intervention activities are proposed for the individual needs of that child. An integrated therapy approach is demonstrated.

1. Deaf readers translate stories using American Sign Language.
2. Deaf readers keep both languages visible (American Sign Language [ASL] and English).
3. Deaf readers are not constrained by the text.
4. Deaf readers re-read stories on a "storytelling" to "story reading" continuum.
5. Deaf readers follow the child's lead.
6. Deaf readers make what is implied explicit.
7. Deaf readers adjust sign placement to fit the story.
8. Deaf readers adjust signing style to fit the story.
9. Deaf readers connect concepts in the story to the real world.
10. Deaf readers use attention maintenance strategies.
11. Deaf readers use eye gaze to elicit participation.
12. Deaf readers engage in role play to extend concepts.
13. Deaf readers use ASL variations to sign repetitive English phrases.
14. Deaf readers provide a positive and reinforcing environment.
15. Deaf readers expect the child to become literate.

Figure 4-1   Principles for Reading to Deaf Children

Source: Copyright © 1996 by David R. Schleper, Pre-College National Mission Programs, Gallaudet University, Washington, DC. Used by permission.

Arlis

Arlis was born with a bilateral, progressive, mild to moderate sensorineural hearing loss. The etiology of his loss is hereditary. His maternal grandmother and mother were born with a bilateral, mild to moderate sensorineural hearing loss that progressed to profound at an early age. Arlis's mother and grandmother use amplification consistently and are oral communicators. Because of the family history of hearing loss, Arlis's hearing was tested, and his hearing loss was identified shortly after birth. At 4 months of age, he was fit with binaural, Phonak behind-the-ear hearing aids. Arlis's parents took sign language classes and were interested in having Arlis learn signs as well as spoken language. By the age of 2 years his hearing loss progressed to profound bilaterally. Because Arlis was doing so well with amplification, it was recommended that he be considered for a cochlear implant. After the candidacy evaluation, Arlis was given a Clarion Cochlear Implant in his right ear at age 2.6.

After Arlis received the implant and the external components were fit, he attended several mapping/programming sessions. During these sessions the speech processor was programmed. While using the implant, Arlis was able to detect all six sounds in the Six Sound Hearing Test (Ling, 1989). He was also seen twice per week for aural rehabilitation. Arlis made excellent progress. By age 3.6 years he had age-appropriate receptive and expressive spoken language skills. His voice quality was good, and he demonstrated production of many age-appropriate speech sounds.

At age 4 years, Arlis's parents enrolled him in a noncategorical preschool program in the public school system. There is one other child with hearing loss in his class, but Arlis is the only child with a cochlear implant.

Assessment

A daily listening check was completed for Arlis's cochlear implant to be sure that it was functioning properly and to establish a "baseline" of auditory functioning. Before assessment and intervention, Arlis's cochlear implant was checked, and the results were compared with baseline data (see appendix B).

Eye Contact.   Arlis was observed during play with children in his class. A time-sampled checklist was used and demonstrated that Arlis looked at the face of his communication partner and would hold eye contact for 10 to 20 seconds. He appeared to attend well during signed and spoken communication. He has been described by his cochlear implant rehabilitationist (CIR), his teacher, and his parents as "very visual." His CIR wants Arlis to depend less on his eyes and more on his ears.

Arlis also was tracked during his reception of sign language and demonstrated good visual skills in that mode. By using short (subject-verb-object) sentences with nouns and objects that the parents indicated were familiar to Arlis, his speechreading was evaluated. He was able to comprehend approximately 50% of the sentences with auditory and visual input.

Facial Expression.   Arlis was asked to identify facial expressions by matching the clinician's facial expression to pictures and then by imitating facial expressions when the clinician pointed to a picture. Finally, Arlis was asked, through speechreading, auditory input, and sign simultaneously to "pretend" different emotions, for example: "Pretend you're very mad!" He was able to identify the basic facial expressions of sadness, anger, happiness, surprise, and sleepiness. It was also noted at this time that Arlis responded appropriately to his mother's angry or happy facial expressions and used both facial expressions as well as sadness (crying).

Turn-Taking.   Observations, using another time-sampled checklist, indicated appropriate turn-taking, both in an individual situation and a small group situation. With his CIR, he was learning to take turns during small group auditory training activities when no visual cues were provided.

Intentions.   Arlis demonstrated all the intentions proposed by Halliday (1977). Some of the gestural intentions were beginning to change to words (e.g., the instrumental gesture of raising his hands to be picked up, became the verbal intention /"up"/). He continued to use pointing regularly to get an object or food. Intentions were evaluated over several different therapy sessions by using a check sheet and indicating whether they were expressed verbally or gesturally.

Auditory Skills.   Arlis was able to detect the Ling six sounds and all the phonemes presented in subtest 1 of the Glendonald School for the Deaf Auditory

Screening Procedure (GASP) (Erber, 1982). He was also able to successfully make sound-object associations using Level I of the Word Association for Syllable Perception (WASP) (Koch, 1999) program that is used at his cochlear implant center. Arlis's parents were asked to complete the Meaningful Auditory Integration Scale (MAIS) (Robbins & Osberger, 1990) to determine how he is using his listening skills/cochlear implant at home. Their responses indicate that Arlis is adjusting well to his implant. They have noted a significant difference in his responses to sounds in his environment compared with when he was wearing conventional hearing aids. Arlis responds to sounds in his environment and has begun to label the sounds that he hears by using signs/words.

Visual Skills.   Arlis's parents arranged for the Public Health Center to administer a vision screening. No vision problems were noted.

Visual-Gestural Skills.   As mentioned earlier, Arlis demonstrated excellent visual skills for reception of sign language. Arlis's expressive visual-gestural skills were well developed and age appropriate, as demonstrated to a sign language interpreter who consults with the school. He has basic vocabulary and is using signs in short sentences in English word order.

Speech/Vocalizations.   Arlis was given Ling's Phonetic Level Evaluation (Ling, 2002). He demonstrated appropriate suprasegmental skills, produced bilabial stops appropriately, produced the vowels appropriately and was able to imitate a continuant breath stream (wh and w) but had distorted sibilants and liquids. Arlis's parents were asked to complete the MUSS (Robbins & Osberger, 1991). His parents indicated that Arlis uses speech to communicate at home and only uses signs when he is not using his cochlear implant (e.g., bath time). They also reported that his speech sounds better while he is using his cochlear implant.

Preliteracy.   Arlis's teacher reported that he enjoys storytime at school; however, he tends to become distracted when it is noisy or when the other children ask questions. The teacher further reported that he seems to attend better when the teacher signs the story in addition to reading it aloud. Arlis's parents reported that at home he is exposed to books and seems to enjoy them; however, his parents report that they do not read to him often.

Intervention Goals

Goals for Arlis include the following:

- Expand his sound repertoire.
- Expand his signed and spoken vocabulary.
- Increase the time he uses speech reading with a communication partner.
- Improve his auditory skills when provided with auditory cues alone.
- Encourage Arlis's parents to read to him at home.

Books will be used during therapy activities. All the areas that were assessed will continue to be monitored throughout the time Arlis is receiving therapy.

Intervention Approach

The following methods and materials are used in one therapy session. A brief period of time (5 to 8 minutes) is given to production of /s/ in syllables. Because Arlis is able to produce vowels, syllables will be practiced that contain a vowel that is used in /s/ words; for example, see, say, sigh. These words are practiced using Visual Phonics (ICLI, 1982) as a cue. Arlis enjoys puzzles, so they are used as reinforcement for accurate production; following each correct production, he is allowed to place a piece of a small jigsaw puzzle.

To facilitate auditory skill development, the words mentioned in the preceding paragraph are used in short phrases. Arlis is instructed to say the name of the object he heard. For example, the clinician using an auditory screen, says "I see a ___ " after pulling a toy retrieved from a bag. For this activity, the toys selected are those that Arlis has demonstrated the ability to verbally label with some accuracy. This activity further develops Arlis's perception-production abilities. This same activity can be used to facilitate his turn-taking skills by having the clinician and Arlis "take turns." After the clinician asks Arlis to verbally identify the toy, Arlis picks a toy from the bag, produces the word behind an auditory screen, and the clinician identifies the word that Arlis produced.

Although many of Arlis's skills are consistent with the prelanguage phase of language learning, his speech skills are actually somewhat consistent with those of hearing children. Because Arlis is able to produce the /s/ correctly when cued with visual phonics, new words with the /s/ are introduced into his vocabulary through a "hide and seek" game. Objects and pictures are hidden around the room. When Arlis finds an object/picture, he shows it to the clinician. The clinician then articulates the word with the visual phonics cue, and Arlis imitates the word. (In future sessions, Arlis will initiate saying the words without clinician model or visual phonics cues.) Because Arlis's preschool class will have a field trip to a local aquarium, words that are included in this activity are those that begin with /si/, /sae/, and /sai/ and follow a theme of terms used at the aquarium (e.g., *seal, salt, sight* [discussing creatures in the dark], *sea,* and others).

The aquarium theme will be followed to facilitate Arlis's speechreading skills. Pictures of various animals, including a skate and a seal, are presented on cards. The clinician uses the word in a sentence, and Arlis identifies the word by pointing to the picture.

Continuing with the aquarium theme, Arlis drew pictures for the following "made up" story about going to the aquarium.

> Our class is going to the Aquarium.
> We will get on the bus.
> We will see fish, dolphins and seals.
> A lady at the Aquarium shows us the animals. She is the guide.
> We will eat lunch at the Aquarium.
> The bus will bring us back to school.

The clinician then reads the story to Arlis, and he is asked to "re-tell" the story by putting the pictures he drew in the proper order, along with the text. Arlis and the clinician put the pictures into a book, which is then sent home. The parents are encouraged to read the story to Arlis and to encourage discussion about the aquarium, both before and after the trip.

Cathy

Cathy is a 3-year-old girl born with a severe to profound bilateral hearing loss. Her hearing loss was identified at birth through the newborn screening program at the hospital, and her parents immediately sought services. Cathy received binaural amplification at 6 months and has been continually amplified since that time. Upon receipt of the aids, she immediately started responding to environmental sounds and to her parent's voice. This initial response led her parents to seek additional services from a speech pathologist and audiologist throughout her early years. Cathy's speech is developing, and although she is receiving some special services, her spoken language skills are developing at a pace that is more often seen by a hard of hearing child. The audiologist has concluded that Cathy has a considerable amount of usable hearing.

Assessment

As might be expected, many of the areas and procedures that were the focus for Arlis were also addressed for Cathy. Results include the following:

Eye Contact and Facial Expression.　Eye contact was poor. Cathy was not observed initiating eye contact. When she was asked to demonstrate eye contact, by turning her head to the speaker, she looked away after 1 to 5 seconds. Comprehension of facial expression could not adequately be evaluated because Cathy had poor eye contact. She appeared to respond auditorally to angry voices from her mother, and her mother reported that she responded to happy and sad voices if they were "loud enough."

Turn-Taking.　Turn-taking was inconsistent as indicated by the checklist used for evaluating. Cathy tended to interrupt with nonverbal (e.g., taking a toy or pointing) behaviors as well as verbal behaviors (syllable productions, one word-utterances such as "no," "dat" (meaning "that"), "mama," and other words of interest to her at the time).

Intentions.　Intentions were informally evaluated through observation of play. Cathy tended to express her intentions through gestures, with these gestures inconsistently accompanied by a one-word utterance (e.g., "dat!" accompanied by pointing to get a book to look at).

Auditory Skills.　Cathy was able to detect each of the Ling six sounds, and all the phonemes presented in subtest 1 of the GASP (Erber, 1982). These comprise primarily the following: vowels, nasals, laterals, and voiced and unvoiced fricatives.

Visual Skills.　No visual testing had been done. Although the parents reported that no problems exist, the recommendation was made to the parents to have a visual screening test for Cathy, especially because her eye contact is poor.

Visual-Gestural Skills. Cathy and her family do not use sign language. Accordingly, no sign language assessment was deemed necessary.

Speech/Vocalizations. The Ling Phonetic Inventory (Ling, 2002) indicated the following: neutralization of vowels and correct production of nasals; inconsistent production of stops, particularly back stops; and distortion or omissions of sibilants, affricates, and liquids.

Preliteracy. Cathy's parents reported that there are reading materials in the home for Cathy to look at—primarily children's books and magazines. They further reported, however, that Cathy does not seem interested in books and rarely initiates reading.

Intervention Goals

Based on the assessment outcomes, a series of long-term goals were established for Cathy. They include the following:

- Increased use of eye contact and turn-taking.
- Use of speech for communication—encourage use of vocalizations instead of gestures.
- Increase production of appropriate vowels and stops.
- Increase eye contact and promote identification of bilabial stops through speech reading

Intervention Approach

Cathy is not enrolled in a preschool program; she attends individual therapy 3 days a week for a 50-minute period. The first activity of each therapy session is to use the Ling six sound test to make sure Cathy's hearing aids are working correctly. Therapy sessions take an integrated form as they did with Arlis. Cathy's mother observes each session and talks with the clinician after each session. Cathy is an only child, and her mother works with her consistently at home but expresses some frustration that progress is slow.

Cathy begins sessions with a 10- to 15-minute period of working on consonant-vowel-consonant (CVC) words with bilabials and different vowels (e.g., pop, hop, or mop). She is able to imitate these words correctly and use the vowels correctly during imitation time. The clinician uses a modified cycles approach (see Hodson & Paden, 1991), in which correctly imitated words are drawn on a card by the child, used for playing games such as "Go Fish" and other similar activities, and new words are probed for the next session. In addition, the child receives auditory stimulation with additional amplification (in Cathy's case, a frequency-modulated [FM] system) during each session. In this auditory training activity, the child is required to listen to a series of words containing segments that are to be emphasized in production. A word list and the cards the child has used during therapy are sent home, and the family is encouraged to say the words on the list and to encourage the child to imitate production of the picture cards. During the next session the probed words that were accurately produced in the previous session are used following the same procedure described above.

Cathy enjoys drawing and has been very responsive to activities that involve drawing. Cathy was given a series of target CV or CVC words containing segments to be practiced and was asked to draw pictures that depict those words. Cathy's pictures are then used during activities aimed to attain goals associated with turn-taking, eye contact, and speechreading readiness. Cathy watches the clinician for a minimum of 7 to 10 seconds (timed by a stopwatch) while the clinician holds the card by her own mouth, points to it, and says the word (quietly, so Cathy cannot hear the entire word). Cathy must respond by producing the word, thus practicing establishing eye contact, production, speechreading, and turn-taking.

The book *Hop on Pop,* by Dr. Seuss, is used as a way to create turn-taking, stimulation of practice words, and encouragement of preliteracy. Cathy is shown that when the reader (in this case, the clinician) stops speaking, it is time to turn to the next page of the book. Cathy and the clinician sit at a table with Cathy directly across from the clinician so she can see when the clinician stops talking and thus is cued to turn the page. To encourage using speech for communication (e.g., answering questions and taking turns), the clinician asks Cathy to name some of the objects and actions in the book, e.g., *Pop, hop,* and so on. If Cathy responds well to the book, it can be sent home with her, along with a brief note about the goal of this activity. Her family can then read to her while Cathy is practicing her newly learned page-turning skills.

Future sessions will proceed in similar ways, expanding production of the bilabials to include additional stops, using other vowels, playing other games that involve turn-taking and eye contact perhaps with some other children Cathy's age), speechreading, and reading. Each session will begin with conversation about something of interest to Cathy (as supplied by either Cathy or her mother) to encourage using speech for communication and turn-taking.

Bridget

Bridget was born with a severe to profound, bilateral, sensorineural hearing loss of unknown origin. The hearing loss was identified at birth after newborn hearing screening. She was fitted with hearing aids at 6 months and wears them all waking hours. Bridget is an only child with hearing parents. Her parents struggled with the diagnosis of her hearing loss and seemed to put a lot of pressure on Bridget and the professionals working with her. Her parents utilized the public school Parent Infant Program and the program provided by the local school for the deaf. However, no sign language has been used with Bridget per her parents' request. In addition, Bridget has received private speech-language services since she was 1 year old. Bridget is now 3 years old and entering a center-based program in her local public school. She is enrolled in a noncategorical preschool class. Bridget is the only child with a hearing loss in the school. Bridget is developing spoken language slowly. She has fair voice quality, evidences some age-appropriate sounds, and speaks in one- to two-word utterances. Her vocabulary is delayed, and she has difficulty following all but the most routine directions.

Assessment

As was shown for Arlis and Cathy, it is necessary to evaluate a range of skill areas to establish appropriate therapy goals. The areas and strategies for assessing them are described in the following.

Pragmatics. Bridget demonstrated consistent eye contact, most likely as a result of past therapy. She responded well to attention mechanisms (e.g., tapping her shoulder), and her comprehension and use of facial expression were excellent. Bridget demonstrated turn-taking in diads, but experienced difficulties following interactions in groups. It was difficult for Bridget to find the speaker, even in a group of three to four, and she became easily frustrated, as evidenced by tears and stamping her foot. Intentions were expressed through use of one- to two-word phrases, with some accompanying appropriate gestures.

Audition/Listening. Bridget was able to correctly identify the vowels using the Ling six sound test but was only inconsistently able to identify the consonants, /s/, /ʃ/ (/ (or /sh/), and /m/. It was also noted that with the use of an FM system Bridget was more consistently able to identify the vowels and the accuracy of /m/ identification also increased. Further analysis of auditory input will be done through evaluative therapy, using the GASP (Erber, 1982).

Auditory/Visual. Bridget had a visual screening at her pediatrician's office, and the parents reported that it was normal. She was beginning to develop speechreading skills as assessed by informal activities and was able to understand routine related statements (e.g., line up and wash your hands).

Speech/Voice. The Ling Phonetic Inventory (Ling, 2002) revealed the following: ability to sustain and vary the duration of a sustained vowel; a tendency to neutralize many vowels; omissions and distortions of back consonants, fricatives, affricates, and liquids; and stimulable but inconsistent production of bilabial and alveolar consonants. From these findings a number of speech goals will be able to be established.

Visual-Gestural Skills. No sign language has been used with Bridget, upon the parent's request. Accordingly, visual-gestural communication was not assessed.

Preliteracy. Bridget's parents reported that a variety of age-appropriate print materials are available in the home. They reported that Bridget enjoys looking at books and spends a great deal of time by herself pointing to the words and using what the mother describes as "gibberish" (vocal sounds that the parents cannot identify).

Intervention Goals

Among the goals established for Bridget are the following:

- Turn-taking in small groups.
- Promote production of age appropriate sounds.

- Develop and refine listening/speechreading skills.
- Develop vocabulary (as indicated by the next level evaluation).

Integrated Therapy Activity (in Classroom)

The speech-language pathologist and the preschool classroom teacher have an ongoing collaborative program with children in their school. Because Bridget is the only deaf child in the school, one of their goals is to educate the other preschool children about her hearing loss. They prepared a program for the other children that included having the children listen to a tape that simulates hearing loss, letting Bridget show the children her hearing aids and letting them listen to similar aids, and using puppets to talk about hearing loss and what the other children can do when they talk to Bridget, as well as each other (e.g., look at her face, tap her shoulder when they want to talk with her instead of just saying her name, and raising a hand when in a group and they want to talk with her).

In addition to educating the other children about hearing loss, the speech-language pathologist also works with the class for a few minutes before each of Bridget's therapy sessions and plays a "sound game" requiring the children's participation. For example, because Bridget is working on production of fricatives, the game "Simon Says" can be used with the children taking turns repeating the instructions of the speech-language pathologist. After the game, the children can discuss what they liked about the game as well as practice raising their hands and looking at each other when they talk. This activity provides the children with the opportunity to practice with Bridget and each other the various strategies needed to most effectively communicate with Bridget.

The preschool teacher and the speech-language pathologist decided on themes to use during the school year. New vocabulary is introduced by the teacher in the classroom, with the speech-language pathologist present. The speech-language pathologist then initiates activities based on these words in her once weekly individual therapy session with Bridget. Pictures of the new words are drawn or cut from a magazine and pasted into a "journal" that Bridget takes home every day. For example, one theme might be the seasons and new vocabulary might be *Fall, Halloween, leaves, pumpkin, orange*. In keeping with the recommendation that new vocabulary words be presented a minimum of 10 times (Nichols & Moseley, 1996), the individual therapy session continues with these vocabulary items, and the parents reinforce the activities at home by playing games with new words.

The vocabulary words are also used for auditory discrimination training and speechreading. For example, Bridget responds well to auditory information of varying syllables (e.g., *Fall* and *Halloween*) and can discriminate between the two-syllable structures. Games, in which the children identify vocabulary through visual or auditory mode only, are encouraged during small group time in the classroom. Utterances vary from one word to two-plus word phrases. Books are also available that focus on various holidays and seasons and can be used to provide additional reinforcement to new vocabulary, auditory and visual information, sound production, and taking turns identifying and discussing the content.

Dion

Dion was born with a severe to profound, bilateral, sensorineural hearing loss. He is the second deaf child born to deaf parents. His hearing loss was identified at birth following High Risk Registry Screening. He was not fitted with hearing aids until he was 12 months old (based on parental interest and follow-up) and now wears amplification inconsistently. Dion is now 3 years old and entering the non-categorical preschool class in his neighborhood school. Dion and his older sister are the only children with a hearing loss in the school. A sign language interpreter is provided in the classroom full time.

Dion's mother is a hearing aid user but his father is not. His sister has slightly more consistent hearing aid use based on the behavioral reinforcement program implemented in a full-day school program. ASL is the language of the home and reportedly both children are developing ASL in an age-appropriate manner. The children are most comfortable communicating in ASL but will voice to the best of their ability when asked.

Dion is developing some differentiated vowel sounds and approximations of the more visible consonant sounds. Some single words are recognizable to familiar listeners. He has vocal quality characteristic of a deaf speaker. He is able to detect all of the Ling six sounds with his new IMPACT frequency transposition hearing aids. Dion is struggling with attention to the face of a speaker for the purpose of speechreading training. His vocabulary in spoken English is delayed.

Assessment and Intervention Goals

Evaluation of Dion's communication involved examination of many of the same areas and with the same tests as were used with the children described earlier in this chapter. An additional evaluation of Dion's sign language was performed, however, so that a complete picture of his language abilities may be obtained. Results include the following:

- Dion exhibited good eye contact during interactions involving communication in sign language. Eye contact is somewhat variable when only spoken language is used.
- Facial expressions were comprehended and used with sign language. Less attention was paid to the face during speech.
- No deficits in turn-taking were observed, even in group situations with other children who sign. However, because of limited use of speech, there was no indication how Dion uses turn-taking during spoken interactions. This area will be evaluated over time when intervention begins.
- Intentions were expressed consistently with sign language. Use of speech was limited, so an evaluation of the types of intentions used in speech could not be accomplished. This area will be evaluated over time when intervention begins.
- Auditory skills were very limited, probably the result of limited usable hearing and inconsistent hearing aid use.

- Visual skills appeared excellent for sign language reception. Speechreading skills are variable at this time with some comprehension evident. A visual screening will be requested when school begins in the Fall.
- A sign language evaluation was conducted by a sign language consultant, recommended by the sign language interpreter who works with Dion's sister. Different areas evaluated were similar to the areas described in this chapter, e.g., eye contact, facial expression, and intentions, in sign language, as well as general vocabulary, phonology, and syntax in sign. Dion's visual-gestural skills appeared well developed and age appropriate.
- Vocalizations were limited, but syllable approximations were noted, as evidenced by an observational analysis. The Ling Phonetic Inventory (Ling, 2002) indicated sufficient breath support for speech, ability to repeat two to three CV syllables, as well as limited use of different vowels and consonants.
- Parents indicated that books and other age-appropriate print materials are available in the home. They further reported that Dion loves to look at books and that they regularly read him stories in sign language.

Treatment Goals

Long term goals for Dion include the following:

- Increasing attention to the mouth and understanding that meaningful information may be derived from the mouth and face when speaking
- Using evaluative therapy aimed to assess turn-taking and expression of intentions through spoken English
- Encouraging consistent use of hearing aids
- Improving auditory skills through work on awareness and discrimination of sounds
- Increasing vocalizations to include meaningful words

Intevention Approach

The varied goals that exist for Dion are amenable to an integrated approach to intervention. The speech-language pathologist working with Dion uses some sign language and can make herself known to Dion with short phrases. The speech-language pathologist thus uses sign language to explain to Dion activities that will take place using spoken English.

Dion is receiving individual therapy twice weekly for approximately 45 minutes. During one of the weekly sessions, Dion and the speech-language pathologist play with some of the favorite toys Dion brought from home: a fire engine, a Fisher-Price™ schoolhouse with people and furniture, two books with large pictures, and a box of the large-sized Lego blocks. This session is used to permit assessment of Dion's use of various intents and evidence of turn-taking during spoken interchanges.

To accomplish this evaluative therapy, the clinician designed a checksheet, listing the intentions described by Halliday (1975) and discussed earlier in this chapter. She also included a place on the checklist to record each time Dion took turns verbally with no interruption during a 5-minute period. This information is used to establish a baseline for Dion's turn-taking behavior and use of intentions during spoken English interchanges.

To ensure that spoken language is accessible to Dion, he is asked to use his hearing aids during the 45-minute session. (Dion's parents had reported he had no problem wearing his aids for a limited amount of time but never asked for them or put them on himself.) The Ling Six Sound Test was performed at the beginning of each session to ensure that the aids were working.

To facilitate attention to the face during spoken interchanges, the clinician greets the child each day with "Hi, Dion" while drawing his attention to her mouth by pointing. (A goal for a later session will be to have Dion respond with "Hi" verbally and eventually initiate "Hi" when he arrives for therapy). Each time an activity is changed, the speech-language pathologist obtains Dion's attention by using his name and pointing to her mouth.

To promote auditory awareness and to enable practice aimed at facilitating discrimination, the following 5-minute activity is used. The clinician initiates vocalization using the words *fire truck* and *book*. Using an audio screen (as described earlier in this book), she will ask Dion to 1) raise his hand when she uses a word to accompany an action (e.g., moving the fire truck or turning a page in the book) and 2) discriminate between a one-syllable word and a two-syllable word presented verbally by indicating whether the words are the *same* or *different.*

After this activity, Dion and the speech-language pathologist again use the Fisher-Price school. The goal is to probe CVC syllables and check stimulability. For example, the Fisher Price characters are given names such as *Nan* the teacher, *Tom* the child, *Mom*, or a friend named *Pat*. During this play period, the clinician may also use the checksheet previously described to record instances of turn-taking and intentions. Dion is also encouraged to use these words consistently and is given many opportunities to produce them through play.

An important aspect of therapy for a child this age is to work with the parents. The speech-language pathologist discusses with the parents the importance of the use of Dion's hearing aids for speech training and for the classroom. The parents are encouraged to record Dion's hearing aid use in a journal. With parental involvement, a program based on the Ski*Hi Model (Watkins, 2004) was designed to encourage Dion's use of the aids.

In addition to working with the parents, the speech-language pathologist keeps the classroom teacher and other teachers who work with Dion (e.g., the art teacher) informed of some of the goals for Dion and encourages their participation. For example, all the teachers can say "Hi" to Dion when they see him and encourage his use of "Hi" verbally in response.

Renee

Renee has a congenital, bilateral, profound, sensorineural hearing loss that was diagnosed at 2 years of age. The etiology is unknown. She is now 3 years old and is enrolled in a center-based preschool supported by her local school district. Renee lives with her mother, father, and one older sister who are all hearing. They moved here from Haiti when Renee was 2 months old. Her parents and sister are bilingual in spoken English and French. The parents want Renee to be oral and to be able to use both English and French. Currently, the family communicates with Renee mostly through gestures.

Renee has recently received binaural conventional hearing aids. Her parents say she does not like to use them and consistently takes them off. Her parents believe she is getting minimal benefit from the aids. Her parents have considered a cochlear implant, but ruled it out because of concerns regarding the surgery. In addition, Renee shows minimal speech and language skills. Her parents report she does not use any of the sounds meaningfully but uses a few vowels from both English and French.

Her parents report that Renee seems inquisitive and interested in the visual aspects of her environment (e.g., she likes to turn lights off and on and appears to enjoy looking at books). Renee becomes frustrated (crying and stamping foot) when she cannot communicate her needs.

Assessment

Evaluation for Renee will be accomplished using many of the same tests and observations that were described for the previous children. The extent of the information needed about Renee argues for a more intensive diagnostic therapy process than was used with the previous children. It was decided that diagnostic therapy would be a more appropriate approach to assessment with Renee. The assessment took place during eight sessions over a 4-week period. Given in the following are the outcomes of that assessment.

Eye Contact.   Eye contact was observed during spontaneous play with her mother and through a time-sampled analysis on two different occasions. Results indicated that Renee was very inconsistent with her eye contact. The time-sampled analysis indicated that 40% of the time, she watched her mother when her mother was talking and did not the rest of the time. Her mother changed back and forth between English and French when playing with her. The clinician's perception was that Renee was very quick to respond appropriately to gestures from her mother, indicating good visual recognition of particular gestures (e.g., pointing, motioning to come here, "sit down," and head shake for "no").

Facial Expression.   Facial expression, as shown through pictures, did not appear meaningful to Renee. She could not match pictures with actual expressions used by the clinician. The clinician's impression was that Renee demonstrated a *flat affect*; she demonstrated unhappiness by crying but did not appear to show happiness or surprise.

Turn-Taking.   Turn-taking was evaluated over all eight sessions. Because Renee had very little language, three aspects of turn-taking were observed: 1) nonverbal turns in play; 2) turn-taking with gestures; and 3) turn-taking when the clinician/parent spoke and Renee gestured. Results indicated that Renee was aware of the turn-taking process. She could roll a ball back and forth appropriately when playing with the clinician. She watched the clinician gesture to her to do things such as "sit down" and then responded with the action. She also responded with an action when her mother spoke to her. For example, her mother said: "Do you want to read a book?" and Renee then walked across the room and picked up a stuffed animal. Although such responses indicated little comprehension, they were consistent enough to indicate that Renee applied some meaning to her mother's mouth movement. The same responses, albeit inappropriate, were observed with speech from the clinician.

Gestures.   Gestural intentions were examined through observation and a checklist over the eight sessions, using Halliday's classification system. Renee showed several examples of use of each type of intention. These intentions, including imaginative, were manifested gesturally. She played by herself quietly and actively. She dressed dolls, moved them around, and made them wave to the clinician. Observations of some of the imaginative actions she attributed to the dolls indicated some use of symbolic play.

Visual-Gestural Skills.   Renee has used no sign language; however, she appeared very interested in the clinician's hand movement when making some simple developmentally appropriate signs (e.g., mother, sit, eat, sleep, more, and so on). These signs were presented very informally during games.

Auditory Skills.   Renee responds to loud environmental sounds and calling her name loudly by turning her head. In presenting various environmental sounds to Renee, she demonstrated awareness of most of them by turning her head. Over the 4-week period, she gradually used her hearing aids for up to 10 minutes during the therapy sessions. She could respond consistently to the vowel sounds of the Ling Six Sound Test.

The observations obtained in the first four areas above indicate that Renee clearly makes use of visual input, especially gestures and mouth movement, even though her eye contact is limited. A visual acuity screening has been recommended to the parents.

Speech/Vocalizations.   Renee shows minimal speech skills. She is able to produce occasional front vowel sounds and a glottal fricative in English, as revealed by a phonetic inventory. The clinician does not know French, so cannot, at this time, identify other sounds that could be French. The parents report that they hear "a few" French sounds when Renee is playing, but many more English sounds.

Preliteracy.   Examples of both French and English print are available in the home. The parents reported that Renee loves to look at the pictures in books; she will sit for a long time and point to the pictures. This is the major time during which they hear the production of some sounds.

Intervention Goals

Long-term goals for Renee include the following:

- One session a week with the parents to discuss issues related to Renee's communication (see next paragraph)
- Increasing eye contact and use of facial expression
- Comprehending words, through speechreading, that demonstrate the intentions Renee uses
- Designing a program for consistent use of hearing aids
- Discriminating and identifying sounds while using her hearing aids
- Initiation of some sign language use (in conjunction with counseling and support of family)
- Stimulation of meaningful syllables: *hi*, *bye*, etc.

The intervention program for Renee moves in a somewhat different direction from that used with the other children. There is more emphasis on working with the parents. The parents have agreed to come to the school and meet with the clinician once a week. Among issues the clinician feels need to be addressed with the parents are the following: 1) use of two languages in the home (Renee does not demonstrate facility in either; it may be important to use only one verbal language.); 2) the possibility of sign language (Renee responds well to visual input and imitates signs and the parents have shared the fact that Renee seems to be "so visual."); 3) a behavioral program for the parents to help Renee use her hearing aids at home; and 4) a variety of activities at home that will provide ongoing and consistent stimulation for Renee.

Intervention Approach

The speech-language pathologist is in the classroom during the 45-minute period she sees Renee. She has shared the goals described earlier with the classroom teacher and has encouraged the teacher to incorporate activities within the classroom aimed toward these goals. When the speech-language pathologist is in the classroom she works with all the children using several games that will promote achievement of Renee's goals, as well as benefiting all the children. Before beginning, the Ling Six Sound Test will be conducted with Renee to make sure her hearing aids are working correctly.

Eye contact is encouraged with a ring toss game in which two teams throw a ring around a free-standing post. Each child must turn to the child in line behind his, look at him, give him the ring, and smile.

All the children play a game in which they match facial expression pictures (line drawings done by a friend of the speech-language pathologist's) with actual facial expressions. Children will sit in a circle and take turns matching the pictures and expressions of the teacher, then of each other.

During play time, the speech-language pathologist stays with Renee and verbalizes what she believes her intentions to be. She points to her own mouth and has Renee look at her. This activity encourages Renee to make connections between what she wants and the words that express that intention. For example, when Renee reaches up on the shelf to get a book, the speech-language patholo-gist might stand beside her, get her attention by tapping her shoulder, and say "want book." Depending on the outcome of the sign language discussion with the parents, the speech-language pathologist may sign the words, ask for imitation, provide hand over hand modeling, or continue to verbalize only.

While still in the classroom, Renee and the speech-language pathologist have "sound time" while the classroom teacher works with the rest of the group. The speech-language pathologist works on auditory skills and sound produc-tion. The auditory activity facilitates discrimination of speech sounds, either the presence or absence of speech. This is accomplished by using the facial expression pictures introduced earlier, covering her mouth with an audio screen, and either saying or not saying the picture she holds up (e.g., happy or surprised). Renee can indicate the presence or absence of sound by putting a block in a box.

Sound production time focuses on imitating vowels; at first the more visible vowels /i/ and /o/ will be presented. The speech-language pathologist uses a voice-activated toy, such as a teddy bear or dancing flower, and Renee imitates the particular vowel being stimulated. The voice-activated toy provides rein-forcement of the verbal behavior.

The program is changed as needed to accommodate decisions made by the parents regarding sign language, use of English and French, and consistent use of hearing aids.

Summary

In this chapter, areas of prelanguage that are necessary for communication are discussed as well as assessment and intervention tools for this level. Five case studies demonstrate some of the different types of programs that may be appro-priate for different types of functioning. As discussed earlier in this chapter, the prelanguage areas may overlap with the needs of children who are older than the children discussed in this chapter. For example, the second grade child, who does not have good eye contact or understand facial expression, may need to work on some of these prelanguage areas. The next three chapters will follow these five children through their school years.

References

Abraham, S., Stoker, R., & Allen, W. (1988). Language assessment of hearing impaired children and youth: Patterns of test use. *Language, Speech and Hearing Services in Schools, 19*(2).

Ammer, J. J., & Bangs, T. (2000). Birth to Three Assessment and Intervention System (BTAIS-2) (2nd ed.). Austin, TX: Pro-Ed.

CADS (Center for Assessment and Demographic Studies). (1991). *Stanford Achievement Test: Hearing-impaired norms booklet* (8th ed.). Washington, DC: Gallaudet University, Gallaudet Research Institute, Center for Assessment and Demographic Studies.

Clark, T. C. & Watkins, S. (1985). *The Ski*Hi Model: Programming for hearing impaired infants through home intervention.* Logan: Utah State University: Ski*Hi Institute.

Delk, L., & Weidekamp, L. (2001). *The shared reading project: Evaluating implementation processes and family outcomes.* Retrieved from http://clerccenter.gallaudet.edu/Products/Sharing-Results/SharedReadingProject/

Dr. Seuss. (1963). *Hop on Pop.* New York: Random House.

Erber, N. (1982). *Auditory training.* Washington, DC: Alexander Graham Bell Association for the Deaf.

Ezell, H. K., Justice, L. M., Mattingly, S. E., & Parsons, D. (2000). *Shared book reading and emergent literacy: From research to practice.* Paper presented at the annual meeting of the American Speech-Language-Hearing Association, Washington, DC.

Goetz, L., Haring, T., & Anderson, J. (1983). *Educational assessment for social interaction (EASI): An observational checklist for measuring social interactions between nondisabled and severely disabled students in integrated settings* (ERIC Reproduction Document ED 242 184, p. 3). San Francisco, CA: San Francisco State University.

Goldin-Meadow, S. (1975). *The representation of semantic relations in a manual language created by deaf children of hearing parents: A language you can't dismiss out of hand.* Unpublished doctoral dissertation, University of Pennsylvania, University Park.

Graney, S. (1998). *Where Does Speech Fit In? Spoken English in a Bilingual Context.* Washington, DC: Gallaudet University Pre-College National Mission programs.

Haliday, M. A. K. (1977). *Learning how to mean.* New York: Elsevier North-Holland.

Haynes, W. O., & Shulman, B. B. (1998). *Communication development foundations, processes, and clinical applications.* Baltimore: Williams & Wilkins.

Hodson, B. W., & Paden, E. P. (1991). *Targeting Intelligible Speech: A Phonological Approach to Remediation* (2nd ed.). Austin, TX: Pro-Ed.

International Communication Learning Institute (ICLI) (1982), Visual Phonics. Edina, MN: Author.

Koch. M. (1999). *WASP (word association for syllable perception).* Timonium, MD: York Press.

LaSasso, D., & Metzger, M. (1998). An alternate route for preparing deaf children for BiBi programs: The home language as L1 and Cued Speech for conveying traditionally spoken languages. *Journal of Deaf Studies & Deaf Education, 3*(4) 265–289.

Linder, T. W. (1997). *Transdisciplinary play-based assessment: A functional approach to working with young children* (Rev. ed.). Baltimore: Paul H. Brookes.

Ling, D. (1989). *Foundationa of spoken language for the hearing-impaired child.* Washington, DC: Alexander Graham Bell Association for the Deaf.

Ling, D. (2002). *Speech and the hearing-impaired child: Theory and practice* (2nd ed.). Washington, DC: Alexander Graham Bell Association for the Deaf.

Lund, N. J., & Duchan, J. F. (1983). *Assessing children's language in naturalistic contexts.* Englewood Cliffs, NJ: Prentice-Hall.

Martin, B. Jr., & Carle, E. (1970) *Brown bear, brown bear, what do you see?* New York: Holt.

McAnally, P. L., Rose, S., & Quigley, S. P. (1994). *Language learning practices with deaf children* (2nd ed.). Austin, TX: Pro-Ed.

Mohay, H. (1997). *Language in situ: Making language visually accessible to deaf children.* Paper presented at the Festschrift for Professor Kay Meadow-Orlans. Washington, DC: Gallaudet University.

Moseley, M. J. & Schick, B. (Producers). (1999). *Deaf parents' strategies for American Sign Language development in their young deaf children.* [Videotape]. Personal communication with M. J. Moseley.

Newborg, J., Stock, J. R., Whek, L., Guidubaldi, & Svinicki, J. (1984). *The Battelle Developmental Inventory—Screening Test (BDI).* Allen, TX: DLM Teaching Resources.

Nichols, M., & Moseley, M. J. (1996). Language skills. In M. J. Moseley & S. J. Bally (Eds.), *Communication therapy: An integrated approach to aural rehabilitation.* Washington, DC: Gallaudet University Press.

Nussbaum, D., & Waddy-Smith, B. (2001). *Kendall demonstration elementary school.* Washington, DC: Gallaudet University Unpublished manuscript.

Power, D. J., & Hollingshead, A. (1982). *Aspects of a communication curriculum for hearing-impaired pupils: Report of the Second National Workshop on Language Curriculum Development.* Brisbane, Australia: Brisbane College of Advanced Education.

Ratner, N. B., Parker, B., & Gardner, P. (1993). Joint bookreading as a language scaffolding activity for communicatively impaired children. *Seminar in Speech and Language, 14*(4), 296–313.

Robbins, A. M., & Osberger, M. J. (1990). *Meaningful Auditory Integration Scale* (MAIS). Indianapolis: Indiana University School of Medicine.

Robbins, A. M., & Osberger, M. J. (1991). *Meaningful Use of Speech Scale* (MUSS). Indianapolis: Indiana University School of Medicine.

Rossetti, L. (1990). *The Rossetti Infant-Toddler Language Scale: A measure of communication and interaction.* East Moline, IL: LinguiSystems.

Schleper, D. R. (1996). *Shared reading project.* Washington, DC: Gallaudet University, Pre-College National Mission Programs.

Snow, C. (1977). The development of conversation between mothers and babies. *Journal of Child Language, 4,* 1–22.

Volterra, V., & Erting, C. J. (Eds.). (1994). *From gesture to language in hearing and deaf children.* Washington, DC: Gallaudet University Press.

Wallach, G. P., & Miller, L. (1988). *Language intervention and academic success.* Boston: College-Hill.

Watkins, E. (Ed.). (2004). *Ski*Hi curriculum: Family-centered programming for infants and young children with hearing loss.* North Logan, UT: HOPE.

Westby, C. (1988). Children's play: reflections of social competence. *Seminars in Speech & Language, 9,* 1–14.

Zinober, B., & Martlew, M (1985). The development of communicative gestures. In M. Barret (Ed.). *Children's single word speech.* Chichester, England: Wiley.

Early Language: Assessment and Intervention

Introduction

This chapter will serve as the bridge from early childhood speech and language concerns to later language assessment and intervention. As previously mentioned the stages presented are guidelines, and there may be overlap in skill areas, tests, and therapy techniques depending on the abilities of the particular child.

The leap from prelanguage to early language is an essential and significant one for children. All of the important prelanguage skills that have been developing are now put to use in acquiring and using language to control the environment. Eventually these language skills serve as the foundation for all academic learning. Children demonstrate their facility or lack of facility with language learning fairly immediately in the school setting. Children who are unable to access the language of the classroom and thus navigate the environment often display mild to severe behavioral issues in response to the inability to manage the academic tasks and social demands of the school environment.

The early language stage often coincides with the child's introduction to a more structured learning setting. Home-based therapy is replaced by classroom-based services and a relatively intimate setting is replaced by a highly stimulating and more populated learning arena. This presents challenges to all children. They must learn the language of the classroom from both an academic and social perspective. The pragmatic, expressive, and receptive language (spoken and signed), speech, and listening/speechreading skills of deaf and hard of hearing children are now integral to success. The deaf or hard of hearing child may find these tasks to be daunting (McNally, Rose, & Quigley, 1994).

ASSESSMENT

For many public school speech-language pathologists (SLPs), the early language age/stage may be the first time they encounter a child with a hearing loss. This may vary from district to district, but often the prelanguage age child may be placed in a preschool program outside her neighborhood school or served in her home. As such, establishing the child's communication and learning abilities is essential to designing an intervention program suited to a given child. First, the SLP would want to obtain as much previous assessment and intervention planning information as possible from previous service providers. Individualized Family Service Plans (ISFPs) should be forwarded to the SLP. If these are not received, requests should then be made to the parent(s), the previous service providers, or both. It is important to gather all relevant reports, including the most recent audiogram, to adequately determine areas that have previously been the focus of intervention and those in need of further work or additional testing. Different school districts and states have different levels of service provision for the preschool child. In addition, families take advantage of different levels of educational services for their children. Some families may utilize only home-based services whereas others may opt for a school-based preschool placement and others choose to enroll their children in both. Regardless of the preschool approach used, gathering all essential documents and information is the first step in programming for children with hearing loss in the public school setting.

After gathering all available information, the SLP must decipher it. Understanding the child's hearing loss (audiogram), residual hearing, and the type of technology/amplification she uses is the first priority. The level of hearing loss and benefit from technology and subsequent residual hearing/access to spoken language as well as the child's communication mode(s) will dictate the type and breadth of assessment and intervention appropriate for that child. If possible, it is also helpful to obtain information in additional areas such as the child's cognition, play, and overall motor abilities. Once all available information is reviewed the SLP can return to the Scope (see Table 3-1 in Chapter 3) to plan the necessary assessments, and establish baseline skills and Individualized Education Plan (IEP) goals.

The assessment and intervention strategies for early language will be discussed as they apply to a variety of children using the representative case studies. It is essential to begin by reviewing the skills in the prelanguage area of the Scope. These skills are essential building blocks for further communication skill development. Once it is determined that the child has mastered the prelanguage skills to a developmentally and age-appropriate level, the clinician can begin assessment of early language skills. The emphasis in the prelanguage stage is on pragmatic skills. These skills remain important throughout the life of the child but often develop to an age/communication mode-appropriate level and are no longer evaluated and addressed. However, any prelanguage skills that are discovered to be absent or delayed will become the initial and priority goals for the child's IEP. An exception to establishing these skill areas as goals would be if the clinician determines, in cooperation with the family and other professionals, that the skill is unlikely to be developed. For example, a child with no residual hearing and no benefit from amplification will not be able to acquire auditory skills such as identification or discrimination.

If the child demonstrates the necessary prelanguage skills, then the baseline goals will be established from the early language assessment of listening skills, speechreading skills, receptive and expressive language (content form and use), speech and voice skills, sign language production, and early literacy.

Listening Skills

As mentioned briefly earlier, it is important to know the level of residual hearing the child has with and without amplification (Northern & Downs, 2002). Once this is determined, it is necessary to determine where on the hierarchy of listening skills the child is currently performing and set appropriate goals for auditory training. The hierarchy of skills includes detection, discrimination, identification, and comprehension (Erber, 1982). This can be done through a variety of formal and informal measures. The Word Association for Syllable Perception (WASP) (Koch, 1999) and Speech Perception Instructional Curriculum and Evaluation (SPICE) (Moog et al., 1995) plus auditory programs mentioned in other chapters are appropriate and highly structured programs for auditory training. Informal measures (e.g., checklists) can also be used to determine the child's current level of functioning and to move her along the hierarchy in therapy. It is important to realize that the child may reach a terminal point in therapy, which is not at the comprehension level of connected speech. Determinations will eventually need to be made about the efficiency of auditory training as a priority in communication therapy for a given child. At the early language stage, however, work should continue to challenge the listening skills of the child. In later stages, prognostic indicators can be considered and decisions made about the priority of listening training in overall therapy.

Speechreading Skills

There are similarities between auditory and visual skill development used for the reception of speech. As children develop their visual skills for communicating, they progress from detection to perception in a manner similar to that described by Erber for auditory development. Accordingly, the protocol and process for determining the current level of functioning or baseline skills in speechreading follow a theoretical framework similar to that for listening skills. In fact the two can be done in tandem by raising and lowering a listening hoop or by adding or removing voice (either by the speaker increasing or decreasing volume or by manipulating the amplification device of the child). The hierarchy is the same for both receptive modes. In addition, a variety of more or less formal tasks can be used to establish baseline. One example is the *Craig Word and*

Sentence Level Lipreading Inventory (Craig, 1964). *Speechreading in Context: A Guide for Practice in Everyday Settings* (Lee, 1997) can be used as a guide for therapy. Any organized, vocabulary-relevant program will be useful in building a child's visual receptive skills, provided visual acuity and processing abilities are within normal limits. It may be necessary to consult with a developmental ophthalmologist/optometrist and an occupational therapist if the child appears to have difficulties receiving or processing visual information for speech (or sign) reception.

Receptive and Expressive Language

A child's expressive and receptive pragmatic, semantic, syntactic, and morphologic knowledge and use in all languages/modes being used must be ascertained and then appropriate goals set. As with other areas to be assessed, a variety of formal tests can be used with adaptations. In addition, informal speech and language sample analysis can be helpful in determining the child's receptive and expressive language abilities. Tests such as the Preschool Language Scale 3 (Zimmerman, Steiner, & Pond, 1992) and the Clinical Evaluation of Language Fundamentals—Preschool (Wiig, Secord, & Semel, 1992) are helpful and can be adapted to sign if necessary. For the very young child this task may be relatively easy because of the more limited language functioning typical of younger children. For older children or children with more sophisticated linguistic systems, perhaps in sign language, the task may be more complex. As mentioned previously, it is essential for the clinician not to assume that language competency is the same for all the languages/modes the child may use. Some children may develop greater linguistic abilities in a foreign spoken language used in the home or through sign language than in spoken English. The goal of assessment should thus be to facilitate the demonstration of as much language knowledge and use as possible in a variety of formal and informal settings. Standardized tests may be required by the school system and will typically quickly provide information that can then be compared to information from the child's peers. Informal, ongoing assessment, however, is often more useful in establishing goals for therapy and for monitoring progress.

Speech/Voice

Spoken language may be an avenue for expressive communication for a child with a hearing loss. It is often difficult to accurately determine the long-range prognosis for speech production skills and voice quality in the early language learner. As a result it is important to consistently assess progress and provide therapeutic intervention designed to maximize the child's skills in a developmentally and practically applicable manner. Among the areas of expressive communication that may need to be assessed and subsequently addressed in therapy are development of age- and gender-appropriate voice quality, accurate lip movements, accurate articulation of sounds in words and sentences, coordination of voice and breathing for adequate speech sound production, or development of adequate breath support for the production of connected speech.

To establish appropriate therapy goals, assessment tools must be utilized to help the clinician determine baseline skills. A number of tools can and have been used successfully to ascertain this information. Ling's Phonetic and Phonologic Level Inventories (Ling, 2002) are probably among the most often used assessment tools designed for use with children with hearing loss. They are particularly useful in establishing therapy goals and monitoring progress. Other options include standardized articulation tests or informal sound inventories derived from speech samples and stimulability exercises. The NTID Speech and Voice Evaluation (Subtelney, Orlando, & Whitehead, 1981) can also guide the clinician in determining voice and breathing goals. The NTID is generally administered using the Rainbow Passage. Depending on the reading ability and age of the child, a more age-appropriate reading passage would be used. The Fundamental Speech Skills Test (FSST) (Levitt, Youdelman, & Head, 1990) allows the clinician to look comprehensively at production skills (breath and articulation), suprasegmentals (i.e., syllabification and stress), and pitch. Any of these tools or informal measures can yield similar information about a deaf or hard of hearing child's speech, although it is important to cover all the areas mentioned previously in the Scope.

Sign Language Production

Sign language ability is more difficult to assess because of the limited set of formal measures and norms that exist. As stated previously it is important to recognize the importance of assessing all languages that might be part of the child's communication milieu. If sign language is a part of a deaf or hard of hearing child's communication world, a qualified professional may be needed to carry out the assessment. Often accurate assessment of sign language will require the collaborative efforts of the SLP, a professional proficient and fluent in sign language, and an occupational therapist who is knowledgeable of motor and visual perceptual issues.

Early Literacy

Early literacy development may be best assessed by observation and collaboration with the classroom teacher and reading specialist. In addition, strategies for promoting literacy skills can be a collaborative effort. It may become evident from observation of the child that an occupational therapist may also have an important role in looking at preliteracy and early literacy skills of the child with hearing loss. Phonologic awareness skills may need to be assessed to see how they may support the acquisition of literacy skills. The Phonological Awareness Test (Robertson & Salter, 1997) can be used to do this assessment.

Associated with literacy development is the ability to reflect on language. This aspect of development, known as metalanguage, is closely associated with many skills needed to attain literacy. Among the metalinguistic areas that one might expect in children at this stage of language development are the ability to ascertain word boundaries, the ability to separate words into syllables, and the ability to play with the sounds of the language.

INTERVENTION

Intervention for children at the early language stage of development can successfully and efficiently be accomplished with an integrated approach. All of the skill areas can be addressed during thematic activities. Therapy activities can maximize strengths while facilitating areas in need of improvement, thus creating a dynamic in which the child experiences success while striving to develop more challenging skills. This balance will help in maintaining the motivation level and cooperation of the child during therapy over time, which is particularly important when skills are slow in developing.

Additionally, therapy for children with hearing loss often has a diagnostic focus as well as serving to remediate errors and foster skill development. Therapy can provide a means of obtaining diagnostic information that is not easily achieved through formal testing. Even modified formal tests are limited in the information they help the clinician derive. For this reason, a diagnostic perspective and conscientious data collection are critical and beneficial aspects of intervention. Information collected on a regular basis will serve the clinician in therapy and IEP planning as well as in establishing appropriate treatment goals.

CASE STUDIES

The following provides suggested approaches for assessment and intervention for each of the five children who were described in the previous chapter.

Arlis

Arlis is a 7-year-old second grader in a mainstream program. There are other children with hearing loss in the school; however, he is the only child using a cochlear implant. His body-worn speech processor was recently replaced with a unit worn behind the ear. Arlis is much more comfortable; however, the batteries do not last as long as they did in the body-worn processor.

It has been noted that Arlis has difficulty understanding spoken language in group discussions and that he struggles to understand his classmates when they respond to questions asked by the teacher. Arlis tends to avoid participating in class even though his speech is relatively intelligible. The teacher and parents have both noted that Arlis has been having a difficult time learning to read and refuses to read aloud in class.

Assessment

It is imperative to begin all assessment/intervention with a listening check to determine whether Arlis's cochlear implant is functioning properly (see appendix B). It is also necessary to check the room acoustics and make any necessary/possible modifications or recommendations. Even though Arlis's visual acuity was evaluated at age 4, a current visual assessment should also be completed before initial evaluation. Visual problems may impede reading and speechreading progress.

Auditory/Listening. Arlis's auditory/listening skills were assessed using the Glendonald School for the Deaf Auditory Screening Procedure (GASP) (Erber, 1982). Results indicated that he has progressed to GASP Subtest 2, which requires the ability to discriminate between words varying in syllable number and type. He was also able to identify open-set single words. The Pediatric Speech Intelligibility (PSI) Test (Jerger & Jerger, 1984) was administered to determine Arlis's ability to use context to help him understand/recognize sentences using listening only. Arlis was able to understand 8 of the 10 sentences presented.

Auditory/Visual Skills. On the GASP Subtest 3 to assess his skills, Arlis was able to comprehend open-set sentences with auditory and visual cues combined. In addition, Arlis's listening and speechreading skills were assessed in the classroom through observation using the Evaluation of Classroom Listening Behavior (VanDyke, 1985). Results indicated that Arlis has little difficulty listening and speechreading when the speaker is at a close distance but does experience some difficulty when the distance from the speaker exceeds 6 feet. Arlis appears to comprehend oral instructions in quiet; however, he has difficulty in noise and when he is unable to see the face of the speaker.

His synthetic speechreading skills were assessed using Bench-Koval-Bamford/Standard American English (BKB/SAE) Sentences (Bench, Koval, & Bamford, 1979) under three conditions: auditory and visual cues combined (in quiet and in the presence of background noise) and visual only. While listening and speechreading in quiet, Arlis scored 80%; in the presence of noise, he scored 60%; and with visual cues only, he scored 50%. The results suggest that when speechreading and listening, Arlis is able to understand *most* of the message even when the material is composed of unrelated sentences. When information is presented in noise or without voice, his abilities drop to understanding *some* of the message. His visual only abilities are not as strong as his listening only skills. Clearly, his visual and listening skills together provide him the most access to and comprehension of spoken language.

Speech/Voice. The Goldman-Fristoe Test of Articulation (Sounds in Words Subtest) (Goldman & Fristoe, 2000) was administered to determine what sounds Arlis produced incorrectly at the word level. Arlis continues to distort sibilant sounds in all positions, with some final consonant deletions. Further examination of his ability to imitate these sounds through the Ling Phonetic Level Evaluation (Ling, 2002), however, revealed that he was stimulable for many of the consonant sounds.

Finally, the CID Picture Speech Intelligibility Evaluation (SPINE) (Monson, Moog, & Geers, 1988) was used to estimate Arlis's overall speech intelligibility. He scored 80% to 89%, indicating that his speech is intelligible.

English Language. Expressive and receptive language testing will also be necessary to determine baseline and weaknesses so that IEP goals can be determined. The Clinical Evaluation of Language Fundamentals—3 (Wiig, Secord, &

Semel, 1995) or a similar comprehensive language assessment tool can be used. In addition, standardized vocabulary tests, such as the Peabody Picture Vocabulary Test–3 (PPVT-3) (Dunn & Dunn, 1997), can be useful to examine Arlis's vocabulary knowledge. It is important to be cautious with all tests including receptive vocabulary tests because the child's access to the presented stimuli will obviously affect the test results. For Arlis's it was possible to confidently determine his access to the spoken stimulus items through listening and speechreading. Because Arlis is not a signer, no modifications were necessary for the expressive single word vocabulary test. For a signing child, modifications in administration will be needed. For Arlis, vocabulary was assessed using the PPVT-3 with only minimal modification (target words were sometimes repeated when access to the information was in doubt).

Test results revealed mild expressive and receptive single word vocabulary delays. Language testing identified difficulties with English syntax and morphology. For example, Arlis failed to use the /s/ or /z/ segment to mark possessives. Because it was previously determined that Arlis can accurately imitate the segments required to produce the possessives, it was concluded that he was unaware of how the /s/ and /z/ segments could be used to mark possessives. Ling (2002) suggests that this would constitute a phonologic problem, requiring therapy aimed to help Arlis recognize when to use these segments to indicate possession.

Sign Language.   Arlis is not using sign language in the classroom, but his parents report that they use an English-based sign language system to communicate at home when Arlis is not wearing his cochlear implant. Arlis's receptive and expressive sign skills were assessed by an outside American Sign Language (ASL) specialist. His sign skills are significantly below his spoken language skills. He has difficulty processing longer utterances presented at a conversational rate without voice. In addition, his expressive signing is slow and lacks fluidity. In general, he uses his voice and the signs tend to be secondary and lack clarity and completeness. His palm orientation, location, and movement in sign production do not show errors. However, he sometimes uses the wrong handshape when producing signs in conversation.

Pragmatics.   Arlis's pragmatic skills were informally assessed to establish a baseline for skills discussed in the prelanguage stage (e.g., turn-taking). In addition, any new areas such as presupposition (the ability to take the listener's perspective when relating information) will need to be assessed as they become developmentally appropriate. Deaf and hard of hearing individuals typically need to exhibit the ability to maintain and shift eye contact to have receptive access to spoken language. Thus, eye contact in one-on-one and group situations needs to be evaluated. Informal assessment through observation and role-play revealed that Arlis struggles to maintain eye contact, tracking of the speaker, and turn-taking in group communication interactions. Additionally, multiple speakers or background noise also adversely affected his receptive communication skills. He sometimes negatively acted out in these situations.

Even when a child exhibits a reasonable level of eye contact, this can become difficult for extended periods of time or in group situations where the communicator changes often and quickly. Strategies for providing breaks for the child to rest may be necessary. Also strategies should be employed for facilitating the deaf or hard of hearing child's ability to track the speaker in group communication settings. Eventually it would be important to foster the child's ability to advocate and employ the strategies himself (rather than through intervention by the teacher or SLP) to enable the child to better follow rapidly changing classroom conversations and dialogues. Similarly, turn-taking skills can be equally important, and challenging and strategies will also benefit the child's conversational abilities.

Literacy.   Because Arlis is having difficulty reading, his reading skills should be formally assessed by a reading specialist. The Test of Early Reading Ability-Deaf or Hard of Hearing (TERA-D/HH) (Reid, Hresko, Hammill, & Wiltshire, 1991) can be administered by the SLP as part of the overall evaluation. In addition, it is important, either formally or informally, to determine Arlis's phonologic awareness skills. Phoneme/grapheme knowledge should be assessed, along with the child's word attack, sounding out, and rhyming skills. The Phonological Awareness Test (Robertson & Salter, 1997) may be helpful in determining these skills.

Arlis exhibited significant difficulties with reading and phonologic awareness skills. He had difficulty with phoneme/grapheme (sound/letter) relationships. Also, he had difficulty identifying and producing differentiated vowels. Arlis did not demonstrate knowledge of the difference between long and short vowels or diphthongs. Additionally, he was unable to break up words by sounds or syllables; nor could he identify words that had been broken up into smaller parts by the clinician. These skills are important to word attack and decoding in reading activities.

Intervention Goals

Arlis should continue to develop his listening, speechreading, and spoken language skills. In addition, because Arlis is having difficulty with reading, therapy should include an emphasis on phonologic processing and decoding/word attack skills.

Intervention Strategies

It is efficient and beneficial to address Arlis's communication therapy both analytically and synthetically. The synthetic therapy activities lend themselves to an integrated therapy approach. This approach encourages working simultaneously on a variety of communication skills, both stronger and weaker, through a single activity.

At the same time it is important to practice specific skills in an analytic or more drill-oriented fashion. The balance of these two approaches offers a well-rounded approach to enhancing Arlis's communication abilities.

As an example, an integrated therapy plan would begin with the therapist working with the classroom teacher to determine upcoming vocabulary to be introduced in the classroom. The identified vocabulary is then taught to Arlis in an individual therapy session. New vocabulary is taught and then presented with and without voice in a variety of game-like activities (for example, a lotto game) aimed to improving his visual and auditory comprehension of the new vocabulary. Arlis can practice producing the vocabulary words in both isolation and in sentences. At the sentence level, the therapist can challenge Arlis to create novel sentences with the target vocabulary (synthetic activity). This activity can include listening, speechreading, literacy, language, and speech. The key to integrated therapy activities is to look for ways to incorporate a range of skill areas into an activity that has been planned for the session.

Another integrated activity might focus on phrases from the classroom and school routine. These would be practiced to ensure that in noisy situations Arlis is still able to understand the teacher's directions. A *constellation* activity can be used for this as well as for other communication situations. To produce a constellation, the clinician would write on the board a phrase describing a communication situation (such as going to the library). Branching from the center of the description the clinician and child would brainstorm words, phrases, and sentences that the child might encounter receptively in that situation (for example, "Do you have a library card?" or "You owe a fine?"). Arlis and the SLP would then create a second set of branches for that same situation that include the child's responses or initiated utterances. Once these constellations have been created the clinician and child can practice to increasing levels of complexity. An easier task might be to have Arlis speechread the sentences from a limited set and respond with an appropriate utterance. More complex would be for him to role play the situation with the clinician or perhaps an unfamiliar speaker or actually have the opportunity to experience the interaction (field trip interactions). Again, many facets of communication can be practiced within this activity.

A more analytical task would focus on articulation. Arlis would be asked to produce the segments he is having difficulty with, at first in simple consonant (C)-vowel (V) and VC syllables. Listening tasks can be included to support the generalization of the skills at a more synthetic level. For example, using the WASP program (Koch, 1998), Arlis, now at Level III, which uses words representing most English consonants in both the initial and medial positions, would practice listening to and identifying/comprehending words presented auditorily only. To do this the clinician would present the words using a listening hoop and Arlis would identify the card containing the word from a set of cards. He would then be asked to say the word (perception-production practice).

Cathy

At 7, Cathy is in a mainstream classroom without an interpreter. Her speechreading skills are developing well. With audition and appropriate assistive technology she is able to function in the classroom setting although with some difficulty. Cathy's spoken language is characterized by sound distortions and omissions. The speech-language clinician has rated her intelligibility as fair even with familiar listeners when the context is unknown. Her intelligibility increases when the context is known. Her reading and writing skills are delayed. She does not know any sign language.

Assessment

A range of receptive and expressive areas were examined. These included listening, visual reception, language skills, and literacy.

Audition/Listening.   Cathy is completely dependent on her assistive technology (hearing aids and frequency-modulated [FM] system). Without working technology, Cathy is unable to function in the classroom; she cannot access any instructional information when her assistive devices are not working. For this reason, it is essential that these devices be well maintained and checked regularly. Cathy will be made a part of this process and participate to a developmentally appropriate extent. She will be taught to clean and maintain her hearing aids, change the batteries, and report any malfunctions immediately. Her listening skills are at the comprehension level, but continued training in more difficult listening situations can be helpful. It is essential to conduct an environment and classroom assessment to make sure the listening and visual environments are optimal for Cathy's learning. In addition, all educators and professionals working with Cathy should be trained to use the technology in the classroom and the therapy room.

It is imperative to ensure Cathy's access to information as much as possible but also to recognize that a child like Cathy will experience gaps in access to classroom instruction and thus in knowledge and use of those missed concepts. Children learn a great deal of information incidentally by hearing it. Whether a child actively learns it through interaction or passively experiences the language through overhearing adults and peers there is a positive impact on the child's language and knowledge acquisition. When children learn new things in school, learning is accomplished more effectively when the child has at least some previous, passive experience with the knowledge, vocabulary, or language form. This is most often not the case for children with Cathy's level of hearing loss.

The Test of Auditory Comprehension (Trammel, 1979) will reveal more precise listening abilities and levels. In addition, the Assessment of Children's Language Comprehension (ACLC) (Foster, Gidan, & Stark, 1973) can be a useful tool for determining how many critical variables Cathy can comprehend. The ACLC looks at 50 vocabulary words. If Cathy begins to have difficulty with any of these closed-set target words, the test is stopped and further levels are not assessed. If she does well with the 50 target words, these will serve as a test vocabulary for evaluating more complex language skills involving phrases and sentences with two, three, or four critical variables.

Language.   The prelanguage skills Cathy worked on, eye contact, facial expression, and intentions, are part of Cathy's communication system at this point in time. Cathy has consistent eye contact skills, understands and uses a variety of facial expressions to express and comprehend affect, and expresses intentions verbally.

Cathy's vocabulary was evaluated using the Expressive One-Word Vocabulary Test—Revised (EOWPVT) (Brownell, 2000) and the PPVT-3 (Dunn and

Dunn, 1997). It should be noted that during the PPVT-3 modifications had to be made to ensure that Cathy had access to the stimulus words. This was accomplished by repeating certain words and having Cathy repeat the word before making a choice. The repetitions were reported in the write-up of the results in the report. The results of this testing indicated significant delays in expressive and receptive vocabulary development.

In addition, the Clinical Evaluation of Language Fundamentals—3 (Wiig et al., 1995) was administered to assess Cathy's receptive and expressive skills in several areas of language. Results indicated delays in both expressive and receptive abilities. Certain syntactic forms were difficult for Cathy. These syntactical structures included less frequently used and more complex forms of English syntax. Additionally, she experienced difficulty understanding some referents. Semantic deficiencies were also observed on this test. The Listening to Paragraphs subtest (not part of the core battery) was also an area of significant difficulty, despite her use of her FM system to optimize access to auditory information.

Pragmatics was also assessed informally. Other than the difficulty with referencing mentioned previously and her lack of facility with taking the listener's perspective, Cathy's pragmatic skills were well developed. Although taking the listener's perspective is an advanced pragmatic skill, Cathy should have developed some skills for providing sufficient background to conversational partners. She is not yet doing this consistently.

Auditory/Visual Skills.   Cathy's parents had followed the early recommendation to have Cathy's eyes checked and discovered she demonstrates normal (20/20) visual acuity. Cathy's speechreading skills were assessed using standardized speechreading assessments for children as outlined for Arlis earlier as well as through informal measures. The informal measures included assessment based on the activities outlined in *Speechreading in Context: A Guide to Practice in Everyday Settings* (Lee, 1997). The results indicated that her speechreading skills are developing well. She is generally able to understand most of the message when the context is known. When the context is unknown or the speaker is unfamiliar her ability to understand through speechreading diminishes. Residual hearing as well as visual lipreading skills and her emerging facility with spoken language all contribute to Cathy's success in comprehending spoken English.

Speech/Voice.   Cathy's articulation and voice were assessed using standardized articulation tests, a conversational speech sample, and the NTID Speech and Voice Evaluation (Subtelney et al., 1981) using a below grade level reading passage. Determining what aspects of articulation, voice, resonance, and pronunciation negatively affect intelligibility is essential to increasing intelligibility. Cathy's speech errors include vowel neutralization, omission and distortion of sibilant sounds, cluster reduction, a weak /r/, and hypernasal resonance.

Visual-Gestural Skills.   Cathy does not know or use any sign language; this area is not applicable at this age.

Literacy. Cathy is having difficulty with both decoding and reading comprehension. These difficulties were reported by the classroom teacher and confirmed by formal reading testing done by the reading specialist and with use of the Phonological Awareness Test (Robertson & Salter, 1997) performed by the speech-language clinician.

Intervention Goals

Among the intervention goals established for Cathy were the following:

1. Re-evaluate the efficacy of the educational placement and services provided. When one is providing services to children with hearing loss, it is important to do this regularly. If it is determined that the child's needs are not being met and that the child is not able to realize her full academic potential, then changes in service provision or placement need to be made immediately. A team of educational specialists along with the child and the parents should work to determine the most appropriate and least restrictive educational environment.

2. Integrating Cathy's language learning into speechreading and listening training is an important feature in providing efficient communication therapy services. This can be accomplished by continuing to follow and expand on the model presented in *Speechreading in Context: A Guide to Practice in Everyday Settings* (Lee, 1997).

3. Vocabulary can become more sophisticated and should come from the classroom and Cathy's own interests. Language forms can become more complex and the chunks of information longer to challenge Cathy. It is also important to explicitly train that which is acquired naturally by other children. The gaps that are manifested in Cathy's language reflect the lack of incidental learning and reinforcement that occurs for children with normal hearing. As a result, vocabulary, morphosyntactic rules, and conventions must be taught explicitly. An example of integrating this explicit teaching is the use of the morpheme *s*. Cathy has difficulty hearing the sound and subsequently distorts or omits it when speaking. As a result certain language forms are produced incorrectly (i.e., plurals, possessives, and third person singular). To address *s*, the clinician can practice saying the sound in words while at the same time addressing pronunciation /s/ versus /z/. Cathy needs to be taught that when the word ends in a voiced sound the sound added is a /z/ and when the final sound is voiceless the sound added is an /s/ and if the final sound is /s/ or /z/ a syllabic /iz/ is added. Linguistically she is being reinforced to mark the plural morpheme and to become aware that other linguistic structures feature the final /s/ sound.

4. When appropriate for training purposes, the clinician may drop her voice or add background noise to ensure that the more visual speechreading skills, and not listening alone, are also being developed. Similarly, tasks can be presented through a listening hoop (which obscures the mouth

but allows sound to pass through the acoustically transparent fabric) to focus on listening development.

Intervention Strategy

Again, it is suggested that an integrated approach to therapy be employed. The clinician can have Cathy use vocabulary words and syntax from the classroom that represent her interests in school. For example, in social studies, an activity might center around a role-play for some historical event, such as the Mayflower arriving at Plymouth Rock. The role-play would involve the use of vocabulary words that have been previously introduced, as well as specific syntactical forms (e.g., plurals). Speechreading and listening can be done by the clinician while first facing Cathy and then turning away during the role-play. Articulation goals that have been previously introduced may also be used in the role-play.

Bridget

Bridget is 7 years old and in the second grade in her local public school. The public school has provided her classroom with an FM system and subsequent training for the teacher. Bridget puts on the FM system independently each day upon arrival. She is beginning to read and enjoys books. Her sound repertoire is approaching an age-appropriate level with some marked distortions and omissions. The high-frequency, low-intensity consonants, such as /s/ and /z/, are distorted in the initial and medial positions and often deleted in the final position. Her language skills continue to be delayed. She has difficulty with phonics and activities such as rhyming. Her voice quality has been characterized as having a cul-de-sac resonance.

Assessment

A range of areas were assessed, including pragmatics, listening, speechreading, speech and voice, and language.

Pragmatics.   At this time Bridget's pragmatic skills appear to be age appropriate.

Audition/Listening.   Bridget is listening at the comprehension level when her amplification systems are worn and working. The ACLC (Foster et al., 1973) or the Test of Auditory Comprehension of Language (Carrow-Woolfolk, 1999) can be used to ascertain more precise levels of comprehension of language. However, informal assessment of Bridget's ability to follow multistep directions and answer a variety of age-appropriate questions presented auditorily only provides similar information concerning Bridget's listening skills.

Auditory/Visual Skills.   Bridget's speechreading skills are developing well, and a variety of formal and informal measures are used to track her skills and maintain an appropriate level of challenge in therapy. Bridget, at this time, demonstrates the ability to augment her listening skills in noisier situations by speechreading. However, larger groups and less structured situations present a greater communicative challenge for her.

Speech/Voice.   Bridget's SLP is using the FSST (Levitt et al., 1990) and informal measures to monitor her speech development. Noted were a small number of misarticulations of high-frequency sounds in the form of omissions and distortions. It is likely that these errors were related to her limited auditory access to these sounds, and the limited tactile, visual, and kinesthetic cues available to facilitate correct production. In addition, the cul-de-sac voice quality of Bridget's speech has been noted as an area that might be addressed in therapy.

Language.   The Clinical Evaluation of Language Fundamentals—3 (Wiig et al., 1995) or the Test of Language Development Primary 3 (Hammill & Newcomer, 1997) can be used with modifications and attention to her access to the stimuli in the test environment to determine receptive and expressive language levels and any deficient areas. It was noted that Bridget's language has shown significant improvement since her last evaluation although she does exhibit some delays in spoken vocabulary. Further Bridget shows difficulties understanding, and producing longer, syntactically more complex utterances.

Visual-Gestural Skills.   Bridget does not use sign language at this time.

Literacy.   According to observation and teacher report, Bridget's literacy skills are developing. It should be noted that the reading specialist does provide supportive services at this time. In addition, the SLP, reading specialist, and classroom teacher are emphasizing and reinforcing phonics and rhyming skills with Bridget.

Intervention Goals

Among the intervention goals that would be appropriate for Bridget are

1. Following multistep directions and answering more complex questions presented through audition alone
2. Speechreading thematic words and phrases in one-on-one and group situations
3. More accurate production of high-frequency segments in all word positions at the phrase and sentence levels
4. Building vocabulary and language skills for social and academic situations
5. Building decoding and comprehension skills for age-appropriate texts

Intervention Strategies

An integrated approach to therapy is recommended. New vocabulary and concepts from the classroom curriculum can be pretaught to Bridget in therapy. This introduction of material from the classroom increases the redundancy of exposure and improves subsequent acquisition of age-appropriate vocabulary and concepts. In addition, the opportunity to practice listening to, speechreading, and producing these new words is beneficial. Furthermore, more complex and sophisticated syntactic forms and age-appropriate morphemes can be taught and practiced in a more explicit manner.

Speech drills may also be effective in fostering the best production possible of the sounds that are currently omitted or distorted. Omissions of sounds may be based on lack of perception and reflect the linguistic function of those sounds in English. The previously mentioned explicit teaching can overcome these gaps in perception and subsequent linguistic knowledge. One strategy for improving voice quality that has been characterized as cul-de-sac is to encourage a more forward focused production of sounds. For example, the child is encouraged to use an exaggerated articulatory style to encourage a resonance at a more anterior point in the vocal tract. The exaggerated postures can be phased out as the resonance improves.

Language skills, both receptive and expressive, can be addressed in integrated therapy activities as well as in more focused activities. Tasks that focus on increasing Bridget's ability to access and comprehend longer and more complex utterances which contain increasing critical variables in listening activities will consequently improve her receptive language knowledge. Providing opportunities for her to practice these skills expressively will improve her expressive language competence.

As mentioned above, rhyming and phonics skills are being addressed based on a collaborative plan among the SLP, reading specialist, and classroom teacher. Earobics (1998), other computer programs, and text-based activities will assist in building rhyming and phonics skills that will be important in literacy development.

Renee

Renee is 7 years old and is enrolled in the public school in her community. She has completed first grade and is now enrolled in a multi-age, first/second grade classroom. The motivation behind this placement was to allow her an opportunity to review first grade academic skills while being afforded some exposure to second grade curriculum. Her parents struggled with the idea of retention and repetition of first grade and compromised on the multi-age first/second grade. A sign language interpreter is provided in the classroom. Since her enrollment in the public school the SLP has helped Renee adjust to the hearing aids; she now wears them consistently.

Assessment

It is important to evaluate a range of communication skills. The assessment areas and approaches used are summarized below.

Audition/Listening. Renee appears to receive some environmental input as well as access to some lower-frequency, higher-intensity speech sounds from the aids. However, she does not comprehend spoken language auditorily.

Auditory/Visual Skills. Speechreading training is done with auditory information included, although as stated previously Renee realizes a limited auditory benefit. Her speechreading skills have been developing slowly because her language skills were significantly delayed when she began school at age 5. Therapy has focused on increasing language concepts in sign and then connecting them to English through print and speechreading. Progress has been slow, and Renee can only discriminate maximally contrastive items in closed sets of two or three. She was not able to correctly identify any items on standardized tests, such as the Craig Lipreading Inventory (Craig, 1964).

Speech/Voice.   Although Renee has had consistent speech training, she has poor breath support, coordination of respiration, and articulation. She can approximate syllable structure and produces a few functional words (mama, thank you, and come), which have neutralized vowels and some consonant distortion. She seldom uses the few words she has obtained outside the therapy room. Renee has consistently struggled with production of speech and is very inattentive during speech sessions. The FSST (Levitt et al., 1990) can be used to determine the extent of Renee's difficulties with speech production and to plan appropriate and realistic intervention goals.

Language.   Receptive and expressive language skills in either English or ASL were and continue to be significantly delayed. Renee lacks all but the very basic vocabulary related to her daily activities. Although progress is being made, her late introduction to accessible language (sign) and the mainstream teaching paradigm—learning through an interpreter—have resulted in continued deficits. Renee is just beginning to connect signs in a conversational way. Her utterances are characterized by seemingly unconnected signs and extraneous gestures. Some vocalizations accompany her utterances but bear no perceivable connection to the English cognates of the sign used.

Visual-Gestural Skills.   Renee has been increasing her sign vocabulary since she began services in the school. Initially, she was slow to connect signs with intentions, concepts, or objects. This connection has improved as evidenced by her increasing expressive and receptive sign vocabularies. She has some difficulty with sign production and a referral has been made to the occupational therapist to look at visual perceptual skills, motor skills, and visual motor integration as it applies to sign language acquisition. Her signing is improving, with the help of a sign language instructor twice a week. It is essential to evaluate Renee's use of the interpreter and the efficacy of the current educational paradigm. It may be necessary to increase the services provided by the SLP and the sign language instructor.

Pragmatics.   Renee's pragmatic skills are not age or communication mode appropriate. She still lacks sufficient attention and eye contact. Her turn-taking skills continue to improve in one to one and group interactions. The school staff and her classmates have also received education on cueing Renee as to changes in the speaker in group situations. She is not yet able to understand the notion of taking the listener's perspective based on her limited language skills. It is still difficult for even the most familiar communicators to ascertain the topics of some of Renee's spontaneous utterances.

Literacy.   Renee is interested in books but is not yet reading because of her limited language skills. She is developing some sight vocabulary but is not yet able to read. She is beginning to generate increasingly comprehensible strings of signs for wordless story books. In addition, she is learning to write her first and last name and all of her letters, upper and lower case.

Intervention Goals and Strategies

A strongly integrated therapy approach with sign as the core is recommended. However, additional sessions to drill and address more analytic abilities in sign, speech, and speechreading will also be beneficial to Renee. The inclusion of text to increase reading and writing skills as well as the connection between sign, the spoken word, and print will be essential to Renee's future academic and linguistic progress. In addition, activities that increase eye contact and turn-taking are important to ensure that she is learning as much as possible during academic times when she is dependent on reception of sign, particularly following an interpreter.

Renee's receptive and expressive sign language abilities must be focused on as well. It is imperative that she begin to understand and produce utterances of increasing length and complexity. This needs to occur in natural and interactive environments. The more natural the experience and subsequent language exposure the more meaningful it will be to Renee. Her placement in the multi-age classroom with an emphasis on stations and learning through hands-on experiences will hopefully facilitate greater language acquisition. In addition, opportunities for Renee to use language to interact with her environment are important. In addition, Renee needs opportunities to interact with other signing people. This includes deaf adults who can be language models and peers who can motivate her conversational skills. Hearing children are not asked to learn language from only one or even a limited set of people. Hearing children interact, either directly or indirectly, with hundreds of language models and partners. At this time Renee is limited to *one* who is fluent in the language she needs to acquire to be successful.

Dion

Dion is 7 years old and in the second grade in his local public school. The public school has provided his classroom with an FM system and training for the teachers in how to use it. However, Dion rarely uses the FM system and his classroom teachers do not encourage its use. He is beginning to read and enjoys books. He interacts well with others in the school but primarily through his sign language interpreter. Some of his classmates are learning to sign, and some interaction occurs without the interpreter. Dion attempts to communicate by speaking, but he is only minimally understood by his peers. He has shown slow, but consistent, improvement in his speech during the past 3 years.

Assessment and Outcomes

A number of areas have been assessed. Each area is described below.

Audition/Listening.   Informal assessment of Dion's auditory discrimination ability reveals that he can attain some success in closed-set discrimination tasks if the alternatives differ significantly and the options are limited to two or three items. He discriminates sounds as the same or different. He can differentiate between speech and nonspeech sounds and words that differ in syllable length. He inconsistently recognizes his own name through audition alone. Dion is very dependent on his hearing aids for access to sounds. Even with his amplification, he appears to have limited ability to identify or understand speech through listening alone.

Auditory/Visual Skills.   Dion's ability to receive speech through speechreading and audition is variable and ranges from awareness to comprehension. His speechreading with listening is improving, however, and he is able to speechread phrases in closed sets comprised of increasing the number and complexity of items. He is also able to accurately speechread routine and highly contextual information, with accuracy increasing when audition is used to supplement speechreading. For example, he can line up, wash his hands, and go to various classroom stations when presented with up to three commands through speech.

Speech/Voice.   His sound repertoire is increasing with significant sound distortions, substitutions, and omissions being observed. His spoken language skills continue to be delayed. He speaks in short phrases at most, and the intelligibility of these utterances is variable. Speech was assessed using the FSST (Levitt et al., 1990). Spoken language skills, particularly voice and articulation, are still quite delayed. Again, lack of access to sounds negatively impact speech production. Voice quality is characterized by an abnormally high pitch for his age and hypernasality.

Language.   As is the case with many deaf and hard of hearing children, development of language skills must consider not only spoken language but also proficiency in reading and writing and sign language. Each of these areas must thus be evaluated. In the following paragraphs the findings for Dion in each of these language forms and modalities are examined.

To evaluate Dion's spoken language abilities, a combination of formal and informal testing was needed. Among the formal tests used were the Grammatical Analysis of Elicited Language, Sentence Level (Moog & Geers, 1979) and the Rhode Island Test of Language Structure (Engen & Engen, 1983). In addition, analysis of a spontaneous speech sample was used employing the procedures suggested by Retherford (2000).

The results of this assessment show significant delays in Dion's receptive and expressive abilities in spoken English. Among the specific problems noted were: limited used of turn-taking, lack of evidence of repair strategies, use of a limited number of grammatical structures, with most restricted to simple subject-verb-object structures, and difficulties with the use of appropriate articles.

Dion's sign language abilities are developing well as observed by the SLP and as reported by the sign language evaluator called in for consultation. His sign production skills and reception are reportedly on target for his age. He evidences language knowledge and use of sign, which surpasses that which is demonstrated in spoken English. He is able to communicate much longer and more sophisticated ideas and concepts in sign language than was evident in his spoken English productions. In addition, he utilizes the interpreter well expressively and receptively as seen in his ability to appropriately engage in classroom conversations and interactions. It should be noted that during longer classroom activities he sometimes fatigues and his attention diminishes.

Pragmatics.   Dion's pragmatic skills are age-appropriate at this time within the framework of interactions facilitated by an interpreter. One noted exception to this is some frustration Dion exhibits regarding the inability to directly communicate with others. When the interpreter is not present or having a conversation with school staff he sometimes acts out his frustration through negative behaviors.

Reading, Writing, and Literacy.   Dion is developing age-appropriate literacy skills. His parents report reading to him every night. He is also beginning to write stories that show good narrative development for his age although some grammatical errors are evident, based on overapplication of sign grammar to writing.

Intervention Goals and Strategies

As a result of Dion's language proficiency in sign language it is important to utilize this knowledge in teaching English language skills. This may require work on certain aspects of language through writing, with the focus being "translation" of ASL to written English. An integrated approach to facilitating development of other skills is still valuable, however, and listening, speechreading, and speaking skills can be integrated and developed in support of each other.

An anticipated aspect of therapy will be the process of helping Dion to differentiate between ASL and English. Toward this goal, activities designed to teach Dion the pattern of English grammar and how it differs from sign can be beneficial. For example, the use of journals with Dion can allow him the opportunity to put down his ideas in written English and then see them reflected back by the teacher, the SLP, and the reading specialist in well-constructed English. This modeling will help him to see how sign language concepts are transformed into written or spoken English. In addition, therapy activities that focus on sentence creation in English can also be beneficial by providing direction about how to generate grammatically correct sentences.

Because Dion's spoken English is quite limited, addressing the difficulties that Dion experiences in spoken English should focus on realistic goals. A determination needs to be made regarding how close Dion's spoken language attempts can get to the target. It may not be realistic to expect flawless production particularly at the connected speech level. Rather, increasing intelligibility should become the goal.

Similarly, his prognosis for listening development is limited, particularly in light of limited hearing aid use. Realistic and appropriate goals concerning development of auditory skills must be made with the family and school staff. This may include goals aimed to increase hearing aid use or the acceptance of the current patterns and adjustments of expectations. Speechreading skills can continue to be developed regardless of speech or listening skills. It is also important to motivate and reinforce Dion despite slow progress. This needs to be done in an honest and straightforward manner.

Finally, some focus on issues such as expanding the grammatical structures used and the use of correct articles would be reasonable goals for improving his expressive language skills, both written and spoken. These can be addressed both through the journal activities mentioned earlier, or through spoken narrative on topics that are related to classroom activities.

Summary

This chapter has discussed areas important for assessment and intervention at the early language area, as discussed in the Scope. The relationship to the previous and following areas of the Scope were addressed as well as assessment and intervention tools appropriate for children at this age and stage of development. Areas discussed were listening skills, speechreading skills, receptive and expressive language, speech/voice, sign language production, and early literacy. The case studies presented in the previous chapter were continued as those children moved into the early language area.

References

Bench, J., Koval, A., & Bamford, J. (1970). The BKB (Bamford-Koval-Bench) sentence lists for partially-hearing children. *British Journal of Audiology, 13*, 108–112.

Biedenstein, J., Davidson, L., & Moog, J. (1995). *Speech perception international curriculum and evaluation.* St. Louis, MO: Central Institute for the Deaf.

Brownell, R. (2000). *Expressive One-Word Picture Vocabulary Test.* Novato, CA: Academic Therapy Publications.

Carrow-Woolfolk, E. (1999). *Test of Auditory Comprehension of Language.* Circle Pines, MN: American Guidance Service.

Craig, W. (1964). *The Craig Lipreading Inventory.* Englewood, CO: Resource Point.

Davis, H., & Silverman, S. R. (1970). Central Institute for the Deaf (CID): Everyday sentences (CHABA). In *Hearing and Deafness,* appendix. New York: Holt, Rinehart, and Winston.

Dunn, L., & Dunn, L. (1997). *Peabody Picture Vocabulary Test—3.* Circle Pines, MN: American Guidance Services.

Earobics. (1998). [Computer software]. Cambridge, MA: Cognitive Concepts.

Engen, E., & Engen, T. (1983). *Rhode Island Test of Language Structure.* Austin, TX: Pro-Ed.

Erber, N. P. (1982). *Auditory training.* Washington, DC: Alexander Graham Bell Association for the Deaf.

Foster, R, Giddan, J., & Stark, J. (1973). *ACLC: Assessment of children's language comprehension.* Palo Alto, CA: Consulting Psychologists Press.

Goldman, R., & Fristoe, M. (2000). *Goldman-Fristoe Test of Articulation* (2nd ed.) (GFTA-2). Circle Pines, MN: American Guidance Service.

Hammill, D., & Newcomer, P. (1997). *Test of Language Development Primary 3.* Circle Pines, MN: American Guidance Service.

Jerger, S., & Jerger, J. (1984). Pediatric Speech Intelligibility Test. St. Louis, MO: Auditec.

Kaplan, H., Bally, S. J., & Garretson, C. (1987). *Speechreading: A way to improve understanding* (2nd ed.). Washington, DC: Gallaudet University Press.

Koch, M. (1999) *Word associations for syllable perception.* Timonium, MD: York Press.

Lee, J. (1997). *Speechreading in context: A guide for practice in everyday settings.* Washington, DC: Pre-College National Mission Programs.

Levitt, H., Youdelman, K., & Head, J. 1990. *Fundamental Speech Skills Test.* Englewood, CO: Resource Point.

Ling, D. (2002). *Speech and the hearing-impaired child: Theory and practice* (2nd ed.). Washington, DC: Alexander Graham Bell Association for the Deaf.

McNally, P. L., Rose, S., & Quigley, S. P. (1994). *Language learning practices with deaf children* (2nd ed.). Austin, TX: Pro-Ed.

Monson, R., Moog, J., & Geers, A. (1988). *CID picture SPINE (SPeech INtelligibity Evaluation).* St. Louis, MO: Central Institute for the Deaf.

Moog, J., & Geers, A. (1979). *Grammatical analysis of elicited language.* St. Louis, MO: Central Institute for the Deaf.

Northern, J., & Downs, M. (2002). *Hearing in children.* Philadelphia: Lippincott Williams & Wilkins.

Reid, D., Hresko, W., Hammill, D., & Wiltshire, S. (1991). *Test of early reading ability—deaf or hard of hearing (TERA-D/HH).* Austin, TX: Pro-Ed.

Retherford, K. S. (2000). *Guide to Analysis of Language Transcripts* (3rd ed.). Eau Claire, WI: Thinking Publications.

Robertson, C., & Salter, W. (1997). *Phonological Awareness Test.* East Moline, IL: Linguisystems.

Subtelney, J., Orlando, N., & Whitehead, R. (1981). *Speech and voice characteristics of the deaf.* Washington, DC: Alexander Graham Bell Association for the Deaf.

Trammel, J. (1979). Test of auditory comprehension. North Hollywood, CA: Foreworks.

VanDyke, J. (1985). Evaluation of classroom listening behaviors. *Rocky Mountain Journal of Communication Disorders, 1,* 8–13.

Wiig, E., Secord, W., & Semel, E. (1992). *Clinical evaluation of language fundamentals—Preschool.* New York: The Psychological Corporation, Harcourt Brace Jovanovich.

Zimmerman, I. L., Steiner, V., & Pond, R. E. (1992). *Pre-school Language Scale—3.* New York: The Psychological Corporation, Harcourt Brace Jovanovich.

CHAPTER 6

Later Language: Assessment and Intervention

Introduction

The later language-learning child who is deaf or hard of hearing is similar to hearing children in that she must continue to expand upon the communication skills already acquired as she progresses through school. Unlike their hearing peers, however, many deaf or hard of hearing children must also focus on speech reception and production skills that require active intervention. This chapter examines those aspects of communication that are often the focus of therapy during the later periods of language development, both those that are typical of hearing children at this age and those that are somewhat unique to the deaf or hard of hearing child. Among the language areas described in this chapter that are typically acquired during this period are lexical development; understanding and use of figurative language; ability to use and understand more complex sentences; verbal reasoning skills; use of discourse in academic and social settings for purposes of narration, conversation, persuasion, and negotiation; and metalinguistic competence. In addition to acquired linguistic features that are normally acquired later, this chapter will also describe assessment and associated intervention strategies to address specific difficulties often encountered in deaf or hard of hearing children of this age. The final portions of the chapter describe strategies for further assessment and intervention with the five case studies that were introduced in previous chapters.

OVERVIEW

During the first few years of life, children undergo a remarkable period of language development. In fact, it appears that most children develop a fairly comprehensive language system by the time they reach 6 or 7 years of age. Although many elements of language have been developed by this age, the child's system is far from complete. The child's knowledge and use of language continue to develop at later ages, with aspects of language development occurring throughout the life span (Nippold, 1998; Vihman, 2004).

As noted in Chapter 1, a number of areas of language refinement occur during the elementary school years. Among the language areas that school-aged children continue to expand upon are the following:

- Lexicon, including
  - Word knowledge
  - Word finding
  - Word definition (a metalinguistic skill)
- Understanding and use of figurative language
- Ability to use and understand more complex sentences
- Verbal reasoning skills
- Use of discourse in social settings for purposes of
  - Narration
  - Conversation
  - Persuasion
  - Negotiation
- Metalinguistic competence

The child who is deaf or hard of hearing also experiences considerable language growth during the later phases of language development. Obviously, to be developing language comparably to his hearing peers, the deaf child must acquire all of the areas mentioned above. In addition, there are other communication areas that many deaf and hard of children in this age range typically experience difficulties with and thus become a focus for therapy. These include the following:

- Speech skill refinement
- Pronunciation skills (the ability to accurately produce words not previously encountered)
- Reading/writing skills
- Sign language development
- Speech reading and auditory development

The next portion of this chapter describes the types of skills that are typically learned and developed during the later language period, along with basic strategies for assessment of these abilities. Areas more specifically of concern for many deaf and hard of hearing children are also discussed.

It should be noted that the suggestions of tests and procedures for evaluating various aspects of a deaf child's communicative functioning are intended to be representative rather than comprehensive. There are other sources of information examining the strengths and weaknesses of tests with deaf and hard of hearing children and of procedures for selecting and using instruments with deaf children (Bradley-Johnson & Evan, 1991; Thompson, Biro, Vethivelu, Pious, & Hatfield, 1987).

LATER LANGUAGE DEVELOPMENT IN HEARING CHILDREN

It is suggested that the reader be familiar with some of the overarching issues associated with assessment that were discussed in Chapter 3. The following sections describe a number of areas commonly addressed in school-aged children who are expanding and refining their language skills.

Lexical Development

Multiple aspects of vocabulary development should be considered in children of this age. These include the development and expansion of vocabulary, the ability to retrieve vocabulary for writing and face-to-face communication, and the ability to define.

Development and Expansion of Vocabulary

The expansion and refinement of vocabulary continues throughout life. As children progress through school, they learn about and begin to use more abstract words, as well as those that are less common or related to specific areas of interest. Unlike earlier stages, however, there is considerable variability in vocabulary development of children at this stage. This is primarily the result of the prominent role of reading in the development of vocabulary (Nippold, 1998). Thus, interests of the child, curricular focus, and other factors may result in children having very different vocabulary content, despite very similar progress toward linguistic competence.

This variability poses significant difficulties in assessing vocabulary at these stages. There are, of course, tools such as the Peabody Picture Vocabulary Test–3 (Dunn & Dunn, 1997) that provide a reasonable snapshot of vocabulary development; it may be necessary to explore vocabulary in a less formal way through interaction with the classroom teacher so that the clinician has a clearer understanding of the functional vocabulary strengths and weaknesses exhibited by the child.

Vocabulary development is not all or nothing, but rather occurs gradually, with the meaning of words changing over time (Nippold, 1998). It is common for children at this stage to exhibit partial lexical knowledge. For example, Miller and Gildea (1987) reported that students between 10 and 12 years of age have only partial lexical knowledge of words such as meticulous, relegate, and redress. This is evident in sentences such as:

I was *meticulous* about falling off the cliff.

I *relegated* my pen pal's letter to her house.

The *redress* for getting well when you are sick is to stay in bed. (Miller & Gildea, p. 99)

McNeil (1970) points out that "words can be in a child's vocabulary but have different semantic properties from the same words in the vocabulary of an older child or an adult" (p. 116). It thus becomes important to understand the lexical knowledge that the child may have beyond simple vocabulary counts.

Retrieval of Vocabulary for Writing and Communication

In addition to lexical knowledge, school-aged children are also challenged to ". . . call up words with speed, clarity and accuracy" (p. 31) (Nippold, 1998). This ability to store ever-increasing vocabulary and to retrieve this vocabulary during spontaneous interchanges develops throughout the school years and has been shown to be positively correlated to reading (Kail and Hall, 1994).

Nippold (1998) suggests that evidence of difficulties with word finding problems in children, adolescents, and adults are often signaled by behaviors such as hesitations, pauses, circumlocutions, or empty fillers (e.g., *things* or *stuff*) during spoken communication. Observation of such patterns in deaf or hard of hearing children during the later language period may thus be indicative of word finding difficulties and may warrant measures aimed at developing strategies to improve word finding abilities.

Word Definition

One final aspect of vocabulary development that becomes increasingly important as children progress through school is the ability to define words. This metalinguistic skill requires that an individual be able to state explicitly what is known implicitly about a word (Watson, 1985). Nippold (1998) cites numerous studies that suggest "The ability to provide a formal definition of a word is closely related to cognitive and linguistic development, literacy and academic achievement in school-age children" (p. 43).

It is recognized that the ability to define words changes and improves during the school years (and into adulthood) and that these changes involve both the number of words that can be defined and the quality of these definitions. In a study by Al-Issa (1969), hearing children's approaches to word definition were described at 1-year intervals between 5 and 10 years of age. Al-Issa found that at the youngest ages, children tend to define words in terms of function (A cat: "It meows") or attribute ("has a tail") while at later ages, children tend to define words in terms of categories ("an animal"). Additional refinements in defining are inclusion of multiple characteristics, more abstract definitions, and expansion of categories used to define words (Nippold, 1998).

A number of both norm-referenced and informal instruments to examine the ability of a child to define are available. Norm-referenced instruments are typically subtests of language or intelligence tests. Nippold (1998) provides a useful analysis of the features reported in these subtests and offers insight into how such tests might be used for clinical assessment of school-aged definition skills. These tests and their characteristics are summarized in Table 6-1.

Table 6-1 Characteristics of Standardized Tests That Examine Word Definitions

1. *Test of Language Development—Second Edition: Primary* (TOLD-2: Primary) (Newcomer & Hammill, 1988)

Subtest	Oral Vocabulary
Age range	4 through 8 years
Words	30 total: 22 nouns, 1 verb, 6 adjectives, and 1 preposition varying in difficulty; concrete and abstract
Scoring	1 point per correct response
Criteria	Must provide a brief explanation, synonym, or two major characteristics (e.g., function, appearance, etc.) of the work, as listed in the manual
Normative data	Mean raw scores from children (N = 2436) ages 4, 5, 6, 7, and 8 years, respectively, were 4, 9, 11, 16, and 18

2. *The Word Test—R: Elementary* (Huisingh et al., 1990)

Subtest	Definitions
Age range	7 through 11 years
Words	15 total: 8 nouns, 2 verbs, and 5 adjectives varying in difficulty; concrete and abstract
Scoring	1 point per correct response
Criteria	Must provide a brief explanation, synonym, or major characteristic (function, appearance, etc.) of the word, as listed in the manual
Normative data	Mean raw scores from children (N = 1359) at each 6-month interval between 7:0 and 11:11. For example, mean = 9.01 at 7:0 through 7:5; mean = 12.21 at 9.0 through 9/5; mean = 13.57 at 11.0 through 11:5

3. *The Word Test: Adolescents* (Zachman et al., 1989)

Subtest	Definitions
Age range	12 through 17 years
Words	15 total: 8 nouns, 3 verbs, and 4 adjectives varying in difficulty; concrete and abstract
Scoring	1 point per correct response
Criteria	Must provide a brief explanation, synonym, or major characteristic (function, appearance, etc.) of the word, as listed in the manual
Normative data	Mean raw score from adolescents (N = 1042), ages 12:0 through 13:11, 14:0 through 15:11, and 16.0 through 17.11, respectively, were 6.62, 8.19, and 10.32

4. *Test of Word Knowledge* (TOWK) (Wiig & Secord, 1992)

Subtest	Word Definitions
Age range	5 through 17 years
Words	32 nouns varying in difficulty; concrete
Scoring	1 or 2 points per correct response
Criteria	1 point from mentioning two correct features of the word; 2 points for mentioning three features, as listed in the manual

(continues)

Table 6-1   (continued)

Normative data | Mean raw scores for children and adolescents ($N = 1570$) at each year from ages 5 through 13; data from ages 14 through 17 years were combined. For example mean raw scores at ages 5, 9, 13, and 14 through 17 years, respectively, were 8.6, 28.5, 41.3, and 47.0

5. *Comprehensive Receptive an Expressive Vocabulary Test* (CREVT) (Wallace & Hammill, 1994)

Subtest	Expressive Vocabulary
Age range	5 through 17 years
Words	25 total: 24 nouns and 1 verb varying in difficulty; concrete
Scoring	1 point per correct response
Criteria	Must provide a synonym of brief description (e.g., characteristic, etc.) of the word, as listed in the record form; some items require two features
Normative data	Mean raw scores for children and adolescents ($N = 1852$) ages 5 through 17 years. For example, mean raw scores at ages 5, 9, 13, and 17 years, respectively, were 4, 12, 18, and 19 (Form A)

6. *Stanford-Binet Intelligence Scale* (Thorndike et al., 1986)

Subtest	Oral Vocabulary
Age range	7 through 16 years
Words	32 total: 14 nouns, 8 verbs, and 10 adjectives varying in difficulty; concrete and abstract
Scoring	1 point per correct response
Criteria	Must provide synonym or brief description (e.g., function, characteristic, etc.) of the word, as listed in the manual
Normative data	Mean raw scores for children and adolescents ($N = 2929$) ages 7 through 16. For example, mean raw scores at ages 7, 10, 13, and 16 years, respectively, were 20, 24, 28, and 32. (These means were obtained by combination scores on Oral Vocabulary with scores on a 14-item Picture Vocabulary task.)

7. *Wechsler Intelligence Scale for Children–Third Edition* (WISC–III) (Wechsler, 1991)

Subtest	Vocabulary
Age range	6 through 16 years
Words	30 total: 15 nouns, 7 verbs, and 8 adjectives varying in difficulty; concrete and abstract
Scoring	1 or 2 points per correct response
Criteria	Must provide a synonym or brief description of the word, as listed in the manual; to get full credit, response must be specific
Normative data	Mean raw scores for children and adolescents ($N = 2200$) ages 6 through 16 years. For example, mean raw scores at ages 6, 9, 12, 14, and 16 years, respectively, were 11.5, 22.5, 33.5, 40, and 44

Although such instruments can be useful in examining the ability of school-aged deaf children to define, Nippold points out some limitations of formal tests in general:

> To discern qualitative aspects of development (of the ability to define), however, it is important to analyze both the semantic content and the syntactic form of the students' responses. The difficulty of words and the classes to which they belong must also be considered when interpreting the results of standardized tests, because performance may be affected by limitations in word knowledge in addition to or instead of limitations in metalinguistic aspects of development. (Nippold, 1998, pp. 55–56)

One informal instrument identified by Nippold (1998) was developed by Feifel and Lorge (1950). This instrument examines a variety of elements of a definition and permits the clinician to develop a fairly extensive description of the ways that a particular child might define terms (Table 6-2).

Table 6.2   Qualitative Classification System Used by Feifel and Lorge

Synonym Category

Synonym unmodified	*Orange* = a fruit
Synonym modified by use	*Straw* = hay that cattle eat
Synonym modified by description	*Gown* = long dress
Synonym modified by use and description	*Eyelash* = hair over the eye that protects you
Synonym qualified as to degree	*Tap* = touch lightly

Explanation Category

Explanation	*Priceless* = it's worth a lot of money
	Skill = being able to do something well

Use, Description, and Use and Description Category

Use	*Orange* = you eat it
Description	*Straw* = it's yellow
Use and description	*Orange* = you eat it and it's round

Demonstration, Repetition, Illustration, and Inferior Explanation Category

Demonstration	*Tap* = (performs action)
	Eyelash = (points to eyelash)
Repetition	*Puddle* = a puddle of water
Illustration	*Priceless* = a gem
Inferior explanation	*Scorch* = hot

Error Category

Incorrect demonstration	*Eyelash* = (points to eyebrow)
Misinterpretation	*Regard* = protects something
Wrong definition	*Orange* = a vegetable
Clang association	*Roar* = raw
	Skill = skillet
Repetition without explanation	*Puddle* = a puddle
Omits	When the word is left out

Source: Reprinted with permission from Feifel, H., & Lorge, I. (1950). Qualitative differences in the vocabulary responses of children. *Journal of Educational Psychology, 41,* 4–5.

Understanding and Use of Figurative Language

For an individual who is deaf or hard of hearing to fully function in the world, he needs to understand those aspects of language that are not literal. Examples of figurative expressions that a child must learn about include metaphors and similes ("The boy grew like a weed"), proverbs ("a stitch in time saves nine"), idioms ("Get off my back"), slang ("a five-finger discount") and ambiguity and humor ("Mine is a long and sad tale!" said the mouse, turning to Alice and sighing. "It is a long tail, certainly," said Alice, looking with wonder at the mouse's tail, "but why do you call it sad?") Lewis Carroll, *Alice's Adventures in Wonderland* (from Fromkin and Rodman, 1988, p. 210).

Hearing children develop the ability to understand and appropriately interpret figurative language through verbal experience with the world. For a child who is deaf or hard of hearing, however, such experiences may be considerably limited, thus leading to limited ability to handle linguistic information that is nonliteral. It thus becomes increasingly important to examine a school-aged child's ability to handle such utterances.

There are a few formal instruments for examining figurative language. Two examples are the Gochnour Idiom Screening Test (Gochnour, 1977) and the Test of Language Competence-Understanding Metaphoric Expressions subtest (Wiig and Secord, 1985). These tests use a multiple choice format to explore a student's ability to identify the correct meaning of an idiom or metaphoric expression, but may not provide a criterion-referenced basis for establishing therapy goals.

Informal evaluation is often the preferred assessment approach in ascertaining a child's knowledge of idioms and proverbs. Given in appendix D are a number of common English idioms, classified according to both their familiarity and transparency (a measure of how literal/nonliteral nature of a particular phrase) (Nippold, 1998). Appendix E provides a description of the transparency of a number of proverbs (Nippold, 1998). This type of information can be a useful means of both informally evaluating and teaching these nonliteral aspects of language. Additional sources of idioms include texts such as the *Dictionary of American Idioms* (Makkai, Boatner, Gates, Boatner & Gates, 2004) or daily comic strips that tend to contain extensive use of idioms.

Ability to Use and Understand More Complex Sentences

As mentioned in chapter 1, the period of later language development marks significant growth in the ability of children to both understand and produce (through reading and writing) more advance sentence structures. These advanced structures affect both the syntax within a sentence and the ability of the child to join sentences (cohesion) in grammatically and syntactically appropriate ways. These aspects of sentential development are described below.

Within-Sentence Development

The school-aged child will begin to exhibit considerable growth in his use of sentences between the ages of 6 and 11. Growth will be evident in the length of the sentences used and the complexity of these sentences. The length of utterances corresponds with grammatical complexity for very young children (e.g. Brown,

Table 6-3	Mean Length of Utterance reported by Leadholm and Miller (1992) for 167 Children Varying in Age during Two Different Speaking Tasks	
Age	*Conversation*	*Narration*
5.40	5.71	6.06
7.10	5.92	7.32
9.10	6.50	8.80
11.10	7.62	9.83
13.00	6.99	9.32

(Adapted from Leadholm, B. J., & Miller, J. F. (1992). *Language sample analysis: The Wisconsin guide.* Madison, WI: Wisconsin Department of Public Instruction.)

1973). Although sentence length continues to grow as children become older, the correspondence between utterance length and the mean length of utterance (MLU) is not as clearly related to complexity. Nonetheless, there is clear evidence that as a child becomes older, the length of utterances (in terms of the mean number of morphemes per complete sentence) increases with age, both in narration and conversation. Table 6-3 provides some normative data for mean length of utterances by different ages of later language learners (Leadholm and Miller, 1992).

In looking at the types of sentence forms that exist in English, one sees that there are a range of sentence forms that the language learner must master. Nippold (1998) suggested that there are three basic forms of English sentences: (1) simple sentences containing a single independent clause (e.g., "Lunch is at noon today."), (2) complex sentences containing one independent clause and at least one dependent clause that are joined by a conjunction such as *so* or *but* (e.g., "It is not snowing today so we will have the test."), and (3) compound sentences containing an independent clause and at least one dependent clause joined by a subordinating conjunction such as *if* or *when* (e.g., "The test will be held on Tuesday if it does not snow.").

It should be noted that the definitions and characterizations of sentence types are not uniform and that the theoretical framework used to characterize sentences, as well as the framework used in a particular setting, may result in sentence types that differ somewhat from those given above. Most important is that a consistent framework be used by the school, classroom teacher, and speech-language pathologist (SLP). A good rule of thumb is to check with the classroom teacher or reading/writing specialist to ensure that a consistent framework is being used to characterize the sentence types that children have or are developing.

Regardless of the schema used to characterize sentence types, these more advanced syntactic structures are increasingly important academically to the child as he is expected to both read text that contains compound and complex syntactic structures, and to incorporate compound and complex sentences into his writing. As noted in Chapter 1, deaf children often exhibit considerable

Table 6-4 Structures and Tasks for the Test of Syntactic Ability	
Structure evaluated	*Type of Task Used to Evaluate*
Negation	Recognition and comprehension
Conjunction	
Conjunction	Recognition and comprehension
Disjunction and alternation	Recognition and comprehension
Determiners	Recognition
Question formation	
W/i- questions	Recognition
Answer environments	Comprehension
Yes/no questions	Recognition
Verb Processes	
Verb sequence in conjoined structures	Recognition
Main verbs, linking verbs, and auxiliaries	Recognition
Passive voice	Recognition and comprehension
Pronominalization	
Possessive adjectives	Recognition
Reflexives	Recognition
Possessive pronouns	Recognition
Forward and backward pronominalization	Recognition
Relativization	
Relative pronouns and adverbs	Recognition
Comprehension	Comprehension
Embedding	Recognition
Complementation	
That-complements	Recognition and comprehension
Infinitives and gerunds	Recognition
Nominalization	Recognition and comprehension

(Adapted from Quigley, S., Steinkamp, M., Power, D., & Jones, B. (1978) *Test of Syntactic Abilities*. Beaverton, OR: Dormac.)

difficulty with these structures (Paul & Quigley, 1994). Linguistic structures that often pose problems for deaf and hard of hearing individuals are those tested by the Test of Syntactic Ability (Quigley, Steinkamp, Power, & Jones, 1978) and summarized in Table 6-4. Because of the prominent role that these advanced syntactic forms play as a child progresses through school, it is important to examine the deaf or hard of hearing child's ability to both generate and understand these types of sentences.

There are a number of useful instruments for evaluating the syntactic abilities of school-aged children that can be used with those who are deaf or hard of hearing (see Figure 3-2). Depending on the child's reliance on audition and speech, one can select instruments that are administered via voice (such as the Test of Auditory Comprehension of Language) or by text (such as the Test of Syntactic Ability).

The Test of Syntactic Ability (TSA) (Quigley, et al., 1978) was developed for and is normed on deaf children. The TSA is composed of 20 diagnostic subtests, as well as two forms of a screening test. The test is designed for deaf children between 10 and 18 years of age and involves analysis of written sentences. The content of the diagnostic subtests, given in Table 6-4, shows that there are a number of subtests that are measuring specifically later emerging, complex, and compound sentences.

Intersentence Complexity

As the child develops, he will also begin to demonstrate growth in his ability to connect sentences through the use of cohesive devices. A number of cohesion types are typically found (Figure 6-1). In many cases, it is best to evaluate the child's use of cohesive devices through analysis of written or spoken discourse. The importance of discourse and narrative skills for the school-aged child will be discussed later in this chapter.

Metalinguistic Competence

Recently, my $7\frac{1}{2}$-year-old daughter (JM) asked me about various meanings the word *fish* might have. After offering one or two meanings (an aquatic animal and the act of catching one of these animals), she in turn noted an additional meaning that I had not thought of (what she did to retrieve her shoe when it fell in the water). This ability to consider aspects of language in much the way one might consider other aspects of the child's experience (such as friends, or pets, or mommy) is referred to as metalanguage. Metalanguage formally means the ability to reflect on language. Much of what a child learns about language after 6 years of age or so is related to development of metalinguistic awareness (Wallach & Miller, 1988). Wallach and Miller elaborate on metalanguage:

> Being metalinguistic involves an appreciation for both the arbitrariness and the custom (of language). Being metalinguistic also involves knowing that language is a code for representation. (pp. 32–33)

As the child grows as a language learner, he develops a multitude of metalinguistic skills and abilities, for example, the ability to understand multiple meanings, figurative language, and verbal humor or an appreciation for the listener's perspective and the use of language appropriate for the listener. A summary of later-occurring metalinguistic skills is given in Figure 6-2. It is evident that much of what has been discussed above and in the following sections relates to the development of metalinguistic abilities.

Use of Discourse

As children mature, the expectation that they will be able to communicate effectively in face-to-face communication is greater. Such communication, or

References: a semantic relation whereby the information needed for interpretation is found elsewhere in the text; cohesion lies in the continuity of reference, as the same thing is referred to more than once in the discourse (Mentis & Prutting, 1987, 9, 96):
  Pronominal: Mary is a teacher. *She* teaches second grade.
  Demonstrative: Tom is in his office. You can find him *there.*
  Comparative: John wore his *red* shirt. His *other* shirts were dirty.

Lexical: a relation that is achieved through vocabulary selection; cohesion is formed by using the same word, a synonym, a superordinate word, and a general item or an associated word.
  Same word: We went to the *store.* The *store* was crowded.
  Synonym: The *boy* is climbing the tree. The *child* could fall.
  Superordinate: Take some *apples.* The *fruit* is delicious.
  General word: I gave *Tom* the keys. The *jerk* lost them.
  Associated word: I told her to call the *doctor.* She was *ill.*

Conjunction: a logical relation expressed between clauses that signals how what is to follow is related to what has gone before; cohesion is achieved by using various connectors that show relationships between statements
  Addictive: I fell. *And* everything fell on top of me.
  Adversative: All the numbers looked perfect. *Yet* the conclusion seemed inaccurate.
  Causal: I did not know. *Otherwise,* I would have stayed away.
  Temporal: She opened the door. *Then* she put her coat away.
  Continuative: You needn't apologize. *After all,* you did not know what happened.
Conjunctive ties include many transitional words that express a variety of relations (as pointed out by Gregg, 1986):
  Consequence: therefore, then, thus, hence, accordingly
  Likeness: likewise, similarly
  Contrast: but, however, nevertheless, on the other hand, yet (adversative)
  Amplification: and, again, in addition, further, moreover, also, too (additive)
  Example: for instance, for example
  Sequence: first, second, finally (temporal)
  Restatement: that is, in other words, to put it differently

Substitution: the cohesive bond is established is established by the use of one word for another but repetition of the first term is avoided. The substituted word has the same structural function as that for which it substitutes (Mentis & Prutting, 1987, p. 96).
  Nominal: I need a bigger *cup.* I'll get *one.*
  Clausal: They've lost them? I regret *so.*

Ellipsis: cohesion is established by the deletion of a phrase or a word or a clause.
  Verbal: Who's eating? I am (eating).
  Nominal: What kind of ice cream do you want? Chocolate (ice cream).
  Clausal: Has she done her exercises? She has (done her exercises).

Figure 6-1.   Cohesive Devices
Source: From Nippold, M. (1998). *Later language development: The school age and adolescent years* (p. 123). Austin, TX: Pro Ed.)

discourse, is an important vehicle for obtaining and sharing information throughout life. In addition, similar skills are needed to ensure that the written discourse of a child is organized and presented effectively. Given in the following are three specific forms of discourse that emerge during later language development: conversation, narration and instructional discourse (Wallach

Ages 6 to 10
- Begins to take listener perspective and use language form to match
- Understands verbal humor involving linguistic ambiguity, e.g., riddles
- Able to resolve ambiguity: lexical first, as in homophones; deep structures next, as in ambiguous phrases ("Will you join me in a bowl of soup?"); phonological or morphemic next (Q: "What do you have if you put three ducks in a box?" A: "A box of quackers.")
- Able to understand that words can have two meanings, one literal and the other nonconventional or idiomatic, e.g., adjectives used to describe personality characteristics such as *hard, sweet, bitter*
- Able to resequence language elements, as in pig Latin
- Able to segment syllables into phonemes
- Finds it difficult to appreciate figurative forms other than idioms

Ages 10+
- Able to extend language meaning into hypothetical realms, e.g., to understand figurative language such as metaphors, similes, parodies, analogies, etc.
- Able to manipulate various speech styles to fit a variety of contexts and listeners

Figure 6-2.   Stages of Metalinguistic Ability in Later Language Learners
Source: Adapted from Wallach, & Miller, 1988).

&Miller, 1988). It should be noted that other taxonomies exist for characterizing discourse types (e.g., see Nippold, 1998); the taxonomy described here provides a fairly comprehensive view of essential discourse skills that develop during the later periods of language development.

Conversation

Although children engage in conversation at a relatively young age (Bryant, 2001), the nature of children's and adults' conversations is quite different. Thus, the language learner must learn a great deal about engaging in adult-like conversation. As the child's conversation proficiency develops, he begins to exhibit skills such as the ability to: consider the perspective of the communicative partner (presupposition), stay on topic, introduce new topics, have protracted dialogues with others, maintain a topic with fewer tangential comments, and increase the number of factually based comments (Nippold, 1998).

There is evidence that children show continued development throughout childhood in skills required to initiate and maintain conversations (Brinton & Fujiki, 1984). In particular, they found that whereas children between 5 and 9 years showed only limited increases in the variety of skills used to maintain conversation, these children did increase the variety of novel utterances used to maintain conversations. Children between 9 years of age and young adulthood, on the other hand, showed increases in the number of relevant skills, including the ability to introduce and reintroduce topics, the ability to maintain topics, and the variety of sentences used to maintain topics.

Other research supports the notion that children gradually develop conversational cohesion skills, particularly during adolescence and young adulthood. For example, (Dorval & Eckerman, 1984) noted that as children matured, their conversations were accompanied by increases in exchanges where one speaker asked a question and another answered, where utterances added new information to the topic, and through increased use of utterances that expressed awareness of the thoughts, feelings, and attitudes of others. These researchers also found a reduction in the introduction of unrelated or marginally related utterances, or abrupt topic switches. There thus appear to be a change, both in early and later portions of language development, that result in improved conversation ability. These improvements in conversational discourse are thus a primary aspect of language learned during later language development.

Narration

Narration is the ability to relate an event or story. Narrative skills are of obvious importance in school settings where children are often asked to describe historical events, convey personal stories, or relate a series of propositions in conjunction with many academic areas. Narration generally involves more sophisticated skills than does conversation. It is thus reasonable that the emergence of narration in school-aged children requires development of more sophisticated syntax and greater organization than does conversation. These additional skills include things such as appropriate sequencing of events, the use of devices that appropriately relate separate elements of the narrative, and the use of linking grammatical forms (e.g., use of conjunctions to achieve cohesion). Additionally, the later language learner will show gradual improvements in production of longer stories with more details and improved organization, creation of a greater number of complete episodes with subplotting, achievement of greater cohesion across episodes, and creation of stories with greater focus on characters' emotions, thoughts, and plans (Nippold, 1998).

A related aspect of narration is the understanding and use of story grammar. Story grammar refers to the rules and constituents of a simple story. One schema for characterizing story grammar is given in Table 6-5.

Instructional Discourse

Although one might assume that discourse in the classroom is a variation of everyday conversation, research suggests that instructional discourse differs considerably from other forms of verbal interaction. Sillman (1984) describes four attributes of instructional discourse that distinguish it from other forms of discourse: (1) general purpose, (2) nature of comprehension activities, (3) coding complexity, and (4) participant assumptions.

The general purpose of instructional discourse is to convey technical or academic information. This contrasts markedly from conversational discourse, which focuses on the regulation of social interactions and interpersonal functions.

Table 6-5	Story Grammar Constituents for Simple Stories
Setting	Introduction of main characters: sets stage, gives context
Initiating event (beginning)	Action that changes the story environment evokes formation of the goal
Internal response	Goal: serves as motivation for later action
Attempt	Overt actions that are directed toward goal attainment
Consequence	Result of an attempt: attainment or nonattainment of goal
Reaction or ending	Emotion, cognition, or end, expressing protagonists feelings about goal generalization to some broader consequence

Source: Adapted from Stein, N., & Glenn, D. (1970). An analysis of story comprehension in elementary school children. In R.O. Freedle (Ed.), *Advances in discourse processing* (Vol. 2). Norwood, NJ: Ablex.

The second attribute, the nature of the comprehension activity, involves the information provided through the interaction, and how that information is used. In the classroom, language typically carries the entire context that is needed for understanding, whereas conversational discourse relies on a variety of contextual cues to aid in understanding. Clearly the less contextualized interactions in the classroom will require greater effort to comprehend. Instructional discourse thus tends to require greater mental effort by the student than does conversation, resulting largely from the reduced context that is typical of instructional discourse.

The third attribute described by Sillman (1984), coding complexity, refers to the complexity of the language that is used in conveying technical information. Language for instruction is typically aimed at developing logical definitions and explanations that are largely disconnected in time and space from the events being described. This language is used to add information that is typically evident from context and the here and now of conversational discourse.

Finally, there is a fairly complex set of assumptions that are made during instructional discourse that rests very heavily on metacognitive and metalinguistic skills. For example, when a teacher asks a child to define a word, inherent in this request is the assumption that the student will grasp the intention of the task—to generate a metalinguistic statement explaining the meaning of a particular word in terms of other work meanings (Wallach & Miller, 1989). Wallach and Miller further suggest that

> . . . much of language arts in the elementary grades requires a child talk about language: words, sounds, letters, sentences, spellings, punctuation. In addition, much of the discourse used to teach language arts assumes that children possess a level of conscious awareness of their own mental processes . . . (and) that children can talk about their problem-solving strategies. (p. 96)

Speech Skill Development and Refinement

Perhaps one of the most remarkable aspects of child development is the ability of children to acquire a fairly complete speech production system by age 4 or 5.

Although children's pronunciation patterns are not yet completely adult-like at age 3, the basic features of the adult phonologic system are present (Menn & Stoel-Gammon, 2001). Despite such progress, the child does have challenges associated with speech development during elementary school (Vihman, 2004). These include things such as the need to develop and expand phonology and to refine articulation. Moreover, the hearing child must also focus on the appropriate use of his production skills in the context of new vocabulary acquired through reading. The ability to regularize pronunciation of English and to use a dictionary to produce unfamiliar words are among those things that constitute a major focus of speech learning amongst hearing children of school age.

LATER LANGUAGE DEVELOPMENT IN THE DEAF OR HARD OF HEARING CHILD

By the time a deaf or hard of hearing child reaches school age, there is usually a clear indication of how effective the child will be in communicating through speech. For some, speech will be used for communication with peers, parents, and teachers. Other deaf children, however, will demonstrate varying degrees of success with spoken communication. It is, of course, necessary to evaluate the specific skills required to effectively communicate. In addition, factors such as auditory capabilities and residual hearing, support of those in the child's environment, the extent of formal and informal speech teaching, and expectations of parents and teachers may play a role in the ultimate level of success that a child has with speech for communication.

Background Information

Although true for children at all ages, examination of a school-aged deaf or hard of hearing child's speech in the context of communication is especially important. Using speech skills for communication reinforces the role of speech as a vehicle for language. Examination of the effectiveness of speech for communication for a school-aged child can also provide useful insight into the prognosis for spoken communication. Because of the potential for a range of communication problems by a deaf or hard of hearing child, selecting communication goals that are reasonable, appropriate, and attainable is extremely important. Failure to consider how the child has developed spoken communication skills thus far can result in considerable effort and frustration if communication goals are selected that are not consistent with current or past progress toward spoken communication.

Establishing appropriate and effective strategies for speech improvement will thus rely on a clear understanding of how the child currently uses speech for communication. If the clinician is unfamiliar with the child, a questionnaire for the teacher or parent might be the most effective way of establishing the child's current functioning. Among the questions that should be posed are the following:

1. What form of communication does the child use with parents (sign, speech, cue, writing, etc.)?
2. What form of communication does the child use with teachers?
3. In what situations will the child most likely be successful communicating through speech?
4. In what situations would you expect the child to have the most difficulty communicating through speech?
5. Has the child demonstrated improvement in speech production during the past year? If so, in what aspects of speech (new segments, more understandable speech, or others)?
6. How intelligible is the child to you?

Speech Skills

As noted in earlier chapters, it is important to have a general notion of the child's overall intelligibility. One approach is to characterize the child's intelligibility on a scale, such as that used at Gallaudet University (Figure 6-3*). Alternatively, it may be useful to examine the number of words in an utterance that are correctly produced. In this approach to assessing intelligibility, a speech sample produced by the child is played to a group of listeners who are asked to write down what they hear. The percentage of total words in the sample that are correctly identified constitutes an intelligibility score. Additional procedures rely on more standardized approaches to gathering speech samples, such as the CID Picture Speech Intelligibility Evaluation (SPINE) (Monsen, 1981; Wold, Evans, Montague, & Dancer, 1994).

It is often the case that school-aged children who are deaf or hard of hearing will present persistent voice and articulation problems that have not been resolved by the time the child enters school. It is important to identify those difficulties in production of both segmental and suprasegmental aspects of speech. In examining the pattern of articulation evidenced by the deaf child, it is important to examine the source of the error. As mentioned in chapter 3, the clinician has to

1. The student is easily understood by the general public. He has no obvious voice and/or articulation errors.
2. The student is easily understood by the general public, but has obvious voice and/or articulation errors. "Good deaf speech."
3. The general public has some difficulty understanding the student initially, but the student can be understood once the listener adjusts to his "deaf speech."
4. The student's speech is very difficult for the general public to understand. He is probably only understood by his family and teachers.
5. The student's speech cannot be understood

Figure 6-3.   Gallaudet Intelligibility Scale

* Note that this scale rates intelligibility differently from the NTID scale in chapter 3 (Figure 3-2, p. 108).

SECTION 1. NONSEGMENTAL AND SUPRASEGMENTAL VOCALIZATION AND VOICE PATTERNS

	Produced spontaneously	Evoked through imitation	Uses with intent to communicate	Uses in familiar words and phrases	Uses appropriately in conversation	Comments and targets
BREATHING						
Adequate breath flow						
VOCALIZATION						
Uses voice						
VOICE PATTERNS						
Duration						
Long (>5 seconds)						
Short						
Varied						
Intensity						
Moderate						
Loud						
Quiet						
Varied						
Whispered						
Pitch						
Moderate						
Low						
High						
Varied						

Figure 6-4. Ling Phonetic Level Evaluation: Nonsegmental and Suprasegmental Vocalizations and Voice Patterns

Source: From Ling, D. (2002). *Speech and the hearing impaired child: Theory and practice* (2nd ed., p. 165). Washington, DC: Alexander Graham Bell Association for the Deaf and Hard of Hearing. Used with permission.)

establish whether an error pattern is the result of an inability to produce a particular pattern (such as a particular vowel or a fricative such as /s/) or rather the result of not knowing the words and utterances in which the pattern should be used. This phonetic (ability to produce motor patterns) versus phonologic (ability to use patterns correctly in words) assessment provides a valuable basis for establishing appropriate goals for improving articulation.

There are tests and procedures available that provide information about phonetic and phonologic level skills. For example, establishing the phonetic level ability to produce a particular pattern can be accomplished through an imitation task in which the child is asked to produce a range of syllables varying systematically in composition and complexity. The Ling Phonetic Level Evaluation (Ling,

SECTION 2. VOWELS AND DIPHTHONGS

	Uses in spontaneous vocalizations	Imitates in repeated syllables	Alternates syllables and words	Uses accurately in familiar phrases	Uses accurately in spontaneous discourse	Comments and targets
Step 1.						
a (pa)						
i (fee)						
u (boo)						
aʊ (how)						
aɪ (eye)						
Step 2.						
ɔ (awe)						
ɔɪ (boy)						
ɛ (red)						
ʊ (look)						
ɪ (fit)						
Step 3.						
æ (cat)						
ʌ (cut)						
ɒ (pot)						
o (toe)						
Step 4.						
ə (again)						
ɝ* (her)						
ɚ** (mother)						

*stressed
**unstressed r-colored central vowels.

Figure 6-5. Ling Phonetic Level Evaluation: Vowels and Diphthongs
Source: From Ling, D. (2002). *Speech and the hearing impaired child: Theory and practice* (2nd ed., p. 166). Washington, DC: Alexander Graham Bell Association for the Deaf and Hard of Hearing. Used with permission.)

2002) offers a systematic approach to exploring such abilities. An example of a portion of this evaluation instrument is shown in Figures 6-4 and 6-5.

Establishing the child's ability to use a particular pattern appropriately in words can best be evaluated through an analysis of spontaneous speech (e.g., see Ling, 2002). Because of the time involved, however, it may not be reasonable for a school clinician to obtain such information immediately. A useful index of such phonologic usage can be obtained through use of standardized three-position articulation tests such the Fisher-Logemann (Fisher & Logemann, 1971) or the Goldman-Fristoe-2 (Goldman & Fristoe, 2000). By comparing performance on the phonetic level evaluation and the three-position test, the clinician can establish areas in need of work and establish the level of skill development needed.

It is also important to examine the suprasegmental error patterns that the child might be exhibiting. Suprasegmentals are those aspects of speech exerting an influence across segments. Suprasegmentals are typically divided into two categories: those that affect prosody and thus communicate meaning (such as intonation patterns and stress) and those that affect speech quality. Among the suprasegmental features affecting speech quality are things such as average fundamental frequency, amplitude, speaking rate, and laryngeal adjustments such as those that result in breathy or strained voice qualities (both often encountered in the speech of deaf children).

There are a limited number of instruments for assessing the suprasegmental aspects of speech. Two useful instruments are the Fundamental Speech Skill Test (FSST) (Levitt, Youdelman, & Head, 1990) and the NTID Voice and Speech Assessment (Subtelny, Orlando, & Whitehead, 1981). Examples of areas assessed by these two instruments are shown in Figures 6-6 and 6-7.

Pronunciation and Vocabulary Development

It was noted earlier that vocabulary development is significant during later language development. Related to vocabulary development in spoken language is the ability to accurately pronounce vocabulary. Indeed the rules of English for pronouncing various words are at times challenging to learn, yet it is often the case that a deaf or hard of hearing child must rely primarily on the written word to expand upon his vocabulary.

There has been increased awareness about the importance of pronunciation knowledge and skills as a vehicle for improving communication (Moseley & Bally, 1996). Among the specific skills needed are knowledge of the rule-based aspects of pronunciation and the exceptions to these rules. It is also important that the deaf or hard of hearing child be able to effectively use the dictionary as an aid to pronunciation. The ability to use the dictionary will affect the child's expansion and refinement of vocabulary; thus, skills related to dictionary use can have a positive effect on both vocabulary development and speech.

One informal instrument for assessing the pronunciation skills of deaf children is the Pronunciation Skills Inventory (PSI) (Bally, 1996). The PSI provides useful information about a child's knowledge of pronunciation rules, strategies the child may have for pronunciation of new vocabulary, and the child's awareness of how to use the dictionary to facilitate accurate pronunciation. The PSI is found in appendix F.

Literacy and Reading and Writing Problems

"Reading and writing are not just very useful practical skills; they are powerful agents in the process of language development" (Perera, 1992, p. 186). The importance of reading, together with the difficulties that many, if not most, deaf children experience with reading (Gentile & Defrancesca, 1969; Trybus & Karchmer, 1977; Allen, 1986; CADS, 1991) suggest that assessment of reading and writing skills of a child who is deaf or hard of hearing is essential. In addition, reading and writing provide an alternative approach to language learning and teaching in addition to conversation. Indeed, Perera (1986) suggested that writing is an ideal way of promoting development of advanced syntactic structures

Sample Profile Form

F S S T™   **Profile Form II**

Birth Date _____
Name _____ M. M.

Age Range: 6 - 9 years
Hearing Level: 96 - 114 dB

Age ___ 8

PRODUCTION SKILLS

Breath Stream Capacity.. <u>47.0%</u>

Elementary Articulation... <u>75.0%</u>

PITCH CONTROL

Average Pitch................. <u>85.4%</u>

SUPRASEGMENTALS

Syllabification............. <u>72.2%</u>

Stress....................... <u>61.1%</u>

Intonation Contours.... <u>41.6%</u>

TOTAL SCORE............. <u>382</u>
(0-600)

Fundamental Speech Skills Profile

Decile	Production Skills		Pitch Control		Suprasegmentals			Total Score	%ile
	Breath Stream	Elem. Artic.	Avg. Pitch M	F	Syllab.	Stress	Intonat. Contours		
10	87.7	87.1	100.0	100.0*	100.0*	88.2	65.1	471	100%
9	74.6	86.1	97.8	100.0*	100.0*	78.9	50.9	447	90% / 80%
8	68.5	79.4	92.1	100.0*	93.2	72.1	32.3	419	70%
7	67.0	74.6	86.4	93.8	89.4	65.6	20.6	398	60%
6	58.4	71.9	77.1	80.3	83.4	58.4	14.0	357	50%
5	50.9	69.3	68.3	74.0	80.6	45.9	9.2	344	40%
4	46.4	65.7	47.7	66.7	73.7	34.5	3.7	313	30%
3	28.0	60.1	33.8	48.0	60.9	20.6	0.0*	285	20%
2	20.5	53.0	15.9	20.9	56.2	10.1	0.0*	256	10%
1	0.0	0.0	0.0	0.0	0.0	0.0	0.0*	0	0%

Evaluator _____
Test Date _____

Figure 6-6.   Sample Profile Form from the Fundamental Speech Skills Test
Source: From Levitt, H., Youdelman, K. & Head, J. (1990). *Fundamental Speech Skills Test.*
Englewood, CO: Resource Point. Used with permission.

Pitch Register: If pitch register is judged to be below optimal, mark rating with a (—).

1. Cannot sustain phonation.
2. Much above or below optimal level.
3. Moderately above or below optimal level.
4. Slightly above or below optimal level.
5. Appropriate for age and sex.

Pitch Control

1. Cannot sustain phonation.
2. Noticeable breaks or fluctuations of large magnitude.
3. Noticeable breaks or fluctuations of small magnitude.
4. Flat with limited speaking range.
5. Appropriate —— satisfactory modulation of pitch.

Loudness: If loudness is judged to be below an appropriate level, mark with a (—).

1. Cannot sustain an audible tone.
2. Much above or below an appropriate level.
3. Moderately above or below an appropriate level.
4. Slightly above or below an appropriate level.
5. Appropriate intensity level.

Loudness Control

1. Cannot sustain audible tone.
2. Noticeable breaks or fluctuations of large magnitude.
3. Noticeable breaks or fluctuations of small magnitude.
4. Flat within limited speaking range.
5. Appropriate —— satisfactory modulation of intensity.

Figure 6-7. Examples of Areas Assessed by the NTID Speech and Voice Evaluation
Source: Adapted from Subtelney, J., Orlando, N., & Whitehead, R. (1981). *Speech and voice characteristic of the deaf.* Washington, DC: Alexander Graham Bell Association for the Deaf and Hard of Hearing. Used with permission.)

"because it allows the language user to deliberate, to review and to correct, without pressure from conversational partners" (p. 518).

The responsibility for addressing literacy issues in deaf and hard of hearing children falls on many professionals, including the SLP (ASHA Ad Hoc Committee on Reading and Writing, 2003). Although language is sometimes viewed as the domain of the classroom teacher in many school systems, the importance of reading and writing for overall communication development of deaf and hard of hearing children of this age argues for the speech-language professional having a significant role in both assessment and intervention related to reading and writing problems. Indeed, the speech and language professional often works with the classroom teacher, reading and writing specialists, and others to both screen and conduct more detailed assessment of reading skills of children.

Among the potentially valuable screening tools for examining the reading and writing skills of deaf and hard of hearing children are the Test of Written Language or TOWL-3 (1996), or the Woodcock Reading Mastery Test (1987). If a reading resource teacher is available, it is highly recommended that a referral be made for a comprehensive assessment of reading and writing skills of school-aged children who are deaf or hard of hearing.

Sign Language Development

One would expect that many, if not all, of the structures and functions evidenced in the spoken English of hearing children would be evident in signed utterances of the deaf or hard of hearing child who is relying primarily on sign language for communication. This is often difficult to assess, however. Most clinicians have limited or no knowledge of and abilities in American Sign Language (ASL). Moreover, few formal instruments are available to assess the signed language skills of children.

It may be helpful to develop a checklist of the types of structures that are expected of children at this age and to work with the classroom interpreter to determine whether the child has any evidence of those structures and forms in ASL. It is evident, however, that for the child whose primary language is ASL, it is necessary to have a sign language expert to assist in evaluating the child's proficiency in that language.

Speechreading and Auditory Development

During the period of later language development, there may still be a need for some aspects of speechreading and auditory development. If significant effort is directed to speech development, then it is appropriate to also focus on parallel aspects of auditory training that address similar aspects of spoken language. For example, if a speech goal is to facilitate the child's production of a broader range of vowels, then it is appropriate to commit some effort to discrimination training that helps the child to both auditorily and visually (via speechreading) distinguish among vowels that will be taught. This will both facilitate the child's receptive skills, and the child's attainment of speech production goals (e.g., Ling, 2002).

An additional skill that is important for effective communication and that is refined during later language learning periods focuses on the use of communication strategies. Communication strategies are the various things that a communicator can do to facilitate, enhance, or repair the communication process (Bally, 1996). The successful use of communication strategies requires that the child have a clear understanding of his own communication strengths and weaknesses, as well as knowledge of various approaches to ensuring that communication is successful. Such strategies include devices such as asking for the communication partner to repeat or rephrase, indicating what is understood or not understood, altering the communication environment to ensure maximum visual or auditory access, or using alternative forms of communication (such as writing) when the situation requires. A communication strategies checklist,

Client Name: _____   Date: _____

Communications Strategies Checklist

Based on observation of a communication interaction, indicate consistent ($\sqrt{}$) inconsistent (+) or absent (—) use of each of the following

DISCOURSE RULES
Client:
_____ readily uses the most appropriate communication mode (for the situation)
_____ attends to various speakers
_____ gets the attention of communication partner
_____ takes turns using appropriate prompts
_____ gives others a turn
_____ follows a topic change
_____ terminates a conversation
_____ utilizes strategies to maintain communication
_____ utilizes strategies to repair communication breakdowns
_____ provides adequate information in response to inquiries
_____ terminates conversations appropriately

EXPRESSIVE REPAIR STRATEGIES
Client:
_____ repeats
_____ partially repeats
_____ confirms/clarifies
_____ rephrases
_____ spells key words
_____ codes key words
_____ writes key word in palm of hand or other available surface
_____ uses universal gestures
_____ writes understandable notes
_____ requests signing/fingerspelling (if appropriate)

RECEPTIVE MAINTENANCE AND REPAIR STRATEGIES
Client:
_____ requeste partial/full repetition ("Say that again please." Or "What did you say about the test on Friday?")
_____ confirms ("Did you say that ____?")
_____ requests rephrasing ("Would you say that again in a different way?")
_____ requests key word ("Could you give me the most important word?")
_____ requests spelling
_____ requests sign/fingerspelling
_____ requests number formatting

ANTICIPATORY OR PLANNING STRATEGIES
INTERPERSONAL
Client:
_____ speaks clearly, using "best" speech during conversation
_____ modifies rate

Figure 6-8. Communications Strategies Checklist
Source: J. Mahshie, modified in 2005.

(continues)

_____ modifies intensity
_____ modifies phrasing
_____ obtains unimpaired view of speaker (speechreading)
_____ requests an interpreter

LINGUISTIC
Client:
_____ anticipates dialogue (or questions)
_____ anticipates sequence of dialogue
_____ anticipates vocabulary
_____ is able to effective role play various situations before they occur
_____ practices speaking and speechreading important vocabulary

ENVIRONMENTAL STRATEGIES
Client:
_____ modifies position relative to the speaker to obtain improved visual field
      for speechreading
_____ recognizes noise sources in environment and take steps to reduce them
_____ reduces environmental distraction
_____ optimizes lighting (by increasing light, altering position to avoid back-
      lighting, etc.)
_____ requests a notetaker
_____ requests appropriate visual aids (handouts, reading list charts, etc.)

APPROACHES TO COMMUNICATION
Behavioral Affect (note overall observed functioning on continuum):

Passive				Assertive				Aggressive	
1	2	3	4	5	6	7	8	9	10

Overall Flexibility (willingness to try/modify strategies with goal of effective communication)

1	2	3	4	5	6	7	8	9	10

ADDITIONAL OBSERVATIONS OR COMMENTS:

_____

_____

_____

_____

_____

_____

_____

_____

_____

Figure 6-8. (continued)

such as that shown in Figure 6-8, provides a useful approach to examining the child's understanding and use of communication strategies during face-to-face communication.

CASE STUDIES

In the following section, the children described in earlier chapters will be discussed. For each child, an overview of assessment procedures and results, together with suggestions for possible goals and outcomes, and intervention strategies, will be given.

Arlis

Arlis is now 11 years old and in the sixth grade. He continues to use his cochlear implant and receives significant benefit. However, he is reluctant to wear his behind the ear hearing aid and tends to only wear it during therapy.

Arlis has continued to develop his auditory skills, as evidenced by his 84% correct score on an open-set word recognition test completed during his last audiologic assessment. He is able to use the voice telephone, but tends to only use it to call his father.

Despite the significant progress that Arlis has shown in his ability to receive and understand speech auditorily, he tends to have difficulty communicating in groups and in noisy situations. As a result he continues to avoid classroom discussions and describes himself to the guidance counselor as "a loner." Arlis's academic performance is below grade level due to the difficulty he continues to have with reading and writing.

Assessment

Arlis's ability to receive speech and to monitor his own productions is obviously tied to the adequate functioning of his cochlear implant. It is thus imperative that his implant be in good working order. Arlis should be taught to test the batteries of his implant and to recharge the implant when needed. In addition, the functioning of the implant should be checked daily using the Ling 6 Sound Test. A functional listening check should be completed each morning and before any assessment and intervention (see appendix B). At this age, Arlis should be actively involved in the troubleshooting and maintenance of his implant. He should be able to report any changes in his hearing sensitivity while using the implant. The clinician and Arlis should use the troubleshooting checklist found in appendix B to problem solve any equipment malfunction.

A related audiologic issue is the ongoing difficulty that Arlis has listening in group settings. It would be appropriate to refer Arlis to an audiologist for consideration of a personal frequency-modulated (FM) system (see chapter 2) that would connect directly to his cochlear implant. This would help improve the signal to noise ratio and perhaps help Arlis to communicate in noisy situations.

Auditory/Visual Skills.   Arlis has continued to show progress in his ability to understand speech through audition and vision. He is able to comprehend open-set sentence level speech through formal activities. Because he continues to have difficulty in less structured activities and in situations where there is competing noise, such as group activities, it is important to establish a baseline of performance in such situations.

One instrument that provides a measure of ability to perceive speech in noise is the Test of Auditory Comprehension (TAC) (1979). The TAC is normed on deaf and hard of hearing children between the ages of 4 and 17 and provides valuable information regarding auditory functioning level. The test assesses a range of auditory skills from awareness of sound to comprehension of speech in the presence of background noise. Earlier subtests assess suprasegmental discrimination, proceeding from gross differentiation between speech and nonspeech stimuli to discrimination among various speech phrases differing in rhythm, stress, and intonation patterns. Subsequent subtests assess discrimination and memory sequencing abilities for messages containing one, two, and four linguistic elements. Later subtests measure comprehension of simple stories by sequencing events and comprehension of complex stories by recalling details. The final subtests assess auditory figure-ground abilities by presenting simple and complex stories in a background of competing speech noise. The TAC could thus provide very useful information about where Arlis begins to experience difficulty in the auditory perception of speech and perhaps provide insight into when therapy might begin to improve his skills in more adverse conditions in less structured settings.

The results of the TAC with Arlis revealed, as suspected, that he has difficulty understanding complex stories, both in quiet and in noise. While he is able to understand simple stories in quiet, his reception is also reduced in noise.

A less formal approach was also employed in which a short story was read to Arlis, and he was asked to respond to a series of questions about the content. This approach was used under a variety of conditions: auditory alone using a listening hoop (an auditory screen to obscure the lips and face), visual alone by asking the child to switch off the aid and implant, and combined auditory and visual input. Arlis exhibited the best reception under the auditory and visual condition (11 of 12 questions answered correctly). He performed less accurately under auditory alone (9 of 12), and did quite poorly under visual alone (4 of 12 correct). The results supplemented the findings of the more formal TAC by providing possible insight into the source of Arlis's receptive difficulty, notably with speechreading. This was reflected in his difficulty understanding speech without the use of his cochlear implant (visual only).

It is also possible to conduct the auditory and auditory/visual portions of this assessment in the presence of background noise. Although this can be done in the therapy room using a tape or CD containing background noise, it would best be done in collaboration with the audiologist to ensure careful consideration of the signal to noise ratio (see p. 54). The goal is to have the background noise at a loudness level comparable to the noise level in the classroom. This would provide information about Arlis's functional listening skills in the classroom.

A functional check of Arlis's communication skills in the classroom was also conducted through observation and consultation with the teacher. Arlis's teacher was asked to complete the Listening Inventory for Education (L.I.F.E.) (Anderson & Smaldino, 1996) to determine the specific listening difficulties Arlis was experiencing in his classes. Arlis was also asked to complete the L.I.F.E. student appraisal of listening difficulty. Analysis of the teacher's responses indicated that Arlis is a successful listener in the classroom; however, he has difficulty following lengthy conversations and that in group settings the children often speak before Arlis has an opportunity to determine who is contributing to the conversation. This results in Arlis's missing significant portions of the interaction. Arlis's responses indicated that he has difficulty listening in noise and often becomes "lost" during classroom discussions.

Speech and Voice.   Arlis's speech and voice characteristics should be evaluated periodically. The FSST (Levitt et al., 1990) can provide useful information about various aspects of speech, including segmental and suprasegmental speech characteristics and speech intelligibility. In addition, the instrument provides norms for children between 6 and 20 years of age. Arlis exhibited breath support, pitch control and suprasegmentals that were in the 90th percentile for children his age with similar degree of hearing. He demonstrated articulation at the 70th percentile, suggesting the need for further articulation assessment. Arlis's articulation was evaluated using the Goldman-Fristoe Test of Articulation-2 (Sounds in Sentences Subtest) (Goldman & Fristoe, 2000). Arlis continues to distort sibilant sounds; however, he is stimulable for correct production.

Pronunciation.   The PSI (Bally, 1996) (see appendix F) was used to assess Arlis's acquisition, understanding, and use of the rules and principles that determine the correct pronunciation of English words, as well as to assess his understanding of the nomenclature. The PSI also was used to assess Arlis's ability to use the dictionary pronunciation key to self-correct pronunciation errors. Arlis demonstrated strengths in the following areas: alphabet, vowel, and consonant identification; vowel and consonant production; phoneme production; and syllabification identification and stress. He had difficulty with the following: production of plurals, past tense, and contractions; grapheme/phoneme differentiation; diagraphs (vowels and consonants); silent letter rules; and dictionary skills.

Language, Reading, and Writing.   Many of the skills that are elements of later language development, such as the use of narrative and understanding of figurative language, are essential elements of a school-aged child's ability to read and write. It is thus important to work closely with the classroom teacher and reading specialist to coordinate both assessment and needed treatment of Arlis's language difficulties.

It was recommended that Arlis receive a comprehensive reading assessment by the reading specialist. Results from that assessment revealed that Arlis continues to have difficulties with decoding and comprehension. In addition, the classroom teacher noted that Arlis's writing is often disconnected and fails to display an orderly structure.

Intervention Goals

Based on the assessment described above, a series of goals were established that were believed attainable during the academic year. Among the goals to be worked on are the following:

- Improved speech reception through speechreading and listening in quiet and in the presence of background noise
- Continued work aimed to reduce articulation errors as well as to improve pronunciation skills (e.g., use of the pronunciation key).
- Language work focusing on areas that will supplement reading and writing, including work to improve narration and expansion of vocabulary through dictionary work (in conjunction with pronunciation drill and practice)

Intervention Strategies

Vocabulary from Arlis's content courses could be used for working on pronunciation, speechreading, and listening. Given a list of new vocabulary words, Arlis will use the dictionary to define and pronounce (using the correct number of sounds, syllables, and stress) the words. Articulation work can also be incorporated into this type of activity by targeting words containing the fricatives that he continues to distort. This is a particularly appropriate level of activity for articulation since he has demonstrated stimulability for these segments.

Arlis will then use the words to write sentences and then read his sentences aloud. The clinician will randomly present the words behind an audio screen. Arlis will identify the word presented. Additionally, the clinician will read aloud a story containing the new vocabulary words in the presence of background noise. Arlis will speechread the clinician and then answer questions about the story.

Cathy

Cathy is fairly typical of oral deaf children that are seen in mainstream settings. At 11, she is showing many speech and language characteristics that are age appropriate. As noted earlier, she has shown significant development in those skills addressed in the prelanguage and early language period. Thus, goals such as establishing eye contact or employing turn-taking are well integrated into Cathy's current communication system. Cathy has also shown significant improvement in many aspects of her spoken communication. She has a fairly complete speech sound system, and although there are persistent errors, her speech is relatively intelligible (a 2 on the Gallaudet Intelligibility scale).

Cathy continues to be a good speechreader, but her difficulties in class suggest that she is having difficulty applying appropriate communication strategies to situations she encounters. Her speech is quite intelligible, although she has some persistent articulation errors that limit her speech intelligibility. Nonetheless, it is clear that her speech intelligibility has improved during the past few years.

Among the persistent misarticulations are distortions of fricatives and the liquid /r/, continued reduction of vowel space, and hypernasal voice quality.

She is experiencing some difficulties in the classroom, however, related to the way that the classroom operates. Because she does not use an interpreter, she must rely on speechreading and listening to get information. When questions are being asked and answered, she often has a hard time following the conversation.

Although her reading comprehension and decoding have improved, problems are still evident in this area. Like many students her age, she is learning about vocabulary and its usage. One area that poses problems to her relates to idioms— her lack of access to the everyday hearing world results in her often having a hard time understanding many nonliteral statements such as "I ran into Aunt Jean yesterday." These skills are seen in both her oral and written production. In addition, her knowledge of narrative structure seems to be emerging, but she still has difficulty organizing her written thoughts into a narrative form that is easily understood, as well as comprehending this type of structure.

Cathy's vocabulary is spotty—she seems to have a good command of vocabulary that one might expect in a child her age, but there are many content-specific words that Cathy has a difficult time understanding and hence using in her written or spoken communication. The teacher has further noted that Cathy exhibits some "unusual" sentence structure in her written communication, although she is doing adequately in assignments requiring writing.

Assessment Strategies

As was the case in assessing younger children, educational placement was re-evaluated and again deemed appropriate for Cathy at this time. She continues to grow academically and appears to benefit from the social interactions in her school. Because of the presenting problems noted above, a series of assessment procedures were employed. These were aimed at assessing her classroom functioning, writing skills, knowledge of idioms, and speech production skills. Assessment of each area is given below.

Classroom Interactions.   One of the first goals was to observe classroom interactions to determine those factors that are controllable in the environment that would improve communication. Using the environmental checklist given in chapter 3, it was noted that many of the activities and interactions that took place in the classroom were less than optimal for a hard of hearing student. The classroom environment was very informal. Students tended to give responses or ask questions, without raising their hands, and this sometimes resulted in a somewhat energetic, but chaotic, interchange within the classroom. This obviously was contrary to Cathy's communication needs. Because Cathy tends to sit in the front of the class, and chairs are organized in rows, she misses many of the interactions that occur.

Written Language.   The TOWL-3 (1996) was used to examine Cathy's ability to organize and present ideas in a narrative form. It was found that she fails to consistently present ideas in a coherent sequence, and her narration often fails to include the key constituents of story grammar (Table 6-5). In addition, her writing was informally evaluated by looking at her use of cohesive devices, those linguistic structures that tie together a narrative structure. She also demonstrated difficulty in the use of referential and lexical cohesion. In therapy, Cathy was given a graphic organizer to help her include the key constituents in stories she generates. A series of picture sequences from the comic pages of the newspaper were used to both determine contexts and situations that Cathy was better able to handle through spoken narrative and also to begin working on improving the structure and form of her narrative productions in both the verbal and written form. This informal approach constituted an ongoing assessment that occurred during the first third of the academic year and that provided a useful basis for both examining what she could do and expanding on her strategies for organizing her narrative structure.

Idioms.   Examination of Cathy's knowledge of idioms was accomplished both formally and informally. The Gochnour Idiom Screening Test (1977) is a formal instrument aimed to examine the areas of knowledge of idioms and other aspects of figurative language that the child possesses. The results of the Gochnour revealed a significant delay in her understanding of figurative language.

In addition to this formal instrument, the clinician used the list of common idioms developed by Nippold (1998) given in appendix D to examine the idioms that Cathy understood, and those that were problematic. This also serves as an excellent source of therapy materials that could subsequently provide a direction for working on idioms.

Speech Skills.   Cathy's speech difficulties were examined initially using a standard articulation test (the Goldman-Fristoe Test of Articulation–2 (Goldman & Fristoe, 2000) and the Ling Phonetic Level Evaluation (Ling, 2002). It was evident from these results that Cathy had continuing difficulty with the production of fricatives. They tended to be fully occluded resulting in an utterance that sounded like a stop consonant. Cathy also tends to produce words containing /r/ incorrectly, as assessed by the Goldman-Fristoe Test of Articulation–2. Further assessment using the Ling Phonetic Level Evaluation, however, revealed that she is able to imitate accurate /r/ production and that her difficulties with /r/ seem to stem from lack of awareness of when the accurate pattern should be used in new words.

To better understand the nature of the nonsegmental patterns observed in Cathy's speech, the FSST (Levitt et al., 1990) was used. The results showed that hypernasal quality was pervasive, although it was found during informal assessment that she was able to produce vowels with reduced nasality when they occurred in syllables that began and ended with plosives. This was clearly an excellent starting point for intervention.

Intervention Goals

Based on the assessment described above, a series of goals were established that were believed attainable during the academic year. Among the goals to be worked on are the following:

- Development of classroom communication strategies and approaches that will enable Cathy to better communicate with her peers in class
- Work on narrative structure in written and spoken communication (through picture sequencing and the use of cohesive devices)
- Increased knowledge of idioms
- Development of fricatives
- Improved accuracy of /r/ production in new words
- Production of vowels with reduced nasality

Intervention Strategy

Cathy is seen twice per week for therapy. The clinician determined that a combination of pull-out and in-class therapy would be appropriate. The pull-out activities were aimed at providing needed information about things such as articulation and the use of communication strategies whereas the in-class activities are more aimed to application of skills learned to real communication situations.

Communication Strategies.   Classroom communication strategies and approaches that will enable Cathy to better communicate with her peers in class need to be developed. Cathy was provided a list of communication strategies, and using role play, she was asked to determine the best and most appropriate strategy to use based on the specific characteristics of each scenario. These included things such as communicating in class, in the school yard, in the cafeteria, and in a fast food restaurant. Among the strategies employed were requests to repeat and rephrase and the use of writing. Once Cathy was able to demonstrate mastery of these skills, she was then asked to employ them in various real-world settings and to record her experiences in a communication notebook that was brought to class. The therapist was also able to monitor her use of appropriate strategies during the classroom-based session each week and discussed these observations with Cathy during the pull-out session.

Additionally, the classroom session involved working with the other children in the classroom to help them better understand Cathy's hearing loss and some common communication strategies that could help Cathy follow conversations in class. This will initially involve working with the teacher to ensure her familiarity with the measures that should be implemented in a classroom with a deaf or hard of hearing child.

The initial session might involve a question and answer activity, perhaps with a quiz about things such as a famous deaf composer (Beethoven) or the origin of the huddle in football (the football team at Gallaudet University). This in turn could lead to a discussion of things that might be harder for a deaf person to accomplish, including a discussion of communication areas. This is a natural entrée to a discussion of the need to help Cathy follow conversations. The classroom teacher may suggest ways in which the class might accomplish this. Hand raising or the teacher pointing to the child talking, could prove effective ways of helping Cathy in these more difficult situations.

Narrative Structure. Work on narrative structure in written and spoken communication was accomplished in the pull-out therapy session through picture sequencing and the use of cohesive devices. Cathy was given a set of cards depicting a sequence of activities and was asked to order the cards to depict a logical sequence. Once arranged, Cathy was asked to describe the sequence, with her description recorded on video tape. Cathy then reviewed the tape with the therapist and was asked to note each time she used or could have used a particular cohesive structure (such as substitution or ellipis) to connect sentences in her "story." The classroom teacher was briefed concerning these activities and was asked to note the child's use of these cohesive structures in written assignments.

Increased Knowledge of Idioms. By using the checklist of idioms (see appendix D), it was determined that Cathy understood some, but not all, idioms with particular difficulty exhibited on those with higher levels of transparency. As a result, these idioms were specifically addressed in therapy. The therapist had collected a series of daily comic strips appearing in her local newspaper that reflected idioms and used these as a basis for discussion. Cathy was asked to describe both the literal and figurative meaning of each idiom and to then use the idiom appropriately. To facilitate carryover, Cathy was asked to try to use the idiom outside of class and to note each use in her communication notebook.

Speech Skill Improvement. Aspects of therapy were aimed toward a number of aspects of speech that are often challenging for a deaf or hard of hearing individual. These include the production of the fricatives, improved production of /r/, and production of vowels with reduced nasality.

With the IBM Speechviewer III©, it was possible to provide visual feedback to Cathy about fricative and /r/ production. Fricatives are particularly difficult for deaf children because they are typically less visible than many sounds and are composed of higher frequency sound components that are inaccessible to many children with hearing loss. Provision of visual feedback offers the child information about her production while the game activities of these devices often provides needed motivation to older children to continue working on these more challenging speech skills.

Finally, working on nasal quality can also benefit from the use of visual feedback devices such as the Nasometer (Kay Elemetrics). This device provides children with visual displays that correspond to the acoustic consequences of nasal tract coupling employed during speech. This acoustic measure, or nasalance, provides a means of quantifying coupling and a visual display that can be useful in helping the child maintain proper velopharyngeal posturing and patterning during production of speech.

Bridget

Bridget is 11 years old and in the sixth grade. In the past 6 months she has demonstrated very inconsistent use of her hearing aids. She cites a number of reasons for not wearing her aids—they are not working, they are lost, or they hurt her ears. She further resists wearing her FM system because it embarrasses her. Her performance in school has declined and she is becoming further behind her hearing peers in language skills, presumably because of the complexity of class work, a greater expectation of independent work skills, and the inconsistent use of amplification. Bridget's parents have requested weekly meetings of all professionals to resolve this issue. Of particular concern to her parents is her 2-year delay in reading skills.

Assessment Strategies

Based on the presenting problems noted above, a series of assessment strategies were employed. These included (1) a review of Bridget's academic performance to ensure that she was at grade level and that her language skills were commensurate with cognitive functioning, (2) reading and writing assessment (in conjunction with the reading/writing specialist and/or classroom teacher), (3) probing of psychosocial issues, which may have resulted in reduced use of her personal amplification system; and (4) speech assessment to establish appropriate goals for therapy. Each of these will be discussed further below.

Academic Performance. By this age Bridget should clearly be achieving many of the language functions described in chapter 3 as typical of later language learners. These skills are important for literacy as well as for many other aspects of academic success. It is important that the clinician work closely with the classroom teacher to identify areas of strength and weakness and to develop strategies for addressing areas that might reasonably fall under the purview of the hearing and speech professional.

It was revealed that many aspects of Bridget's language performance, as identified by the classroom teacher, were below grade level. As a result, the SLP-t explored a number of language areas. These included vocabulary (Peabody Picture Vocabulary Test-3, Dunn & Dunn, 1997), syntax (Test of Syntactic Ability, Quigley et al., 1988), and broad aspects of written discourse (TOWL-3, 1996). This additional assessment permitted establishment of a series of language goals that converged with the academic goals of the teacher.

Reading and Writing. Clarification of those areas that Bridget experiences as difficulties in reading can then be incorporated into therapy. In Bridget's school, all reading areas are evaluated through the reading specialist assigned to the school. As a result of the reading assessment, it was found that Bridget is experiencing comprehension difficulties. Because these areas reflect the kinds of problems identified by the classroom teacher and examined further by the SLP, areas for focus in the classroom, as well as through speech-language therapy, were identified.

Exploration of Issues Affecting Amplification Use. Children in mainstream settings often experience a considerable amount of difficulty adjusting to the hearing school environment. The need to fit in, to make friends, and to be accepted often take precedence over the need to wear amplification. Through interactions in therapy, the clinician can sometimes explore the issues that are leading to reduced use of amplification. Once the issues are identified then it may be possible to explore strategies for increasing usage. It should be stressed, however, that the psycho-social issues involved may be complex, and it may be necessary to make appropriate referrals to a counselor, social worker or psychologist.

Speech Assessment.   For Bridget, it is important to monitor her speech production skills and to address any errors in articulation, voice, and resonance that may persist. As described for the other children, a combination of a standard three-position articulation test, such as the Goldman-Fristoe Test of Articulation–2 (Goldman & Fristoe, 2000) or the Fischer-Logemann (1971) tests and an imitation task such as the Ling Phonetic Level Evaluation (2002) can provide needed information on both the pattern of misarticulations and the bases for the patterns observed. Bridget's clinician also opted to examine suprasegmental aspects of the child's speech using the FSST (1990).

The results of testing revealed continued distortions of many speech sounds. However, these patterns are inconsistent, and Bridget is highly stimulable for the error patterns identified. The results of the FSST revealed few problems. One area of concern was the use of proper intonation patterns to signal questions.

Intervention Goals

The following goals were established for Bridget:

- Improve her ability to accurately construct imbedded sentences
- Increase her vocabulary, particularly related to geography and science
- Promote increased amplification use
- Improve articulation and intonation at the phrase and sentence level

Intervention Strategies.   At this stage, therapy should incorporate increased levels of classroom-related content. The SLP and classroom teacher(s) should collaborate to provide the most relevant support to Bridget. Pull-out therapy can still be done through an integrated approach in which new concepts are introduced and all skill areas are addressed. Another important technique to be utilized is preteaching of the classroom academic concepts. Hearing children learn a great deal incidentally; deaf children do not. Hearing children, when presented with many new ideas, recall overhearing terms or ideas from a variety of media. Thus, these "new" concepts become solidified, clarified, or overlaid onto a rough framework. Preteaching in the weeks before new lessons are introduced can prepare the deaf or hard of hearing child for the upcoming lesson. This serves to approximate the incidental learning that hearing children are afforded. Thus, the deaf child is able to process the new incoming information in a more manageable way.

Dion

Dion is 11 years old and in the sixth grade. He is a consistent hearing aid user, although he has begun to refuse to use the classroom FM system that has been provided. Strategic seating and an acoustically treated room improve the listening environment to some degree. Dion depends, instead, on the interpreter for access to most communication in the classroom. He has developed some close friendships among the hearing children in the classroom, and they tend to communicate through a combination of speech and sign. His academic performance in school in all subjects is at or near grade level, except for subjects that rely heavily on writing. Dion's writing skills are progressing well, but he does show some writing errors typical of second language learners. Although Dion's speech skills have improved, he is difficult to understand unless the listener is familiar with his speech.

Assessment and Outcomes of Assessment

The SLP determined that the primary areas to assess were the following: speech and voice skills, pragmatic skills during spoken interactions, and narrative structure during both writing and spoken communication. Each of these will be discussed below.

Speech and Voice.   To assess Dion's articulation, both a phonetic and phonologic level assessment were used. The Goldman-Fristoe Test of Articulation–2 (Goldman & Fristoe, 2000) provided useful information about the Dion's ability to produce various segments in words. In addition to this information, the clinician felt it important to assess whether or not any of the error sounds were the result of limited articulatory skills, or the consequence of limited knowledge of when to use a particular articulatory pattern. As a result, the Ling Phonetic Level Evaluation (Ling, 2002) was used to determine how well Dion could imitate phonetic elements in syllable contexts. The results of this assessment revealed that Dion's repertoire of vowels was limited and that he has difficulty producing fricatives and semivowels. It was encouraging, however, to note that Dion was using nearly all sounds that he could produce in the three-position test. This suggested good ability to generalize production skills to actual word usage.

To assess Dion's suprasegmental and voice skills, the FSST (1990) was again used. This revealed that Dion had difficulty coordinating respiration and phonation. Additionally, he showed difficulty producing the correct intonation pattern to indicate questions. His pitch was generally appropriate though he lacked the ability to vary it. He was able to vary his loudness but tended to use a louder than appropriate volume. Dion also still demonstrates a hypernasal vocal quality. His overall intelligibility is fair when the listener is familiar and the subject is known.

Pragmatic Skills.   The primary area of concern was Dion's difficulty negotiating face-to-face conversations involving spoken language. Informal assessment revealed that he often appeared to panic and not have an idea of how he might communicate in these situations. The clinician decided that through evaluative therapy she would examine Dion's knowledge of and ability to use communication strategies during spoken face-to-face interactions.

Narrative Structure.   To assess Dion's ability to construct stories both through the air (spoken and/or signed) and in writing, he was shown two pictures and asked to write a story about one and to tell a story about the other. Both the through-the-air and written samples derived from the pictures lacked the level of syntactic structure, and vocabulary, that one would expect in a sixth grade student. Additionally, Dion sequenced the events but did not include any transitions. The stories consisted of formulaic sentences stating events. Dion did name his character and used that name to begin all of his sentences. The through-the-air story was slightly longer than the written one, but evidenced many of the same characteristics as his face-to-face narrative.

Intervention Goals and Strategies

Dion's three main areas for therapy at this time consist of the following:

- Addressing difficulties negotiating face-to-face spoken only communications situations
- Generating more sophisticated narratives
- Improving articulation and voice quality

Although these skills should all be addressed individually, they also lend themselves to work in an integrated fashion.

Drill on the erred sounds, speechbreathing exercises, and work to improve voice quality will supplement the integrated activities. Communication strategies can be taught to Dion and then practiced within the integrated activities. Dion's teacher will certainly need to be involved in the facilitation of narrative development. It is possible that the more analytic work will be done in the classroom.

Several types of integrated activities are possible to foster the skills Dion needs to develop. If there is a drama program in the school it might serve to have Dion be a part of it. It would allow him opportunities to negotiate a variety of face-to-face interactions and use newly learned communication strategies. Additionally, the nature of the stories and performing them will help to build Dion's understanding of story-ness and improve his expression of those stories. His interpreter would still be important especially to allow Dion to learn and express stories in his more comfortable mode (sign). At times, however, Dion would benefit from learning and practicing spoken stories. The other students in the group and the teacher would provide a variety of challenges and opportunities for Dion to improve his speech and communication strategy use.

Another integrated therapy idea is a dialogue journal group. This could even be an offshoot of the drama group. The children could communicate with each other online through instant messaging and with the teacher and or SLP. Dion would be encouraged to create and expand on stories alone and with others. This would allow practice as well as modeling and would allow him to work on his written narrative skills and his overall syntactic skills in English.

Renee

At 11 years of age, Renee is a fifth grader. She continues to be in speech therapy at her parents' request. She continues to have very little interest in speech and does not like to come to therapy. Her parents still hope she will learn to use oral speech (English) to communicate with them. The family does not sign, although her mother knows a few signs. Communication at home is mainly gestural and now includes some writing.

Renee is reading and writing at school but continues to fall behind her class-mates in content material. She is experiencing reading problems in both decod-ing and comprehension and is unable to write a coherent story or text without considerable individualized instruction. She continues with a sign interpreter at school, but no longer has a sign language instructor.

Assessment

Renee presents a set of communication difficulties not uncommon among deaf and hard of hearing school-aged children. Although she is experiencing some speech problems, the language areas, particularly related to narrative and acade-mic activities, appear to be a significant problem.

Audition/Listening. Renee has not obtained any functional use of residual hearing and often does not wear her hearing aids. She will wear them for com-munication therapy if encouraged. She is independent in the care and mainte-nance of her hearing aids.

Auditory/Visual Skills. As Renee's sign language and subsequent under-standing of spoken English increase so, too, do her speechreading skills. The integrated therapy approach allows her to make the connections between signs, print, and spoken language representations on the lips and face. In addition, as she acquires more language she is able to better use contextual strategies. She is now able to function in the classroom for short periods without the interpreter. For example, she is able to follow the routines of the classroom by speechreading the teacher or her classmates. Also, she is able to have some successful one on one conversations. However, beyond brief, highly contextualized situations with familiar speakers she is unable to effectively process spoken English.

Speech/Voice. Renee's speech continues to be unintelligible to all but the most familiar speakers. Even with family and close friends the context is very important to her being understood by others. In addition, her vocal quality is poor, and the sounds she makes when attempting to sign and voice at the same time do not match her intended message. This makes her even less intelligible at times. A more detailed assessment of her speech skills through the FSST revealed that her breathstream and elementary articulation skills were in the 20th percentile for children her age with similar degrees of hearing and that she had numerous suprasegmental errors related to syllable identity, stress, and the appropriate use of intonation patterns.

Language. Renee's language skills in sign have improved dramatically over the past several years. She is now able to communicate a variety of social and aca-demic ideas more effectively. She still demonstrates difficulty with reception of longer, more complex, signed utterances. This was noted, and strategies were implemented to ensure that concepts presented in class were reviewed with Renee. The speed of the classroom instruction through the interpreter remains too quick and fleeting for Renee to grasp all of the material. As a result, preteaching and review strategies are incorporated. The interpreter was provided training to allow her to tutor Renee. It is important to note that the tutoring occurs outside of the therapy room, and the role is clearly shifted from interpreter to tutor. Within the classroom environment the interpreter adheres to her role as interpreter. Renee has become more confident and interactive within the classroom. After training for the teacher, the interpreter, and Renee's classmates, the dynamic of the classroom has been modified to allow for increased wait time between questions and the students' answers. This has benefited all the children in the classroom. More children participate and answers tend to be more thoroughly thought out. Additionally, if a question is going to be directed to a child (including Renee) the child is called on and notified that the next question will be hers. This increases attention to the question as well as preparation of an appropriate answer.

Although Renee is still behind her peers in many aspects of language, she is demonstrating marked improvement. With continued services, the professionals working with her hope to "catch her up."

Visual-Gestural Communication.   As stated in the language section, Renee is acquiring more and more sign language everyday. It should also be noted that she is no longer demonstrating any sign production errors. The biggest issue related to Renee's sign language development remains her limited access to signers. There have been attempts made by the school to facilitate interactions, and these have been successful. Unfortunately, Renee's family remains reluctant to learn sign or to interact with the deaf community outside of the school setting. The SLP is working with the family to coordinate Renee's participation in a summer school program at the state school for the deaf. Although hesitant, the family may acquiesce and allow Renee to attend an 8-week residential summer school program.

Pragmatics.   Renee's pragmatic skills also show improvement. Her eye contact and turn-taking skills are age appropriate. In addition, her ability to take the listener's perspective is improving. The SLP and the classroom teacher implemented strategies for Renee to use to ensure that she included enough information for the listener to understand her stories. She was instructed to assess her communication partner as a stranger, new friend, or old friend. These designations allowed her to anticipate the level of background information she needed to include. After some practice, Renee has learned to use this strategy with increasing facility.

Literacy.   Recent assessment of Renee's literacy skills show that she is solidly reading at the third grade level. This is still behind age level expectations but reflects improvement.

Intervention Goals and Strategies

Intervention techniques should continue to incorporate an integrated approach to therapy, focusing on strengths as well as areas of improvement. Additionally,

Renee, her parents, and the SLP need to negotiate more realistic speech goals. The SLP hopes to convince Renee's parents that it is time for Renee to turn off her voice and focus on improving her ability to accurately mouth words and phrases to improve her communicative efficiency in interactions with unfamiliar hearing people. There has been little improvement in voice or articulation in the past few years. This is related to Renee's residual hearing and her lack of motivation.

Therapy should be focused on increasing Renee's facility with school language, reading, and writing. Activities would include comprehension of narrative and expository text and increased written language skills. Collaboration among the SLP, classroom teacher, and literacy specialist would benefit Renee. The professionals would evaluate her classroom texts for complexity of grammar, complexity and use of figurative language, understanding and use of cohesive devices, advanced vocabulary, and discourse structure and then implement support services to facilitate her ability to manage these more sophisticated language forms.

Summary

This chapter has addressed a number of areas that are important to assessment and intervention with deaf children that are later language learners. Discussed were a range of areas that are typical of later language learning of hearing children. In addition, specific areas that are often the focus of therapy with deaf children are explored. Finally, the five cases presented earlier were examined, this time as they might appear as later language learners. The following chapter will explore a number of assessment and treatment issues that might affect deaf adolescents.

References

ASHA Ad Hoc Committee on Reading and Writing. (2003). Knowledge and skills needed by speech-language pathologists with respect to reading and writing in children and adolescents. *ASHA Leader, 8*(7 Suppl), 93–102.

Al-Issa, I. (1969). The development of word definition in children. *Journal of Genetic Psychology, 114,* 25–28.

Allen, T. (1986). Patterns of academic achievement among hearing impaired students. In A. Schildroth & M. Karchmer (Eds.), *Deaf children in America* (pp. 161–206). Boston: Little, Brown.

Anderson, K. L., & Smaldino, J. (1996). *Listening Inventory for Education (LIFE), an efficacy tool.* Retrieved Month April 2005, from Educational Audiology Association Web site: www.edaud.org.

Bally, S. J. (1996). Pronunciation skills. In M. J. Moseley, & S. J. Bally (Eds.), *Communication therapy: An integrated Approach to aural rehabilitation.* Washington, DC: Gallaudet University Press.

Bradley-Johnson, S., & Evans, L. (1991). *Psychoeducational assessment of hearing-impaired students.* Austin, TX: Pro-Ed.

Brown, R. (1973). *A first language: The early stages.* Cambridge, MA: Harvard University Press.

Brinton, B., & Fujiki, M. (1984). Development of topic manipulation skills in discourse. *Journal of Speech and Hearing Research, 27,* 350–358.

Bryant, J. B. (2001). Language in social contexts: Communicative competence in the preschool years. In: J. B. Gleason (Ed.), *The development of language,* (5th ed.). Boston: Allyn & Bacon.

CADS (Center for Assessment and Demographic Studies). (1991). *Stanford Achievement Test,* (8th ed.). *Hearing impaired norms booklet.* Washington DC: Gallaudet University, Gallaudet Research Institute, Center for Assessment and Demographic Studies.

Dorval, B., & Eckerman, C. (1984). *Developmental new in the quality of conversation achieved by small groups of acquainted peers.* Monographs of the Society for Research in Child Development, 49 (2 Serial No. 206).

Dunn, L. & Dunn, L. (1997). *Peabody Picture Vocabulary Test–3.* Circle Pines, MN: American Guidance Services.

Feifel, H., & Lorge, I. (1950). Qualitative differences in the vocabulary responses of children. *Journal of Educational Psychology, 41,* 1–18.

Fisher, H. B., & Logemann, J. A. (1971). *Fisher-Logemann Test of Articulation Competence.* Austin, TX: Pro-Ed.

Fromkin, V., & Rodman, R., (1988). *An introduction to language* (4th ed.). New York: Holt, Rinehart and Winston.

Gentile, A., & Defrancesca, S. (1969). Academic achievement test performance of hearing impaired children in the United States. *Spring* (Series D, No. 1). Washington, DC: Gallaudet College Office of Demographic Studies.

Gochnour Idiom Screening Test (1977). Upper Saddle River, NJ: Prentice Hall.

Goldman, R., & Fristoe, M. (2000). *Goldman-Fristoe–2 Test of Articulation.* Circle Pines, MN: American Guidance Service.

Kail, R., & Hall, L. (1994). Processing speed, naming speed, and reading. *Developmental Psychology, 30,* 949–954.

Leadholm, B. J., & Miller, J. F. (1992). *Language sample analysis: The Wisconsin guide.* Madison, WI: Wisconsin Department of Public Instruction.

Levitt, H., Youdelman, K. & Head, J. (1990). *Fundamental Speech Skills Test.* Englewood, CO: Resource Point.

Ling, D. (2002). *Speech and the hearing impaired child: Theory and practice* (2nd ed.). Washington, DC: Alexander Graham Bell Association for the Deaf.

Makkai, A., Boatner, M. T., & Gates, J. E. (2004). *A dictionary of American idioms* (4th ed.). New York: Barron's.

McNeil, D. (1970). *The acquisition of language: The study of developmental psycholinguistics.* New York: Harper & Row.

Menn, L., & Stoel-Gammon, C. (2001). Phonological development: Learning sounds and sound patterns. In: J. B. Gleason, Ed., *The development of language* (5th ed.). Boston: Allyn & Bacon.

Miller G. A., & Gildea, P. M. (1987). How children learn words. *Scientific American, 257,* 94–99.

Monsen, R. B. (1981). A usable test for the speech intelligibility of deaf talkers. *American Annals of the Deaf, 126,* 845–852.

Moseley, M. J., & Bally, S. (1996). *Communication therapy: An integrated approach to aural rehabilitation.* Washington, DC: Gallaudet University Press.

Nippold, M. (1998). *Later language development: The school age and adolescent years.* Austin, TX: Pro Ed.

Osberger, M. J., Robbins, A. M., Todd, S. L., & Riley, A. I. (1994). Speech intelligibility of children with cochlear implants. *Volta Review, 96,* 169–180.

Paul, P., & Quigley, S. P. (1994). *Language and deafness.* Clifton Park, NY: Singular.

Perera, K. (1986). Language acquisition and writing. In: P. Fletcher & M. Garman (Eds.), *Language acquisition: Studies in first language acquisition* (2nd ed.). Cambridge, England: Cambridge University Press.

Perera, K. (1992). Reading and writing skills in the National Curriculum. In: P. Fletcher & D. Hall (Eds.), *Specific speech and language disorders in children: Correlates, characteristics and outcomes* (pp. 183–193). London: Whurr

Quigley, S., Steinkamp, M., Power, D., & Jones, B. (1978). *Test of syntactic Abilities.* Beaverton, OR: Dormac.

Sillman, E. (1984). Interactional competencies in the instructional context: The role of teaching discourse in learning. In: G. P. Wallach & K. G. Butler (Eds.), *Language learning disabilities in school-age children.* Baltimore, MD: Williams & Wilkins.

Subtelney, J., Orlando, N., & Whitehead, R. (1981). *Speech and voice characteristic of the deaf.* Washington, DC: Alexander Graham Bell Association for the Deaf.

Test of Written Language-3 (1996). Austin TX: Pro-Ed.

Test of Auditory Comprehension TAC. (1979). North Hollywood, CA: Foreworks Publishers.

Thompson, M., Biro, P., Vethivelu, S., Pious, C., & Hatfield, N. (1987). *Language assessment of hearing-impaired school age children*. Seattle, WA: University of Washington Press.

Trybus, R., & Karchmer, M. (1977). School achievement scores of hearing-impaired children: National data on achievement status and growth patterns. *American Annals of the Deaf, 122,* 62–69.

Vihman, M. M. (2004). *Later phonological development*. In J. E. Bernthal & N. W. Bankson (Eds.), *Articulation and phonological disorders* (5th ed.). Boston: Allyn & Bacon.

Wallach, G. P., & Miller, L. (1988). *Language intervention and academic success*. Boston: College-Hill

Watson, R. (1985). Towards a theory of definition. *Journal of Child Language, 22,* 211–222.

Wiig, E., & Secord, W., (1985). *Test of Language Competence–Expanded Edition*. San Antonio, TX: Harcourt.

Wold, D. C., Evans, C. R., Montague, J. C., Jr., & Dancer, J. E. (1994). A pilot study of SPINE test scores and measures of tongue deviancy in speakers with severe-to-profound hearing loss. *American Annals of the Deaf, 139,* 352–7.

Woodcock, R. (1987). *Woodcock Reading Mastery Tests—Revised*. (1998). Circle Pines, MN: American Guidance Service.

Adolescent Language: Assessment and Intervention

Introduction

This chapter describes a framework for providing useful and relevant assessment and intervention services to deaf and hard of hearing adolescents in the high school setting. High school is a very challenging time for most students. It may be challenging not only for the student but also for family and the professionals working with the student at school. At this stage, the student is searching for identity, trying to answer questions about place in her family and trying to identify models and friends, while also determining what to believe in and what the future holds (Head, Long, & Stern, 1991). In addition, these students are also faced with the responsibility of doing well on standardized or informal tests to graduate with a high school diploma (instead of a "certificate of completion") and to get accepted into college (e.g., College Board testing [SAT/ACT]).

The adolescent must develop the linguistic proficiency and communicative competence to succeed in high school and prepare/plan for her future in college or the work environment. Many deaf and hard of hearing adolescents will demonstrate varied communication skill levels. As explained in previous chapters, each student will move through the various skills and levels presented in the Scope at different rates. The clinician should review the skill areas in the previous developmental stages in the Scope, as they are "building blocks" for further communication skill development/refinement. For example, a student may have mastered the prelanguage skill area of turn-taking nonverbally by the time she is in high school; however, she may still have not mastered turn-taking during spoken interactions. She may have difficulty carrying on a verbal conversation using appropriate turn-taking in one-to-one and/or group situations.

The high school student may also still be working on many of the skill areas addressed in the chapter on later language, such as nonliteral language, and the use of more complex verbal and written language forms. It is also important to keep in mind that by this stage in development, some skill areas may have reached a terminal level. For example, when working with a student who does not have intelligible speech and depends primarily on sign language for communication, it may not be advisable to continue to work on speech skills if the student is not planning to use speech as a mode of communication. It may, however, be more beneficial for this student to modify this goal area and work on other communication skills that would facilitate communication with nonsigners.

Before modifying goals, the clinician must first determine how the student/parents view the student's communication skills. Often the student/parents may have a different perception of the student's communication skills and potential for improvement. It is very important that the clinician provide honest feedback to the student. Too often, students are told by their clinicians that they have "good" speech, only to experience surprise and frustration when they are not understood by an unfamiliar listener (Mahshie & Allen, 1996). Parents may also have unrealistic expectations. Once the student develops more realistic expectations, perhaps she will be able to better discuss her communication needs with her parents. The clinician, however, must keep the parents informed of any changes in communication goals and provide a rationale.

In addition to understanding the student's perception of her communication skills, the clinician must understand the student's internal and external motivation for improving her communication skills. Linguistic/communication competence is acquired during a life-long learning process and assumes not only an ability to learn but also an adequate motivation on the part of the learner. If the student is not personally motivated to receive communication services, or if motivation does not internalize during the early therapy process, therapy outcomes can be affected in terms of prognosis, learning rate, and personalized applications of learning (Whitehead & Barefoot, 1992).

Before beginning assessment and intervention, the clinician must first gather and decipher all available information. The information should include the following: the student's hearing ability (auditory access), technology use (e.g., hearing aid(s)/cochlear implant; assistive listening devices, or visual technologies) and benefit; communication mode (e.g., spoken language/sign language/use of an interpreter in the classroom); and educational and communication history (individual education plan (IEP) as well as past therapy reports/progress). In addition, the clinician needs to assess the listening and visual environments of the school/classrooms/therapy room to understand the challenges the students face in their "communication" environment.

SERVICE DELIVERY

The types of speech-language services provided in a high school may be different from those provided in elementary and middle schools. Often the high school clinician works on language and communication skills in the classroom or provides services in small groups as opposed to providing individual therapy. For this type of programming to be effective, the clinician must establish a working relationship with the classroom teachers (CRTs) to plan communication goals for a specific student. As discussed earlier in this text, this relationship can either be collaborative or consultative. Collaboration requires more direct interaction between the clinician and the CRT outside and inside the classroom (e.g., planning/teaming). The clinician may work with the student(s) in the classroom on communication goals or supplement comprehension of the material being covered in the class. Using a consultative model, the clinician would take the role of an observer and not participate. In the high school setting the clinician may collaborate with some CRTs (e.g., English class) and consult with other CRTs (e.g., health class). In addition to collaboration/consultation, the clinician might also see students individually or in small groups in the therapy room. Figure 7-1 presents suggestions for implementing a collaborative model and Figure 7-2 presents suggestions for implementing a consultative model for working with deaf and hard of hearing adolescents in the mainstream. These models provide the clinician with a functional approach to working with deaf and hard of hearing high school students outside in addition to inside the therapy room (Reinstein & Moseley, 2001).

If the clinician has implemented a collaboration or consultation program in lieu of and/or in addition to "traditional" pull-out therapy, it is imperative that the parents be provided with information and a rationale. Parents may have questions about the value of this type of programming especially if they have requested individual therapy during an IEP meeting. If at all possible, the clinician should arrange for a meeting with the parents. Figure 7-3 presents information and a rationale for the collaborative model, and Figure 7-4 presents information and a rationale for the consultation model that should be shared with parents (Reinstein and Moseley, 2001).

ASSESSMENT

Given below are a number of areas that are important to evaluate in a deaf or hard of hearing adolescent.

Attitudes and Motivation

One of the primary goals of intervention with deaf and hard of hearing high school students is for them to develop an understanding/perception of their own communication skills. If a student does not demonstrate an understanding of her communication skills or has an unrealistic perception, the clinician needs to provide an information base regarding communication strengths and weaknesses. In addition, the clinician needs to determine the student's internal and external

Implementing a Collaborative Model

- Determine the number of students receiving speech-language services in a particular classroom.
- Choose a class in which she demonstrates a certain level of mastery (e.g., English).
- Present the classroom teachers with specific information related to the student's speech-language needs as they relate to the student's academic needs and overall classroom functioning.
- Communicate expectations clearly.
- Schedule time for collaborating with the students in the classroom as well as a specific time to meet with the teacher(s) monthly.

Figure 7-1. Suggestions for Implementing a Collaborative Model

Implementing a Consultative Model with Teachers

- Don't expect the teacher to modify his/her lesson plan.
- Observe but do not participate or encourage students in any way.
- Observe not only the student(s) you are working with, but also the other members of the class; some observations may yield more information than others.
- Focus on the interactions rather than just observing the students asking/answering questions in class.
- Remember that consultation also incorporates feedback from other students, teachers, professionals, and parents.
- Seeing a student in her class is NOT adequate for determining progress.
- Each observation actually represents a "snapshot" of the student's communication functioning.
- Make sure to ask the student(s) being observed for feedback after the observation.

Figure 7-2. Suggestions for Implementing a Consultative Model with Children

motivation for improving her communication skills. The best way to determine how the student perceives her communication skills and her motivation to improve is to conduct a communication information interview. The communication information interview provides the clinician with an opportunity to establish a rapport with the student as well as insight into the student's attitudes and motivation toward therapy and oral/aural communication. A list of interview questions taken from The Gallaudet University Hearing and Speech Center Intake for Communication Therapy form have been modified and are presented in Figure 7-5. The student's responses will reveal her understanding of her background information (e.g., age of onset, etiology, the student's understanding of her hearing loss and benefit from technology, educational/career goals, and so forth), as well as

Information Sharing with Parents: A Collaborative Model

- Reinforces academic material; provides students with strategies to master material in a specific content area
- Allows the students additional opportunities for practice and reinforcement of skills
- Allows for additional time to be spent on remediation of a problem skill area
- Monitors a student's progress
- Reinforces and encourages positive communication interaction in multiple contexts.

Figure 7-3. Strategies for Information Sharing with Parents Using a Collaborative Model

Information Sharing with Parents: A Consultation Model

- Allows monitoring of a student's progress and performance in the classroom
- Does not require the students to miss time out of class
- Allows the clinician to have greater understanding of the student's communication needs in multiple contexts
- Allows the clinician to gain additional insights into teaching methodologies used in the student's various classes

Figure 7-4. Strategies for Information Sharing with Parents Using a Consultative Model

identify those skill areas she is most interested in improving. If the student uses spoken language to communicate her answers, the clinician will also be able to informally judge the student's speech intelligibility. If the student uses sign language to communicate her answers and the clinician is a fluent signer, then the clinician will also be able to informally judge the student's sign language proficiency. If an interpreter is used, the interpreter may be able to provide information regarding sign language proficiency; however, it is recommended that a sign language specialist perform a formal evaluation. Figure 7-6 presents a framework for determining communication needs and establishing functional therapy goals. This model depicts a system for assessing communication skills that considers both the student's perception and the clinician's perception. The student's perception of her skills/abilities is often based on communication experiences, as well as on feedback received from family, friends, and previous clinicians. The clinician's perception of the student's communication skills is based upon the interview, observation, and formal and informal assessment. This approach to assessment and negotiation of therapy goals will help the student develop a more realistic view of her skills and become better able to self-evaluate in various communication situations (Wilson & Scott, 1996).

Communication Information Interview

Name: Date:
Class: D.O.B.:

Communication Interests and Needs

1. What do you want to do after you graduate from high school?
2. Do you have a part-time job?
3. What extracurricular activities are you involved in?
4. Have you had speech therapy/communication training before? What did you practice? Do you feel you improved because of this training? Did you enjoy therapy/training?
5. Why are you interested in improving your communication skills?
6. Which communication skills would you like to improve? The following are some of the communication skills we can work on in therapy:

SpeechVoice	Telephone/TTY
Pronunciation	Vocabulary
Voice	Communication Strategies
Speech	readingListening
Written Language	Understanding Idioms

Technology Background

1. What is your hearing ability (e.g., deaf, hard of hearing, dB average)?
2. Do you know the reason why you are deaf or hard of hearing?
3. How old were you when your parents found out you had a hearing loss?
4. Has your hearing changed over the years or has it stayed the same?
5. Do you experience or have you ever experienced the following:
   —ear infections:
   —tinitus/ringing in your ears:
   —dizziness:
6. Do you use a hearing aid/cochlear implant? How often do you use it?
7. How old were you when you got your first hearing aid/you were implanted?
8. Are you satisfied with your hearing aid/cochlear implant?
9. Tell me the communication technologies that you currently use at home, school/work, and for recreation (e.g., alerting devices, telecommunication devices, FM).

Communication Mode/Perceptions

1. How do you communicate with your family?
2. How do you communicate with your friends?
3. How do you communicate in class?
4. How do you communicate with hearing people who do not know sign language/Cued Speech?
5. How do you feel when you have problems communicating?
6. What do you do when you have problems communicating?

Figure 7-5. Communication Information Interview Used at the Gallaudet University Hearing and Speech Center

(continues)

7. Using a scale from 0–10 with 0 representing no skills and 10 representing excellent skills, how would you rate yourself for the following communication skills:
—Using American Sign Language
—Using English-based sign language
—Talking
—Speechreading
—Understanding speech by listening
—Using the voice telephone
—Using the TTY/pager/Instant Messaging
—Understanding magazines and newspapers
—Writing
—Repairing communication when it is not successful

Figure 7-5. (continued)

Assessment of Skills and Abilities

The goals of assessment are to establish the student's communication strengths and weaknesses, whether attitudes and motivation are consistent with the aims for improvement, and a set of reasonable and realistic therapy goals. As depicted in the model in Figure 7-6, assessment includes an interaction of both formal and informal evaluation measures. Assessment should include the communication information interview (as discussed above), skill assessment using traditional tools, observation of the student in various communication contexts (e.g., classroom and lunch), role-play, and analysis of the student's overall communicative competence (Wilson & Scott, 1996).

Assessment of the student's skills and abilities (upper left-hand box of Figure 7-6) can be accomplished through the use of both formal and informal assessment tools as discussed in previous chapters. Expressive skill areas include speech intelligibility (articulation/voice quality and pronunciation), writing, production of signs, and communication strategies. Receptive skills include listening and speechreading skills, reception of signs, reading/test-taking strategies, and communication strategies.

Assessment of most of the communication skill areas appropriate for this stage were discussed at length in chapter 6 with the exception of test-taking skills/strategies. Test taking skills/strategies refer to the student's ability to demonstrate what she has learned in a given subject area by responding appropriately to comprehension tasks on standardized and informal tests. Test-taking abilities can be assessed by administering comprehension tasks. These comprehension tasks should include question and nonquestion tasks. The questions and responses should be communicated through the air (conversationally) using the student's preferred mode of communication (e.g., signs, finger spelling, Cued Speech/language, or oral methods) and in print. Questions should vary in terms of question

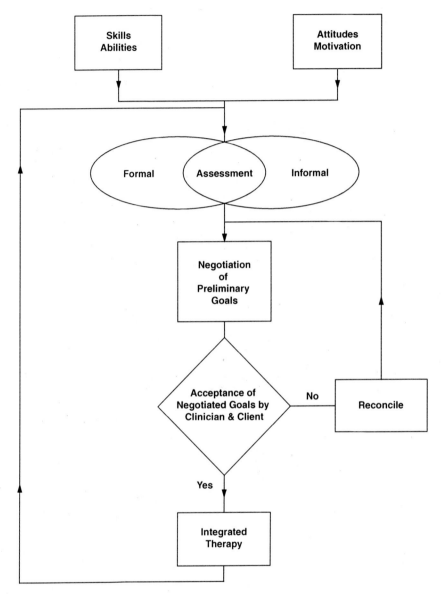

Figure 7-6.   Framework for Determining Communication Needs and Establishing Functional Therapy Goals

Source: Reprinted with permission from Wilson, M., & Scott, S. M. (1996). An integrated therapy model. In: M. J. Moseley & S. J. Bally (Eds.), *Communication therapy: An integrated approach to aural rehabilitation.* Washington, DC: Gallaudet University Press.

types (e.g., wh- or incomplete statement stems), response formats (e.g., multiple choice, short answer, or essay), testing conditions (e.g., timed vs. untimed or look-back vs. no-lookback), and types of information sought (e.g., main idea, support-ing detail, time and setting of stories, characterization, and sequence of events) (LaSasso, 1999). A good source of materials for developing question classification systems related to type of information can be found in reading methods textbooks. The SAT/ACT test preparation software and test booklets are also a good resource for materials for assessment/intervention.

Assessment of communication skill areas can provide important information, but it may not provide information about other factors that have a significant effect on the student's communicative competence. As discussed earlier, the clin-ician needs to observe the student in other communication contexts (e.g., class-room and extracurricular activities) to assess skills in a functional environment. The clinician can also set up a role-play situation between the deaf and hard of hearing student and her hearing peers to assess the types of communication strategies the student uses if communication is not successful.

Negotiation of Preliminary Goals

Once the communication information interview and assessment are completed, the student and the clinician arrive at the point of negotiation of preliminary goals (middle of Figure 7-6). The clinician must consider the relationship between the assessment results and the student's communication needs, motivation, atti-tudes, and interests to establish functional communication goals. In addition, the clinician should consider the following: (1) intervention should be directed toward development of functional skills toward more immediate communication (e.g., class presentation and job interview); (2) therapy should be directed toward refinement of skills for which the student has some demonstrated capability; (3) the student should be aware of how best to use the skills currently acquired; (4) specific skills (e.g., speechreading, articulation, voice, and others) should be addressed to the extent that each area impacts on the student's overall communi-cation; and (5) therapy should be ultimately directed toward integrated actual communication (Mahshie & Allen, 1996). The student and the clinician should then discuss these preliminary goals. If the student does not agree, further dis-cussion and negotiation must occur to reconcile and establish another set of pre-liminary goals (middle right-hand box of Figure 7-6). If the student agrees with the preliminary goals, it is time to proceed with integrated therapy.

Integrated Therapy

The integrated therapy model was described in chapter 3. In this approach, sev-eral aspects of communication are integrated and based on specific situations (e.g., class activity or job interview). Rarely does therapy focus on one receptive or expressive communication area. Communicative effectiveness is enhanced through overall skill development and the use of appropriate communication strategies, technology, and informational counseling. This type of approach allows for greater carryover of skills into real life situations.

CASE STUDIES

In this section, assessment and intervention are discussed as they apply to the students in the representative cases used in the previous chapters. For each case the following information will be provided: responses from the communication information interview; pertinent areas for assessment; assessment results; examples of analytic intervention where appropriate; and an example of an integrated therapy activity.

Arlis

Arlis is now 16 years old and a junior in high school. He continues to use his cochlear implant in class. Arlis's academic performance has improved; however, he scored poorly on the SAT. In class, he has become more assertive and is participating more; however, the level of participation is not comparable to that of his peers. Arlis joined the football team in his freshman year. While at practice and during games, he does not use his cochlear implant. He has a very difficult time understanding the coach and his teammates. Arlis has a girlfriend who is deaf and communicates using American Sign Language (ASL). When Arlis is with his girlfriend he does not use his cochlear implant and uses ASL only. His mother is concerned that he will loose his speech skills. She has contacted the school to arrange a meeting with the speech-language pathologist.

Arlis is now at an age where he should be able to report any changes in the functioning of his cochlear implant; however, before assessment and intervention, the clinician should perform a map check.

Assessment of Attitudes and Motivation

During the communication information interview, Arlis was able to provide accurate background information (as compared with the information provided in his school file). He reported that he is very interested in attending Gallaudet University upon graduating from high school; however, he is undecided on a major. He plans to apply to Gallaudet as well as other universities. He demonstrates excellent oral/aural communication skills (while wearing his cochlear implant); however, he most recently has developed a strong interest in deaf culture and ASL. He will be taking the SAT I for the second time this year and is very concerned about doing well since he did not do well the first time he took the test. Arlis reported that he does not use his implant during football practice and games and has a difficult time communicating. He also has stopped using his cochlear implant outside of the classroom, especially when he is with his girlfriend who is deaf. His mother has expressed concern about Arlis not using his cochlear implant and his possible loss of his speech skills. Arlis is not concerned about losing his speech skills but is concerned about the difficulty he has communicating while playing football. He therefore wants to work on improving his communication skills without the use of his cochlear implant. He stated that he feels that his speech is intelligible and is not concerned with his ability to use speech for communication regardless of what his mother thinks.

Based on Arlis's stated interests and concerns the following communication skills should be assessed: speechreading (with and without his cochlear implant), receptive vocabulary, and use of receptive and expressive communication strategies.

Assessment of Skills and Abilities

The CID Everyday Sentences Test of Speechreading Ability (Davis & Silverman, 1970) was used to assess Arlis's speechreading skills with and without the use of his cochlear implant. He scored 100% while using his cochlear implant, indicating that he is able to understand all the message; however, he only scored 40% without the use of his implant.

The Peabody Picture Vocabulary Test-Revised (PPVT-R) (Dunn & Dunn, 1981) was used to assess Arlis's receptive vocabulary skills. Arlis wore his cochlear implant and the words were presented using auditory and visual cues combined. He was asked to repeat the word presented to monitor his understanding of the stimulus word. Arlis repeated two of the stimulus words incorrectly. Upon a second presentation he was able to correctly identify the word. He obtained a stand score equivalent of 82, a percentile rank of 11% and a stanine of 2.5 which places him in the moderately low range.

Negotiation of Preliminary Goals

The therapist and Arlis agreed that he would work on the following communication skills: speechreading with and without the use of his cochlear implant, receptive vocabulary/test-taking strategies, and appropriate use of receptive and expressive communication strategies.

Intervention Approach

Arlis requires treatment aimed at both individual skills as well as the integration of these skills in communication. Accordingly, analytical and integrated approaches to intervention are discussed separately below.

Analytic Intervention. Arlis would benefit from improving his word attack skills. It is recommended that the SAT preparation book be used to focus on vocabulary used, test-taking strategies, and critical thinking. These skills can be addressed in a small group with other students who are also preparing for the SAT.

Because Arlis has difficulty communicating when not using his cochlear implant, he was instructed to turn off his implant for the following tracking activity (DeFilippo, 1988). The clinician read from a text (short phrases at a time), and Arlis had to repeat verbatim what was read by the clinician. If Arlis was unable to understand the clinician, he was to use a strategy to get the information he missed. Results from this tracking activity indicated that Arlis uses a limited number of communication strategies. He asked for repetition and if unsuccessful, he would ask that the clinician write down the word or phrase he missed.

These findings suggest that Arlis should be taught appropriate communication strategies for difficult communication situations. A good source of this information could be found in *Communication Therapy: An Integrated Approach to Aural Rehabilitation* (Moseley & Bally, 1996).

Integrated Therapy.   Arlis should identify a difficult communication situation (e.g., communicating during a football practice session while not using his cochlear implant). The clinician and Arlis should brainstorm all the possible vocabulary and language that is used during practice. Arlis should then practice speechreading the vocabulary words, phrases, and sentences that are used. Role-playing the situation with Arlis will probably promote expanded use of appropriate communication strategies.

Cathy

At 16, Cathy is functioning well in the classroom and is showing speech and language skills that are age appropriate. At the same time, she has begun to balk at wearing her hearing aids in class and has refused to ask the teachers to use the frequency modulated (FM) system that is provided by the school system. She has indicated to her parents and the guidance counselor that she is tired of being considered special and is embarrassed by the special attention that comes with wearing hearing aids. Although she knows how much she relies on audition for receiving information, she insists that she functions well without the hearing aids and that she would feel much more comfortable with her hearing peers if she did not have to wear them.

Assessment of Attitudes and Motivation

During the communication information interview it became evident that Cathy has an unrealistic perception of her communication skills while unaided. When questioned about her background, Cathy was unable to explain her hearing ability with and without amplification. She also denied that she has trouble communicating in noise and has refused to use the FM system in the classroom. Cathy is not interested in working on her spoken language skills because she feels that she does not have difficulties communicating. However, classroom observation and teacher report have indicated the opposite to be true.

Assessment of Skills and Abilities

Cathy needs to be encouraged to participate in an evaluation of her skills in the aided and unaided conditions. If Cathy agrees to participate in assessment, her hearing aids and FM system should be checked and a functional listening check performed (see appendix C). Areas for assessment include speechreading (with and without amplification), listening skills (with amplification in quiet and in the presence of background noise), communication strategy use, and speech intelligibility. Cathy would also benefit from informational counseling for her to better understand her communication skills (strengths and weaknesses).

The CID Everyday Sentences Test of Speechreading Ability (Davis & Silverman, 1970) was administered to assess Cathy's speechreading skills. While aided Cathy scored a 98% (with auditory and visual cues combined in quiet). While aided and in the presence of background noise, Cathy scored a 68%. In the unaided condition (with visual cues alone), Cathy scored a 44%. These results indicate that Cathy receives significant benefit from amplification. She is able to understand the entire message when presented in quiet. Cathy does have difficulty understanding in noise, but scored the poorest when no auditory cues were provided.

The CID Everyday Sentences were administered using auditory cues alone in quiet. Cathy scored 72%. Another list was presented (auditory only) in the presence of background noise. Cathy was unable to understand any of the sentence in this condition. The same list was presented again while she wore her FM system coupled to her hearing aids. Cathy scored 72% with the FM system, showing that she receives significant benefit from her hearing aids and the use of an FM system even when noise is present.

The Speech Perception in Noise (SPIN) Test (Kalikow, Stevens, & Elliott, 1977) was administered while Cathy wore her hearing aids to assess her ability to use the context of the sentence to determine the key word in the presence of noise. Cathy scored a 75% for the high predictability sentences and 50% on the low predictability sentences. These scores indicate that Cathy has difficulty understanding speech in the presence of noise even when the context is known.

Cathy's teachers were asked to complete the Listening Inventory For Education (L.I.F.E) (Anderson & Smaldino, 1996) to determine the specific listening difficulties Cathy was experiencing in each of her classes. Cathy was also asked to complete the L.I.F.E. student appraisal of listening difficulty.

Analysis of the teacher responses indicated that Cathy's listening behavior has changed since she has refused to use the FM system in class and now she is considered a "minimally successful listener." Cathy's responses were very different from her teacher's responses. She indicated that she "sometimes" has difficulty listening in the classroom and in the additional listening situations; however, she does not feel that the hearing aids and FM system would improve her listening success.

Cathy's speech intelligibility was informally assessed after a recorded spontaneous conversation between Cathy and a peer (with normal hearing). Overall, Cathy's speech was intelligible; however, she did mispronounce several words. The clinician noted her errors and instructed Cathy to use the dictionary to assist in improving pronunciation. Cathy demonstrated difficulty in using the dictionary to self-correct without the support of clinician modeling.

Because Cathy is refusing to use her FM system in the classroom and does not want to wear her hearing aids outside the classroom, her use of communication strategies was evaluated in the unaided condition. Cathy and the clinician participated in a videotaped thematic role-play of a noisy restaurant. Cafeteria noise was played in the background, and the clinician assumed the role of the waitress. Cathy used a limited repertoire of strategies. She only asked the clinician to repeat or write down information when she did not understand. The clinician/waitress had some difficulty understanding Cathy due to Cathy's mispronunciation of some of the items on the menu and the presence of background noise. Cathy would only repeat the word the clinician/waitress missed and did not use any other strategies to help her listener understand (e.g., she did not compensate for the background noise by increasing her vocal loudness). It was further noted that Cathy became very frustrated during this assessment.

Cathy was given the Communication Scale for Deaf Adults (Kaplan, Bally, & Brandt, 1991) to complete for homework. Interpretation of the scale supports the clinician's original understanding that Cathy has an unrealistic perception of the impact that her hearing loss has on her daily life. Cathy does not perceive that she has a problem in her communication functioning.

Negotiation of Preliminary Goals

Before integrated therapy can begin and functional goals can be established, Cathy needs informational counseling. Using the picture audiogram, the clinician should explain Cathy's unaided and aided thresholds. Speech audiometry results should also be explained (e.g., open-set word recognition scores). Results from the communication skills assessment should then be reviewed as well as the videotaped role-play. Cathy should be encouraged to ask questions and discuss her feelings about the test results. Cathy should then be asked to describe her communication skills and needs before functional goals for therapy are established. If Cathy is still unwilling to use her hearing aids and the FM system, it is likely that factors are contributing to this reluctance that might be better handled by the psychologist. If Cathy is willing to use her hearing aids during therapy, the following is an example of an integrated therapy activity.

Intervention Approach

Integrated Therapy.   Before participating in an integrated activity, Cathy demonstrated the following. When given examples of various difficult communication situations [e.g., activities from *Speechreading: A Way to Improve Understanding* (Kaplan, Bally, & Garretson, 1987], Cathy showed an understanding by providing examples of appropriate communication strategies that could be used, and when given a list of unfamiliar multi-syllabic words, Cathy correctly used the dictionary pronunciation key to pronounce the words.

During a conversation with an unfamiliar speaker/listener in the presence of background noise, Cathy was asked to use appropriate receptive communication strategies (e.g., repair and maintenance) and expressive communication strategies (e.g., correct pronunciation) to successfully communicate. The clinician videotaped the conversation, observed, and kept data. Later the videotape was viewed by both Cathy and the clinician and feedback was provided.

Bridget

Bridget is 16 years old and currently a sophomore in her local high school. She is now a year behind her same age peers after repeating sixth grade. Bridget is currently a consistent hearing aid and FM user; however, for several years (from sixth to eighth grades) she used her aids inconsistently. This period of inconsistent use of amplification has resulted in a significant decrease in Bridget's speech and language skills. Because Bridget's primary mode of communication is through speech and speechreading (she does not know sign language), the decrease in her aural/oral skills has had an impact on her academic performance. Her reading comprehension and writing skills are delayed. Bridget avoids classroom discussion, because she is very self-conscious of her speech and has difficulty understanding her peers. Bridget's favorite subject is math for which she receives average grades. She is involved in a few extracurricular activities, but is not very socially active. She is still receiving speech and language services.

Assessment of Attitudes and Motivation

During the communication information interview, Bridget demonstrated a good understanding of her background information by responding accurately. She consistently wears her hearing aids and FM system and is aware of the benefit she receives for receptive and expressive communication. Bridget is a member of the math club and the yearbook staff. She reported that she has difficulty communicating sometimes during the math club meetings but does not assert herself and ends up missing a lot of information. This is the second year she has been working on the yearbook staff. She has noticed that the freshman students sometimes have a difficult time understanding her (she is a photographer for the yearbook staff). When communication is not successful, she often feels embarrassed and frustrated. Bridget indicated that she wants to attend college after graduating from high school and later become an accountant; however, she is concerned about taking the SAT. She is also concerned about her writing skills. Even though she gets average grades on her classroom writing assignments, she feels that it is always a struggle and that she does not write as well as her peers. Bridget has also reported that often she is misunderstood by people who are unfamiliar with her speech. She is aware of the limited speech skills and is very interested in working to improve her speech and voice quality.

Another concern and motivation for therapy is to improve her understanding of idioms and figurative language. Often when she reads the newspaper, magazines, or novels, she finds that she has difficulty comprehending the text.

Assessment of Skills and Abilities

Bridget's hearing aids and FM system should be checked to be sure they are working properly and a functional listening check performed (appendix C) before assessment and intervention. Areas for assessment include speechreading (in the aided and unaided conditions), listening skills; communication strategies; reading/test-taking strategies, and speech intelligibility (speech, voice, and pronunciation).

The CID Everyday Sentences (CHABA) (Davis & Silverman, 1970) were used to assess Bridget's speechreading skills with and without amplification. Bridget scored 54% (auditory and visual combined) while using hearing aids and a 48% when unaided (visual only). These results indicate that Bridget is able to understand about half of the message with difficulty. The insignificant difference in her scores with and without amplification may be due to the fact that she has recently started using her hearing aids again.

The Binnie Lipreading Test (Binnie, Jackson, & Montgomery, 1976) was used to assess Bridget's ability to identify speech sounds that look the same on the lips (visemes). Fifty consonant-vowel (CV) syllables were presented with auditory and visual cues combined (the aided condition). Bridget was able to correctly identify the syllable or viseme (e.g., if the clinician said /ba/ and she responded /ma/ it was scored as a correct response) with 68% accuracy indicating that she has fair analytic speechreading skills.

The Monosyllabic, Trochee, Spondee Test (MTS) (Erber & Alencewicz, 1976) was administered to assess Bridget's ability to identify words in a closed-set format. The MTS was presented using auditory cues alone while Bridget wore her hearing aids. Bridget scored 48% for identification and 88% for pattern perception. These results indicate that while aided, Bridget is able to discriminate between monosyllabic versus multisyllabic words and stress patterns.

Bridget's teachers were asked to complete the L.I.F.E. (Anderson & Smaldino, 1996) to determine the level of listening difficulty Bridget experiences in their classes. Most of Bridget's teachers reported that she is a successful listener while she is using her hearing aids and FM system. If Bridget is not using the FM system, she is minimally successful. Bridget completed the student version of the L.I.F.E. Her responses indicated that she sometimes has difficulty listening in the classroom and always has difficulty listening in other listening situations (e.g., small groups, gym, and school assembly).

Bridget's articulation skills were assessed at different stages in her development (see previous chapters); however, because she was not using amplification for a period of time and is currently using hearing aids, articulation skills were assessed again for comparison. The Fisher-Logemann Test of Articulation Competence (Sentence Test) (Fisher & Logemann, 1971) was administered to assess Bridget's articulation skills at the sentence level. Bridget continues to omit final consonants and substitutes voiceless for voiced cognates (e.g., k/g and t/d) in all positions in words. These results are consistent with results obtained in previous evaluations.

The Pronunciation Skills Inventory (PSI) (Bally, 1996) was used to assess Bridget's acquisition, understanding, and use of rules and principles that determine the correct pronunciation of English words, as well as to assess her understanding of related nomenclature. The PSI also was used to assess Bridget's ability to use the dictionary pronunciation key to self-correct pronunciation errors. Bridget demonstrated strengths in the following areas: alphabet, vowel, and consonant identification; vowel and consonant production; and syllabification identification. She had difficulty with the following: production of plurals, past tense, and contractions; phoneme production; grapheme/phoneme differentiation; digraphs (vowels and consonants); silent letter rules; syllabification/stress and dictionary skills.

Bridget's speech intelligibility and voice quality were assessed using The NTID Voice and Speech Examination (Smith, 1975).

The clinician and Bridget engaged in a spontaneous conversation and then Bridget read aloud the "Rainbow Passage." Using the Gallaudet University intelligibility rating scale, Bridget's conversational speech intelligibility was judged to be a "3," indicating that her speech is difficult to understand; however, once the listener becomes familiar with her speech intelligibility improves. Bridget's speech intelligibility deteriorated while reading the passage. She was rated a "4"; however, intelligibility could have been negatively affected by her problems with reading and pronunciation.

Bridget's voice quality is somewhat breathy and tense and she has difficulty coordinating respiration and phonation (deficient air expenditure) at the conversational level. Her pitch is moderately above an appropriate level and her resonance is characterized as cul-de-sac. Bridget's cul-de-sac resonance quality may result from resonance in the pharyngeal area, possibly related to the retraction of the tongue toward the pharyngeal wall (Subtelny, Whitehead, and Subtelny, 1989).

Results from previous evaluations have indicated that Bridget's vocabulary skills are several years below those of her her peers. She also experiences difficulty with figurative language (comprehension and use). Deficits in both vocabulary and figurative language have impacted Bridget's reading and writing ability.

Bridget's language and literacy skills were informally assessed through observations in various classes as well as through reading a cross section of Bridget's writing samples, including journal writing.

Negotiation of Preliminary Goals

The assessment results were discussed with Bridget. It was jointly decided that she should focus on the following skills: speechreading and communication strategies, listening skills; overall speech intelligibility (e.g., articulation, pronunciation, ar and voice quality); and language and literacy.

Intervention Approach

Analytic Intervention.   To improve speechreading skills, the clinician and Bridget will review the list of viseme groups (see Kaplan et al., 1987, *Speechreading: A Way to Improve Understanding*). When presented with a list of one-syllable words, Bridget will correctly identify the viseme group for the initial sound in the word presented. These skills could be practiced in a small group with other students who are working on the same goal.

The clinician and Bridget should review the L.I.F.E. suggestions for improving classroom listening for each situation she indicated as difficult. Bridget should then determine how she will self-advocate to improve her listening success.

To improve voice quality and articulation, Bridget needs to become aware of production goals. The clinician and Bridget should review the anatomy and physiology of respiration as a starting point for improved production. Bridget should then be instructed to use diaphragmatic breathing and a supportive posture for speech production. Once a supportive posture is established, Bridget needs to develop a cognitive and sensory awareness of the phonemes in error (Mahshie & Allen, 1996). To do this, she and the clinician should generate a list of cognate pairs (e.g., p/b, t/d, and f/v). For each phoneme, Bridget should identify voicing, manner, and placement. This can be accomplished by using a worksheet such as the one presented in Figure 7-7 (p. 271, Mahshie & Allen, 1996). After correct identification, Bridget should then produce each of the phonemes. To establish sensory awareness, the clinician should provide auditory (aided hearing), visual (mirror/computer software), and tactile kinesthetic cues when appropriate. Bridget should practice correct production/approximation of the phonemes in

Voicing - Manner - Placement Worksheet

NAME: AB Client   DATE: _____

	Voicing		Manner				Placement					
	Voice	No Voice	Nasality	Stops	Continues	Glides	Teeth	Lips	Tongue	Hard Palate	Soft Palate	Nose
b	✓			✓				✓				
d	✓			✓					✓	✓		
f		✓			✓		✓	✓				
g	✓			✓					✓	✓	✓	
h	✓			✓					✓	✓		
j	✓			✓	✓			✓	✓	✓		
k		✓		✓					✓			
l	✓ ✓ ✓			✓	✓				✓	✓		
m	✓ ✓		✓		✓			✓	✓			
n	✓ ✓		✓	✓					✓ ✓ ✓	✓ ✓ ✓		
p		✓		✓				✓	✓	✓		
r	✓			✓		✓			✓	✓		
s		✓ ✓		✓			✓		✓ ✓ ✓	✓ ✓ ✓		
t		✓ ✓		✓			✓		✓ ✓	✓ ✓		
v	✓ ✓ ✓				✓		✓	✓	✓ ✓ ✓	✓ ✓ ✓		
w	✓				✓	✓		✓	✓ ✓ ✓	✓ ✓ ✓		
y	✓					✓			✓ ✓	✓	✓	✓ ✓
z	✓				✓		✓		✓			
ch	✓			✓					✓	✓		
ng	✓ ✓		✓						✓ ✓		✓	✓ ✓
sh	✓ ✓			✓ ✓			✓		✓ ✓	✓		
th	✓						✓		✓			
TH	✓								✓			

Note: Checked areas are used by this client to produce each sound.
Source: Therapy material developed by Scott Bally and Paula Bohn. Gallaudet University.

Figure 7.7. Worksheet for Examining Articulatory Features (Manner, Place, Voicing) Various Sound Segments

Source: Therapy material developed by Scott Bally and Paula Bohn, Gallaudet University.

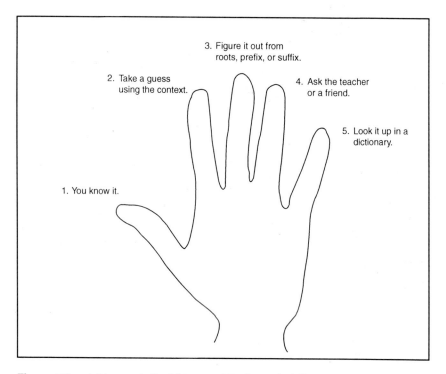

Figure 7.8. A Mnemonic for Addressing Word Attack Skills

Source: Nichols, M. & Moseley, M. J. (1996). Language skills. In M. J. Moseley & S. J. Bally (Eds.), *Communication therapy: An integrated approach to aural rehabilitation* (p. 326). Washington, DC: Gallaudet University Press.

isolation, in syllables (CV/VC) and in words (initial, medial, and final positions). The accuracy of articulation should be based on clinician judgment (e.g., Bridget may not be able to produce some of the phonemes with 100% accuracy). The goal is for Bridget to approximate correct production in words to improve intelligibility.

To address literacy, Nichols and Moseley (1996) suggest a strategy for figuring out word meaning during reading. This strategy has a strong visual component and gives the student a series of choices for figuring out the meaning of an unknown word when it is encountered in a text (see Figure 7-8). This "five-finger" method suggests the following choices:

- Recognize the word/idiom.
- Guess what the word/idiom means from the context and keep reading.
- Figure out what the word means from root, prefix, or suffix.
- Ask a friend or teacher what the word means.
- Look it up in the dictionary.

The clinician and Bridget reviewed the above strategy and then Bridget had an opportunity to practice it using a reading assignment for her English class.

Integrated Therapy Activity.   This activity will demonstrate the integration of reading and writing skill enhancement. The clinician works collaboratively in the English literature class. Students choose books they want to read and then write in peer reading journals. Peer reading journals (Mettler & Conway 1991) are journals in which students have written conversations with peers about the books they have selected to read. The clinician/teacher reads the entries, responds in writing, and develops a three-way reading journal. The clinician/teacher can also suggest the kinds of questions the students might ask each other and/or periodically join the written conversation to encourage deeper thinking about a topic or lead the conversation in a different direction (Nichols & Moseley, 1996). The clinician/ teacher does not correct grammar/syntax; however, studies have shown that the use of interactive conversational writing about experiences with no correction of syntax resulted in an improvement in the use of syntactic skills (Harrison, Simpson, & Stuart, 1991).

Dion

Dion is 16 years old and currently a junior in his local high school. Dion remains a consistent hearing aid user and is a skilled speechreader. He has become much more assertive at advocating for himself in a number of settings. He is involved with a variety of extracurricular activities and is doing well in school. He is still receiving speech and language services. The focus of services is to continue to promote speech, speechreading, and writing skills. He is interested in college and hopes to become a teacher of the deaf.

Assessment

An interpreter was used during the communication information interview. Dion reported that he is enjoying high school, especially because many of his friends know ASL. He wants to do well this year in school, and hopes to enter college when he graduates. During the interview, Dion was able to report background information accurately. He is a consistent user of his AVR IMPACT hearing aids. He feels that he receives significant benefit from his hearing aids. While aided he is aware of conversational speech and environmental sounds; however, he reports not being able to understand speech without speechreading. Dion feels that his hearing aids also allow him to better self-monitor his speech. He is very interested in working on his spoken language skills to facilitate his communication with nonsigners. Dion is aware that the clinician has limited sign skills but feels that communication during his therapy sessions will better simulate communication in the "hearing world." He also expressed concern about his writing skills and feels his writing is not comparable to that of his peers.

Assessment of Skills and Abilities

Before assessment and intervention Dion's hearing aids were checked and a functional listening check was performed. Dion was able to identify all Ling Six sounds.

Because the clinician has limited sign skills, speech with some sign support is used during communication therapy sessions. Dion's speechreading skills and speech intelligibility were informally assessed to determine how well Dion was able to understand the clinician as well as how well the clinician was able to understand Dion. The clinician read a list from the CID Everyday Sentences (CHABA) (Davis & Silverman, 1970), and Dion had to write down what he understood. Dion scored 68%, indicating that he was able to understand most of the message. Dion then read a different list (one that was unfamiliar to the clinician), and the clinician had to write down what she understood. The clinician was able to understand 52%, indicating that she was able to understand with difficulty most of the message.

Another list of sentences was used to assess Dion's use of receptive communication strategies. The clinician read part of a sentence, and Dion had to repeat verbatim (using speech and sign) what the clinician said. When he did not understand a word/phrase, he had to use a strategy to get the information he missed. Dion used a limited number of strategies (e.g., repetition and writing). He became frustrated and resorted to asking the clinician to write down most of what he missed. To assess Dion's use of expressive communication strategies, Dion read another list of sentences to the clinician and the clinician had to repeat (using sign-supported speech) what Dion had said. If the clinician was unable to understand a word/phrase, Dion had to use a strategy to help her understand. Dion used some appropriate expressive communication strategies to help his listener (repeated, verbally spelled, and slowed down his rate); however, he again became frustrated and resorted to writing. These results indicated that Dion would benefit from training in expanding his repertoire of communication strategies.

Because Dion's writing continues to be an area of concern, the clinician should work collaboratively with the classroom teacher(s) to assess areas of weakness. As discussed in the previous case (Bridget), the clinician and Dion can engage in journal writing, specifically a dialogue journal, to expand and refine Dion's writing. A dialogue journal is a written conversation between the student and the clinician/teacher about a student-selected topic. Spelling and grammar are not corrected; however, the clinician/teacher models correct English grammar, syntax, and spelling with the hope that over time, changes in the student's written English occur (Bailes, Searls, Slobodzian, & Staton, 1986).

Intervention Goals

Based on Dion's interests and concerns the following areas were focused on in therapy: communication strategies, speech intelligibility (functional speech), and written language. These goals will be addressed in individual therapy as well as being used as a collaborative model in the classroom(s).

Dion would benefit from a review of receptive and expressive communication strategies. His current repertoire of anticipatory, repair, and maintenance strategies needs to be expanded. It will be important to begin by generating an inventory of his successful strategies. Additional strategies can be introduced once Dion is able to talk about why and when to use various strategies. Employing the teaching approach outlined by Kaplan, Bally, & Garretson (1985) to increase his expressive and receptive communication strategies will probably be effective in improving overall communication in spoken English. These activities will also increase his ability to talk about his communication, analyze the effectiveness of his communication, and generate ideas for improving communication. Along with teaching strategies will be the need to determine Dion's reaction and approach to communication difficulties. Again, following the approach of Kaplan et al. (1985), the clinician will help foster Dion's use of an assertive approach. The final step will be to encourage and facilitate Dion's use of a wider set of strategies. This can occur initially by setting up role-play situations and culminate with real world opportunities for him to use his new skills (i.e., field trips).

Dion still struggles to produce all the sounds of English in connected speech. Analytic work on specific sounds will continue to be a routine part of therapy. The clinician and Dion should strive to achieve sound productions or approximations that are as correct as possible. Practicing these sounds in isolation and at the word, sentence, and conversational level should continue. Further practicing specific phrases and sentences appropriate to situations that Dion is likely to encounter would be beneficial. This can be done as part of an integrated activity focusing on speechreading and speech training of theme-based constellations. These constellations based on relevant activities (e.g., lunch room or physical education) will allow Dion to practice not only what he might see/hear others say but also the utterances he would in turn respond to them. This affords an opportunity to incorporate speech skills that might be worked on into daily communication that is relevant to specific situations.

The clinician should also work closely with the classroom teacher to facilitate improvement of Dion's written language skills. The clinician can emphasize parts of speech that Dion sometimes omits from his writing as well as work to help Dion self-identify aspects of written language with which he struggles.

Whereas the classroom teacher can focus on more technical or academic writing, written language for communication purposes is an area the clinician can work on with Dion. Written language for communication can include working on writing for TTY and Instant Messaging (IM) as well as face to face written messages. Again relevant situations can be generated and role-played. The clinician can also set up IM sessions with the client. This will allow the clinician to model written English as well as assess Dion's progress.

Because Dion wants to attend college and become a teacher, he would benefit from SAT preparation (see Arlis).

Intervention Approach

An integrated approach to intervention will be beneficial in addressing Dion's goals for communication. However, additional intervention to address specific goals will be necessary as well. For example, in a role-play conversation with the clinician or a fellow classmate, Dion will use appropriate receptive communication strategies (e.g., speechreading, maintenance, and repair strategies) and expressive communication strategies (e.g., slowing down his rate of speech, "A mouthing" words appropriately, and writing) during a conversation with an unfamiliar speaker/listener. The clinician will observe and keep data on strategies used. After the conversation, the clinician and Dion will evaluate the conversation. Based on the conversation specific skills can be identified for focus during one-one-one therapy.

Dion's goals of increasing speechreading, communicative effectiveness, speech intelligibility, and written English skills lend themselves to be woven into integrated activities. In addition, role-playing can serve as an important transitional activity to bringing these skills into real-life interactions. His therapy should focus on developing highly effective communication skills for a variety of settings. Additionally, the activities for therapy need to ready Dion for his transition from high school to his choice of vocational endeavors beyond high school. Because college is a goal for Dion, objectives and associated activities should focus on developing skills that will facilitate his enrollment in college and serve him well once he is there. Written language practice can include college application essays. Spoken communication role-plays can include college interviews. Communication strategies can focus on preparing for and learning in a lecture hall environment.

The intervention approach for Dion should be practical and focus on effectiveness of communication in a wide variety of communication situations. Because services for Dion will probably end with high school graduation, it will be essential for the clinician to look beyond high school to help Dion develop life skills. Dion will need to leave high school with the best communication skills he can have as well as the ability to analyze his own communication and make adjustments when necessary. The clinician's job will be well done if Dion can communicate the best way he can but also if he can continually grow and improve as a communicator beyond the therapy room and without the support of the clinician.

Renee

Renee had dropped speech therapy for 3 years before turning 16. Her sign language skills have continued to improve. Her reading and writing have also continued to improve; however, they are around the fourth grade level. She has had difficulty making the adjustment to high school because of the increased academic responsibilities, although she appears to be enjoying her social life. There are several other students at the high school who sign and Renee interacts with them almost exclusively. Renee's parents are pushing her, again, to work on her speech in school. They are concerned about what she will do when she graduates. She continues to interact with her parents through gestures and relies more on written communication than in the past. Her teachers are mainly concerned about her overall general knowledge and her low reading and writing skills.

Assessment of Attitudes and Motivation

Renee reluctantly participated in the communication information interview. She is not interested in being seen for "speech" therapy. The clinician (who is a fluent signer) explained to Renee that communication is much more than speech and that she will be an active participant in her "communication therapy" planning. Renee became more cooperative and interested so the interview continued. She was unable to provide the clinician with detailed information about her background. Renee considers herself to be deaf and has no interest in using amplification. She is satisfied with using an interpreter in the classroom; however, feels that she is still missing a lot of the information. Renee reports that she is sometimes "lost" and does not understand her assignments. She usually does not ask the teacher for help because she is too embarrassed. She knows her reading and writing skills are not at grade level; however, she does not seem motivated to improve her skills. When asked what she wanted to do after graduation, Renee responds that she wants to work with deaf and hard of hearing children in a day-care situation.

Assessment of Skills and Abilities

Renee's use of receptive and expressive communication strategies were informally assessed through a role-play (e.g., ordering food at a fast food restaurant). The clinician played the role of the food server. Renee attempted to mouth the words of the items on the menu. If the clinician was not able to understand, Renee became very frustrated and tried pointing to items on the menu on the wall behind the server. Renee understood little of what the clinician said and did not use any strategies to try to get the missed information.

Assessment of Renee's reading and writing skills has been ongoing. She continues to be behind her peers and is below grade level. Because Renee communicates with her parents and nonsigners through writing, an informal writing evaluation was performed using observation, recording, and interpretation of what Renee was saying and doing during the writing process. Writing for communication was assessed for the following writing tasks: writing an emergency message; using the TTY; writing in a journal; and writing an email message. For each writing task, the clinician evaluated the (1) intent or purpose of the communication, (2) the intended audience or receiver of the message, (3) the effectiveness of the communication, (4) how well Renee was able to determine whether the written communication was effective, and (5) what repair strategies she used to improve the written message (Horn, Mahshie, Wilson, & Bally, 1983). For the emergency message, Renee was not specific and did not provide the important information. During the TTY conversation, Renee was not able to demonstrate correct use of the TTY protocol or formulate or answer questions clearly. Writing in a journal is used in the classroom and Renee continues to demonstrate problems with vocabulary and the mechanics of writing. Renee seemed to have an easier time while writing an email, but her message still lacked clarity.

Renee's pragmatic skills were assessed during signed communication interactions and spoken communication interactions. Assessment was completed through observation of Renee's ability to use elements of discourse such as social versus nonsocial speech/sign; turn-taking and talking/signing time; conversation and topic initiation; maintenance and termination; on-topic exchanges (contingency); and/or conversational repairs (Nichols & Moseley, 1996).

Renee's pragmatic skills were also evaluated during a signed conversation with a peer and during a nonsigned role-play with the clinician. The clinician videotaped the conversation and the role-play. While viewing the videotape, the clinician used a checksheet to indicate whether the above elements of discourse existed regularly, part of the time, or not at all (Deyo & Hallau, 1983; Putting & Kirchner, 1987; Wiig & Bray 1984). Renee was not able to maintain the topic during a conversation in either modality (sign/speech). She also was unable to repair communication when a breakdown occurred.

The informativeness of Renee's message as well as the ease with which her message was conveyed (taking the receiver's perspective) was also evaluated through the use of a barrier game (Hughes & Moseley, 1988). A barrier was erected between Renee and the clinician, and each person was given a set of identical pictures. Renee was asked to describe one of the pictures for the clinician to correctly identify the picture. She described one of the pictures using sign language and another picture using writing. The clinician was able to ask for clarification as needed (in sign or writing). During the signed description of the picture, the clinician needed to ask for clarification and was unable to correctly identify the picture. This was due to Renee's inappropriate use of adjectives. During the written description, Renee did not use the appropriate cohesive devices to accurately describe the picture. She had the most difficulty with pronominalization (pronouns specify a previously used referent).

Negotiation of Preliminary Goals

Based on Renee's interests and concerns the following areas will be focused on in therapy: informational counseling, communication strategies, reading comprehension, writing, and pragmatics. She would benefit from the clinician taking a collaborative role in the classroom and then working with Renee either individually or in a small group. The clinician should also involve Renee's parents in the therapy process as much as possible. Renee's parents may need informational counseling regarding Renee's potential for using speech for communication and help in developing realistic expectations.

Intervention Approach

Analytic Intervention.   Renee needs to develop an appreciation for the use of cohesion in English, particularly pronouns. Wallach and Miller (1988) suggested having the student analyze text used in the classroom. Renee should read through the text and circle the pronouns. A chart can be developed to categorize vocabulary and pronouns specific to the text. For example, "In this story, Mary is referred to as a child, the girl, she, her, the baby, etc." (Nichols & Moseley, 1996). Another analytic activity would involve direct instruction of each of the syntactic/linguistic devices found to be indicators of the ability to take the receiver's perspective, for example, teaching different types of adjective classes (size, color, shape, and texture) and how they are used in relation to nouns.

Integrated Therapy.   The clinician should work collaboratively with the classroom teacher(s) to focus on reading and writing skills. As discussed earlier dialogue journals as well as peer reading journals may be beneficial tools. In addition,

Renee would benefit from watching stories signed in ASL and then reading the same story in English. Later, she should be asked to watch a story in ASL and then write the story in English on her own. The clinician would then provide feedback on Renee's writing of the story.

To further improve Renee's written and conversational skills, the visual/conceptual approach could be used to help Renee provide adequate information to her receiver. According to Hughes and Moseley (1988) the visual/conceptual approach is an effective tool for working with students who have overall difficulties in receptive and expressive language (sign/spoken/written). These students may also have difficulty formulating their thoughts into sign or on paper and responding appropriately to questions, have a limited vocabulary, and seem to have no strategies to repair communication when it is not successful. This approach is based on systematically describing the similarities and differences between two pictures. Similarities include identification of the main idea/topic of each picture (e.g., similar people, objects, space, or color). Differences include the identification of emotions, body characteristics (e.g., hair color, overall height of the individual, and body position), clothing descriptors, location of the picture, texture of objects, angle of the camera (e.g., aerial, lateral), and so on (Nichols & Moseley, 1996).

Renee should identify the kinds of things she is being asked to describe in the pictures. New vocabulary could then be introduced and practiced (e.g., writing a sentence using the new vocabulary, learning the sign, and trying to use the correct mouth postures to produce the word). Renee would be videotaped signing the description of the similarities and differences between two pictures. Later the clinician and Renee would view the videotape and use a checksheet to indicate the use of cohesive devices and differences and similarities.

Summary

This chapter has described relevant assessment and intervention strategies for deaf and hard of hearing adolescents. Adolescent language was discussed as it pertains to students in high school.

The primary focus of this chapter has been on how the clinician could work collaboratively with the students, classroom teachers, and parents to enhance communication skills and improve language and literacy. The representative case studies provided examples of how the clinician working collaboratively, could help the adolescent develop the communicative competence to be successful in and outside of the school environment as well as help the student prepare for her communication needs after graduation.

References

Anderson, K., & Smaldino, J. (1996). *Listening inventory for education (L.I.F.E.): An efficacy tool.* Tampa, FL: Educational Audiology Association.

Bally, S. J. (1996). Pronunciation skills. In M. J. Moseley, & S. J. Bally (Eds.), *Communication therapy: An integrated approach to aural rehabilitation.* Washington, DC: Gallaudet University Press.

Bailes, C., Searls, S., Slobodzian, J., & Staton, J. (1986). *It's your turn now!: Using dialogue journals with deaf students*. Washington, DC: Gallaudet University, Laurent Clerc National Deaf Education Center.

Binnie, C. A., Jackson, P. L., & Montgomery, A. A. (1976). Visual intelligibility of consonants: A lipreading screening test with implications for aural rehabilitation (The Binnie Test). *Journal of Speech and Hearing Disorders, 41,* 530–539.

Davis, H., & Silverman, S. R. (1970). Central Institute for the Deaf (CID) Everyday Sentences (CHABA). *In hearing and deafness,* appendix. New York: Holt, Rinehart, and Winston.

DeFillipo, C. (1988). Tracking for speechreading training. *Volta Review, 90*(5), 215–239.

Deyo, D., & Hallau, M. (1983). *Communicate with me: Conversation strategies for deaf students*. Washington, DC: Gallaudet University, Laurent Clerc National Deaf Education Center.

Dunn, L., & Dunn, L. (1997). *Peabody Picture Vocabulary Test–3*. Circle Pines, MN: American Guidance Service.

Erber, N. P., & Alencewicz, C. (1976) Audiologic evaluation of deaf children. *Journal of Speech and Hearing Disorders, 41,* 256–267.

Fisher, H. B., & Logemann, J. A. (1971). *The Fisher-Logemann Test of Articulation Competence*. Boston: Houghton Mifflin.

Harrison, D. R., Simpson P. A., & Stuart, A. (1991). The development of written language in a population of hearing-impaired children. *Journal of the British Association of Teachers of the Deaf, 15,* 76–85.

Head, J., Long, M., & Stern, V. (1991). Speaking and listening behaviors of hearing-impaired adolescents. *The Volta Review, 93*(5), 23–40.

Horn, R., Mahshie, J., Wilson, M., & Bally, S. (1983). *Audiologic habilitation with the hearing-impaired adolescent/adult: An integrative approach*. Miniseminar presented at the American Speech-Language-Hearing Convention, Cincinnati, OH.

Hughes, M. C., & Moseley, M. J. (1988). *A descriptive pragmatic inventory for deaf adolescents: Implications for intervention*. Miniseminar presented at the American Speech-Language-Hearing Association, Boston, MA.

Kalikow, D. N., Stevens, K. N., & Elliot, L. L. (1977). Development of a test of speech intelligibility in noise using sentence materials with controlled word predictability. *Journal of the Acoustical Society of America, 61,* 1337–1351.

Kaplan, H., Bally, S. J., & Brandt, F. (1991). Communication self-assessment scale for deaf adults. *Journal of the American Academy of Audiology, 2*(3), 164–182.

Kaplan, H., Bally, S. J., & Garretson, C. (1987). *Speechreading: A way to improve understanding* (2nd ed.). Washington, DC: Gallaudet University Press.

LaSasso, C. J. (1999). Test-taking skills: A missing component of deaf students' curriculum. *American Annals for the Deaf, 144,* 35–43.

Mahshie, J., & Allen, A. (1996). Speech and voice skills. In M. J. Moseley, & S. J. Bally (Eds.), *Communication therapy: An integrated approach to aural Rehabilitation*. Washington, DC: Gallaudet University Press.

Mettler, R., & Conway, D. (1991). Peer reading journals: A student to student application of dialogue journals. In: M Abrams (Ed.), *Perspectives in education and deafness*. Washington, DC: Gallaudet University, Laurent Clerc National Deaf Education Center.

Moseley, M. J., & S. J. Bally (Eds.). (1996). *Communication therapy: An integrated approach to aural rehabilitation*. Washington, DC: Gallaudet University Press.

Nichols, M. & Moseley, M. J. (1996). Language skills. In M. J. Moseley & S. J. Bally (Eds.), *Communication therapy: An integrated approach to aural rehabilitation*. Washington, DC: Gallaudet University Press.

Prutting, C. A., & Kirchner, D. M. (1987). A clinical appraisal of the pragmatic aspects of language. *Journal of Speech and Hearing Disorders, 52,* 105–119.

Reinstein, R. & Moseley, M. J. (2001). A model collaboration program with deaf and hard of hearing adolescents in the mainstream. Presented at the American Speech-Language-Hearing Association, New Orleans, LA.

Smith, J. D. (1975). Speech and Voice Therapy at NTID. *Journal of the Academy of Rehabilitative Audiology, 8,* 110–122.

Subtelney, J., Whitehead, E. & Subtelney, J. (1989). Cephalometric and cineradiographic study of deviant resonance in hearing-impaired speakers. *Journal of Speech and Hearing Disorders, 54,* 249–263.

Wallach, G., & Miller, L. (1988). *Language intervention and academic success.* Boston: College Hill Press.

Whitehead, B. H., & Barefoot, S. M. (1992). Improving speech production with adolescents and adults. *The Volta Review, 94,* 119–134.

Wiig, E. H., & Bray, C. M. (1984). *Let's talk: Intermediate level.* Columbus, OH: Merrill.

Wilson, M., & Scott, S. M. (1996). An integrated therapy model. In: M. J. Moseley & S. J. Bally (Eds.), *Communication therapy: An integrated approach to aural rehabilitation.* Washington, DC: Gallaudet University Press.

A Resource List of Books for Use in Joint Bookreading with Language-Disordered Preschoolers

VERB STRUCTURES

I. Present Progressive

Book: Bill Martin, Jr. *Polar Bear, Polar Bear What Do You Hear?* (Henry Holt Co.), 1991.
Theme: Zoo animals
Sample phrase: "I hear (animal) (sound) ing in my ear."

Book: Bill Martin, Jr. *Brown Bear Brown Bear What Do You See?* (Henry Holt Co.), 1967.
Theme: Colors and animals
Sample phrase: "I see x looking at me."

Book: Mirra Ginsburg. *The Chick and The Duckling* (MacMillan), 1972
Theme: Animal activities
Sample phrase: "I am digging."
               "I am going."
               "I am taking a walk."

II. Copula

Book: Eric Carle. *The Very Busy Spider* (Philomel Books), 1984
Theme: Animals
Sample phrase: "She was very busy."

Book: Eric Carle. *The Very Hungry Caterpillar Spider* (Philomel Books), 1969
Theme: Food, numbers and the days of the week
Sample phrase: "But he was still hungry."

Book: Noelle Carter. *My House* (Penguin Books), 1991
Theme: Animal homes
Sample phrase: "I am an x."

III. Contracted Auxiliary/Modal

Book: Margot Zemach. *The Little Red Hen* (folk tale) (Farrar, Straus, & Giroux), 1983
Theme: Flour—fowl planting a grain of wheat to make a loaf of bread
Sample phrase: "'Then I'll do it myself,' said the little red hen."

Book: Ann Jonas. *Where Can It Be?* (Greenwillow Book), 1986
Theme: Looking for things
Sample phrase: "I'll look in my (location)."

Book: Nancy Carlstrom. *I'm Not Moving, Mama* (MacMillan), 1990
Theme: Family moving
Sample phrase: "I'm not moving."

Book: Paul Galdone. *The Gingerbread Boy* (folk tale) (Clarion Books), 1975
Theme: Gingerbread boy eludes the hungry grasp of everyone until he meets the fox
Sample phrase: "I've run from the x."

Book: Janet Slater Redhead. *The Strange Loud Noise* (Scholastic TAB Publishing)
Theme: Suspense
Sample phrase: "I'll find out myself."

Book: Joy Cowley and June Melser. *One Cold Wet Night* (Shortland Publishing)
Theme: Animals
Sample phrase: "I'm going to be warm tonight."

IV. Do-Support

Book: Margot Zemach, *The Little Red Hen* (folk tale) (Farrar, Straus, & Giroux), 1983
Theme: Flour—fowl planting a grain of wheat to make a loaf of bread
Sample phrase: "'Then I'll do it myself,' said the little red hen and she did."

V. Regular Past Tense

Book: Joy Cowley and June Melser. *One Cold Wet Night* (Shortland Publishing)
Theme: Animals
Sample phrase: "The x jumped."

Book: Nancy Tafuri. *The Ball Bounced* (Greenwillow Books), 1989
Theme: Action words
Sample phrase: "The ball bounced."
　　　　　　　　　"The dog barked."

VI. Contracted Copula

Book: Margaret Wise Brown. *Where Have You Been?* (Scholastic TAB Publishing), 1952
Theme: Animals
Sample phrase: "That's where I've been."

Book: Scharlaine Cairns. *Oh No!* (Rigby Education)
Theme: Spills
Sample phrase: "There's a spot on my x."

VII. Modals

Book: Robert Lopshire. *Put Me in the Zoo* (Random House), 1960
Theme: Imaginary animals
Sample phrase: "I can put them x."

Book: Joy Cowley. *To Town* (Shortland Publishing)
Theme: Vehicles
Sample phrase: "I will go to town."

Book: Joy Cowley. *The Monster Party* (Shortland Publishing)
Theme: Action words
Sample phrase: "It can x."

INTERROGATIVES

I. WH-Questions

Book: Thomas and Wanda Zacharias. *Where Is the Green Parrot?* (Delacorte Press/Seymour Lawrence), 1968
Theme: Colors

Sample phrase: "But where is the green parrot?"

Book: Bill Martin, Jr. *Polar Bear, Polar Bear What Do You Hear?* (Henry Holt Co.), 1991
Theme: Zoo animals
Sample phrase: "What do you hear?"

Book: Bill Martin, Jr. *Brown Bear, Brown Bear What Do You See?* (Henry Holt Co.), 1967
Theme: Colors and animals
Sample phrase: "X What do you see?"

Book: Margot Zemach, *The Little Red Hen* (folk tale) (Farrar, Straus, & Giroux), 1983
Theme: Flour—fowl planting a grain of wheat to make a loaf of bread
Sample phrase: "Who will (action) this (object)?"
              "Who will harvest this wheat?"
              "Who will plant this wheat?"

Book: Masayki Yabuuchi. *Whose Footprints?* (Philomel Books), 1940
Theme: Animals
Sample phrase: "Whose are they?"

Book: Margaret Wise Brown. *Where Have You Been?* (Scholastic TAB Publishing), 1952
Theme: Animals
Sample phrase: "Where have you been?"

Book: Janet Slater Redhead. *The Strange Loud Noise* (Scholastic TAB Publishing)
Theme: Suspense
Sample phrase: "What is that strange loud noise?"

Book: Robert Kraus. *Whose Mouse Are You?* (Scholastic TAB Publishing), 1970
Theme: Family
Sample phrase: "Where is your x?"

Book: Janet and Allan Ahlberg. *Peek-A-Boo* (Penguin Books), 1981
Theme: View of a baby's world
Sample phrase: "What does he see?"

Book: Brenda Parkes. *Who's in the Shed?* (Rigby Education)
Theme: Animals
Sample phrase: "Who's in the shed?"

Book: June Melser and Joy Cowley. *Yes Ma'am* (Shortland Publishing)
Theme: Animals

Sample phrase: "What did you feed my x?"
                "How did you feed my x?"

Book: Masayki Yabuuchi. *Whose Baby Is It?* (Philomel Books), 1940
Theme: Animals
Sample phrase: "Whose baby is it?"

Book: Jean Marzollo and Jerry Pinkney. *Pretend You're a Cat* (Dial Books for Young Readers), 1990
Theme: Animals
Sample phrase: "Who else can you do like a x?"

Book: Margaret Miller. *Who Uses This?* (Greenwillow Books), 1990
Theme: Naming
Sample phrase: "Who uses this?"

Book: Robert Lopshire. *ABC Games* (Thomas Y. Crowell), 1986
Theme: Alphabets and naming
Sample phrase: "Which one will x?"
                "Where is the x?"

Book: Paul Galdone. *Henny Penny* (folk tale) (Ticknor and Fields), 1968
Theme: Animals fear, the sky is falling
Sample phrase: "Where are you going?"

Book: Joy Cowley. *Who Will Be My Mother?* (Shortland Publishing)
Theme: Animals
Sample phrase: "Who will be my mother?"

Book: Joy Cowley. *The Monster Party* (Shortland Publishing)
Theme: Action words
Sample phrase: "What can this little monster do?"

Book: Robert Kalan. *Jump Frog Jump* (Greenwillow Books)
Theme: Pond life
Sample phrase: "How did the frog get away?"

Book: Yoshi. *Who's Hiding Here?* (Picture Book Studio), 1987
Theme: Animals
Sample phrase: "Who's hiding here?"

Book: Nicki Weiss. *Where Does the Brown Bear Go?* (Greenwillow Books), 1989
Theme: Animals
Sample phrase: "Where does the x go?"

Book: Sue Williams. *I Went Walking* (Harcourt, Brace, and Jovanovich Publishing), 1989
Theme: Colors and animals
Sample phrase: "What did you see?"

Book: Pamella Allen. *Who Sank the Boat?* (Coward-McCann, Inc.), 1982
Theme: Animals and boating
Sample phrase: "Who sank the boat?"

Book: Mercer Mayer. *What Do You Do?* (Scholastic Magazines)
Theme: Ridiculous situations
Sample phrase: "What do you do?"

Book: Ann Rockwell. *In Our House* (Thomas Y. Crowell), 1985
Theme: Naming objects and actions
Sample phrase: "What do we do?"

Book: Robert Lopshire. *Put Me in the Zoo* (Random House), 1960
Theme: Imaginary animals
Sample phrase: "What can you do?"

II. Yes/No Questions

Book: Eric Carle. *The Very Busy Spider* (Philomel Books), 1984
Theme: Animals
Sample phrase: "Want to (action) in the (location)?"
            "Want to run in the meadow?"
            "Want to roll in the mud?"

Book: Masayki Yabuuchi. *Whose Footprints?* (Philomel Books), 1940
Theme: Animals
Sample phrase: "Can you guess?"

Book: Jean Marzollo and Jerry Pinkney. *Pretend You're a Cat* (Dial Books for Young Readers), 1990
Theme: Animals
Sample phrase: "Can you x?" (action verb)

Book: Nancy Hellen. *The Bus Stop* (Orchard Books), 1988
Theme: Waiting
Sample phrase: "Can you see the bus yet?"

Book: P. D. Eastman. *Are You My Mother?* (Random House), 1960
Theme: Baby bird's search for his mother
Sample phrase: "Are you my mother?"

Book: Rose Greydanus. *Double Trouble* (Troll Associates), 1981
Theme: Boy's mischief
Sample phrase: "Was it Tim?" "Was it Jim?"

Book: Shigeo Watanabe. *Where's My Daddy?* (Philomel Books), 1982
Theme: Searching
Sample phrase: "Have you seen my daddy?"

III. Do Insertion

Book: Dr. Seuss. *Green Eggs and Ham* (Random House), 1960
Theme: Try something new
Sample phrase: "Do you like them?"

Book: Stan and Jan Berenstain. *The Spooky Old Tree* (Random House), 1978
Theme: Suspense
Sample phrase: "Do they dare____?"

Book: June Melser and Joy Cowley. *Yes Ma'am* (Shortland Publishing)
Theme: Animals
Sample phrase: "Did you feed my x?"

Book: Shigeo Watanabe. *How Do I Put It On?* (Philomel Books), 1977
Theme: Clothing
Sample phrase: "Do I put them on like this?"

Book: Mary Serfozo. *Who Said Red* (MacMillan), 1988
Theme: Colors
Sample phrase: "Did you say x?"

NEGATIVES

I. Uncontracted Negatives

Book: Dr. Seuss. *Green Eggs and Ham* (Random House), 1960
Theme: Try something new
Sample phrase: "I do not like them."

Book: Mirra Ginsburg. *Four Brave Sailors* (Greenwillow books), 1987
Theme: Fear
Sample phrase: "They do not fear."

Book: Janet Slater Redhead. *The Strange Loud Noise* (Scholastic TAB Publishing)
Theme: Suspense
Sample phrase: "That noise is not x."

II. Contracted Negatives

Book: Charles G. Shaw. *It Looked Like Spilt Milk* (Harper and Row), 1974
Theme: Animals
Sample phrase: "It wasn't x."

Book: Eric Carle. *The Very Busy Spider* (Philomel Books), 1984
Theme: Animals
Sample phrase: "The spider didn't answer."

Book: Marilyn Sadler. *It's Not Easy Being a Bunny* (Random House), 1983
Theme: Animals
Sample phrase: "I don't want to be a x."

Book: Paul Galdone. *The Gingerbread Boy* (folk tale) (Clarion Books)
Theme: Gingerbread boy eludes the hungry grasp of everyone until he meets the fox
Sample phrase: "They couldn't x."
            "You can't x."

Book: Joy Cowley. *Who Will Be My Mother?* (Shortland Publishing)
Theme: Animals
Sample phrase: "I can't x."

Book: Joy Cowley and June Melser. *Hair Bear* (Shortland Publishing)
Theme: What is making the noise?
Sample phrase: "I don't care."

Book: Joy Cowley. *The Monster Party* (Shortland Publishing)
Theme: Action words
Sample phrase: "I can't."

Book: Uri Shuleintz. *One Sunday Morning* (Aladdin Books), 1967
Theme: Adventure
Sample phrase: "But I wasn't home?"

PREPOSITIONS

Book: Atsuko Morozunu. *One Gorilla* (Farrar, Straus, & Giroux), 1990
Theme: Numbers and animals
Sample phrase: N/A. Each page has a different group of animals in a new location
which is preceded by a different preposition.

Book: Ruth Brown. *A Dark Dark Tale* (Dial Books)
Theme: Suspense

Sample phrase: "In the woods there was a house."
             "On the house there was a door."
             "Behind the house there _____."

Book: Ed Emberly. *Klippity Klop* (Little Brown), 1974
Theme: A knight's adventure
Sample phrase: "Across the field."
              "Through the field."
              "Over the bridge."

Book: Phyllis Bartel. *Cat and Mouse* (Riverside Publishing Co.)
Theme: Cat and mouse running through the house
Sample phrase: "From the attic."
              "Around the flower pot."
              "Over the chairs."

Book: Ann Herbert Scott. *On Mother's Lap* (McGraw-Hill), 1972
Theme: Sharing mother's affection
Sample phrase: Approximately every third sentence includes the phrase "On Mother's lap."

Book: Stan and Jan Berenstain. *The Spooky Old Tree* (Random House), 1978
Theme: Suspense
Sample phrase: "One with a light."
              "One with a rope."
              "One with a stick."

Book: Stan and Jan Berenstain. *Bears in the Night* (Random House), 1971
Theme: Suspense
Sample phrase: "Under the bridge."
              "Around the lake."
              "Between the rocks."

Book: Robert Kalan. *Jump Frog Jump* (Greenwillow Books)
Theme: Pond life
Sample phrase: "Under the fly."
              "After the frog."
              "Into the pond."

Book: Pat Hutchins. *Rosie's Walk* (MacMillan)
Theme: Animal's walk
Sample phrase: "Around the lake."
              "Through the fence."

PRONOUNS

Book: Bill Martin, Jr. *Brown Bear Brown Bear What Do You See?* (Henry Holt Co.), 1967
Theme: Colors and animals
Sample phrase: "I see x looking at me."

Book: Eric Carle. *The Very Busy Spider* (Philomel Books), 1984
Theme: Animals
Sample phrase: "She was very busy."

Book: Eric Carle. *The Very Hungry Caterpillar* (Philomel Books)
Theme: Food, numbers, and days of the week
Sample phrase: "But he was still hungry."

Book: Eric Carle. *The Very Quiet Cricket* (Philomel Books), 1990
Theme: Insects
Sample phrase: "The little cricket wanted to answer, so he rubbed his wings together, but nothing happened."

Book: Masayki Yabuuchi. *Whose Are They* (Philomel Books), 1940
Theme: Animals
Sample phrase: "They belong to (animal)."

Book: Masayki Yabuuchi. *Whose Baby is it?* (Philomel Books), 1940
Theme: Animals
Sample phrase: "It belongs to (animal)."

Book: Robert Kraus. *Herman the Helper* (Prentice-Hall Books), 1974
Theme: Family members
Sample phrase: "He helped his (family member)."
                 "He helped the (person)."

Book: Joy Cowley. *Who Will Be My Mother?* (Shortland Publishing)
Theme: Animals
Sample phrase: "I am x."
                 "I can't x."

Book: Ann Herbert. *On Mother's Lap* (McGraw-Hill), 1972
Theme: Sharing mother's affection
Sample phrase: "Back and forth, back and forth they rocked."

Book: Janet and Allan Ahlberg. *Peek-A-Boo* (Penguin Books), 1981
Theme: View of a baby's world
Sample phrase: "He sees his x."

Book: Nicki Weiss. *Where Does the Brown Bear Go?* (Greenwillow Books), 1989
Theme: Animals
Sample phrase: "They are on their way home."

I. Reflexive Pronouns

Book: Margot Zemach, *The Little Red Hen* (folk tale) (Farrar, Straus, & Giroux), 1983
Theme: Flour—fowl planting a grain of wheat to make a loaf of bread
Sample phrase: "Then I'll do it myself,' said the little red hen."

Book: Janet Slater Redhead. *The Strange Loud Noise* (Scholastic TAB Publishing)
Theme: Suspense
Sample phrase: "I'll find out myself."

II. Possessive Pronouns

Book: Eric Carle. *The Very Quiet Cricket* (Philomel Books), 1990
Theme: Insects
Sample phrase: "The little cricket wanted to answer, so he rubbed his wings together, but nothing happened."

Book: Bill Martin and John Auchambault. *Here Are My hands* (Henry Holt), 1985
Theme: Body parts
Sample phrase: "Here are my (body parts) for (verb) ing and (verb) ing."

Book: P. D. Eastman. *Are You My Mother?* (Random House), 1960
Theme: Baby bird looking for his mother
Sample phrase: "Are you my mother?"

Book: Joy Cowley. *Who Will Be My Mother?* (Shortland Publishing)
Theme: Animals
Sample phrase: "Who will be my mother?"

Book: Robert Kraus. *Whose Mouse Are You?* (Scholastic), 1970
Theme: Family
Sample phrase: "Who is your x?"

Source: Used with permission from Ratner, N. B., Parker, B., & Gardner, P. (1993). Joint bookreading as a language scaffolding activity for communicatively impaired children. *Seminar in Speech and Language, 14*(4), 296–313. © Thieme Medical Publishers.

Troubleshooting Technology

HEARING AIDS

Prior to troubleshooting note the following:

- Style of the child's hearing aid(s) (e.g., BTE, ITE)
- Type of hearing aid (e.g., analog, digital, transpositional)/make and model
- Battery size (e.g., 675, 13)
- Consistency of use
- Information on how to contact the audiologist

Equipment needed for troubleshooting kit:

- A picture of a hearing aid with the parts labeled
- A battery tester
- Hearing aid stethoscope
- Spare batteries
- Earmold air blower
- Brushes, wire loop (for removing wax)
- Antibacterial hand sanitizer and Audioclenz pads

Visual Check

1. Turn **off** the hearing aid and remove it from the child's ear.
2. Inspect the **earmold.** Check for any wax in the canal end of the mold. If wax can be seen in the opening of the earmold, remove it with the **wire loop.**
3. Examine the **tubing** leading from the earmold to the tone hook. If there are any cracks in the tubing or the tubing is yellow or brittle, it needs to be replaced.

4. Examine the **tone hook.** A cracked tone hook will cause acoustic feedback.
5. Inspect the hearing aid. Look for cracks in the **case** or other signs of abuse.
6. Check the **controls** on the hearing. If the hearing aid has a volume control, be sure that it is at the appropriate setting. Make sure the hearing aid is set on the "M" when the child is using it.
7. Look at the **battery compartment.** (There may be a battery lock on the compartment. You will have to open the lock to check the battery/or the battery compartment.) Be sure the battery is properly inserted and that there is no corrosion on the battery or inside the compartment.
8. Check the **battery.** Remove the battery, place it in the appropriate slot of a battery tester, and check according to tester instructions. If the indicator on the tester says the battery is dead, replace the battery with a new one.

Listening Check

1. Place the stethoscope in your ear and put the tip of the earmold into the rubber tip of the stethoscope. Set the volume control to the lowest setting and turn the aid on (for most hearing aids "M" stands for microphone, which means the aid is on). Rotate the volume control up and down. Using running speech, talk into the microphone and listen for a steady increase in loudness as the volume is raised. Note that some digital hearing aids do not have a volume control. They have a set volume level.
2. While listening through the aid, rotate the volume control up and down while you say the Ling Six-Sound Test (ah, ee, oo, s, sh, m). Listen for the clarity. There should not be any crackling, buzzing, or hissing sound, cutting in or out, or any dead spots.
3. Shake the hearing aid gently and tap on the case to see if the aid cuts off.
4. Performing a listening check daily will allow you to become accustomed to the sound of the child's hearing aid. It will then be easier to note any change in the sound quality, which could signal a malfunction.

Behavioral Check

1. Place the hearing aid on the child with it set on "M" and the volume level set where she/he regularly uses it.
2. Make sure the earmold is properly inserted and there is no feedback. If the earmold is inserted properly, but you still hear feedback:
   —Take the earmold out of the child's ear.
   —Turn the volume of the aid all the way up.
   —Put your finger over the canal end of the earmold. If the feedback stops, the earmold is too small for the child and will need to be remade.
3. Using running speech, talk to the child to determine the level at which she/he can detect the presence of your voice. If the child is unable to

detect your voice while you are speaking at a loud conversational level, discontinue the behavioral check and go back and check the hearing aid.

4. Present the Ling Six Sound Test using auditory cues alone. (You can cover your mouth with an acoustic screen, have the child close her/his eyes so she/he can't speechread, or stand behind the child.) Present the sounds in random order, varying the time between presentations. Ask the child to raise her/his hand each time she/he hears a sound.

ASSISTIVE LISTENING DEVICES

Visual Check

Transmitter:

1. Is the transmitter on and set appropriately (e.g., correct frequency for frequency modulation [FM])?
2. Are the microphone and microphone cord in good working order?
3. Is the battery charged?

Receiver:

1. Is the receiver on and set appropriately?
2. Is the receiver on the correct frequency (FM)?
3. Is the hearing aid in good working order and coupled to the receiver appropriately (direct audio input [DAI], neckloop)?
4. Is the battery charged?
5. Is the DAI cord plugged into the hearing aid; is the cord broken?
6. Is the audio shoe/boot attached to the hearing aid (for DAI) correctly?
7. Is the patch cord plugged into the cochlear implant processor; is the cord broken?
8. Is the FM receiver case cracked?

Listening Check/Behavioral Check

- Check the child's hearing aid using the above procedure.
- If the child's hearing aid is functioning normally, couple it to the assistive listening device (e.g., FM receiver) via DAI or neckloop.
- Connect the hearing aid to the stethoscope.
- If the child is using a neckloop to couple the hearing aid to the assistive listening device, be sure the hearing aid is set on "T" or "MT".
- If the child is using direct DAI coupled to the assistive listening device, be sure the hearing aid is set on "M".
- Perform the hearing aid listening check (above) by talking into the microphone connected to the transmitter.
- Perform the hearing aid behavioral check by talking into the microphone of the transmitter. Stand at a distance from the child. You may also want to add background noise.

COCHLEAR IMPLANTS

Before troubleshooting note the following:

1. The type of cochlear implant:
   - Advanced Bionics
   - Cochlear Corporation
   - Medical Electronics
2. Speech processor settings:

   - volume: _____

   - sensitivity: _____
3. Program settings:

   #1_____

   #2_____

   #3_____

   #4_____
4. Information on how to contact the cochlear implant center and "mapping" audiologist

Systems Check

Obtain information about the specific implant system from the child's audiologist or from the manufacturer.

Program/Map Check

Because you cannot listen to a cochlear implant, it is important that you do a behavioral listening check daily. This can be done in the same manner that you do a hearing aid behavioral check. Using the Ling Six Sounds present each sound (with auditory cues only) and check to see if the child can detect and/or identify each sound. The child should be able to detect and/or identify all six sounds. Record the child's responses and use this information as a baseline. If there is any change in the child's performance, it may indicate a need to have the program/map checked.

Behavioral Observations/Changes

In addition to the above listening check, it is important to document any change in the child's behavior that might suggest the need for Program/MAP adjustments. The following are behaviors to look for:

1. Gradual reduction in distance listening
2. Child consistently alters sensitivity setting by more than 2 numeric levels
3. Increased requests for repetition or use of "What?" or "Huh?"

4. "Slushy" production of formerly mastered speech sounds
5. Emergence of persistent disruptive or withdrawn behavior
6. Diminished response to environmental sounds
7. Change in frequency of vocalization, voice quality, and/or vocal intensity
8. Omission or confusion of consonants that were formerly present and discriminable
9. Neutralized vowel production
10. Presence of physical symptoms such as an eye or facial muscle twitch

REFERENCES

Brasham, J. (2001). *Update on cochlear implant technology for the educational audiologist.* Presented in Columbia, MD, October 19, 2001.

Compton, C. L. (2000). *Assistive technology for receptive communication.* Annapolis, MD: Single-handed Productions.

Estabrooks, W. (Ed.). (1994). *Auditory-verbal therapy.* Washington, DC: The Alexander Graham Bell Association for the Deaf.

Johnson, C. D., Benson, P. V., Seaton, J. B. (1997). *Educational audiology handbook.* Clifton Park, NY: Singular.

Koch, M. (1998). *Bringing sound to life: Principles and practices of cochlear implant rehabilitation.* Baltimore, MD: York Press.

Ross. M. (1996). Pediatric amplification: Use and adjustment. In F. N. Martin and J. G. Clark (Eds.). *Hearing care for children* (pp. 233–248). Boston: Allyn & Bacon.

COCHLEAR IMPLANT MANUFACTURERS

Advanced Bionics/Clarion System
Mann Biomedical Park
25129 Rye Canyon Loop
Valencia, CA 91355
(800) 678-2575 (V)
(800) 678-3575 (TTY)
E-mail: hear@advancedbionics.com
Web: www.advancedbionics.com

Cochlear Americas/Nucleus System
400 Inverness Parkway, Suite 400
Englewood, CO 80112
(800) 523-5798 (V/TTY)
(303) 792-9025 (fax)
E-mail: info@cochlear.com
Web: http://www.cochlear.com

MED-EL Corporation
2222 East Highway. 54 Beta Building, Suite 180
Durham, NC 27713
(888) 633-3524
(919) 572-2222 (V/TTY)
(919) 484-9229 (fax)

AUDITORY LEARNING RESOURCES

Anderson, K. L., & Smaldino, J. J. (1998). *Listening Inventories for Education (L.I.F.E)*. Available from Educational Audiology Association, 4319 Ehrlich Road, Tampa, FL 33624; (800) 460–7322.

Estabrooks, W. (1994). *Auditory-verbal therapy for teachers and parents*. Washington, D.C.: Alexander Graham Bell Association for the Deaf.

Firszt, J. & Reeder, R. (1996). *Guide for Optimizing Auditory Learning Skills (GOALS)*.

Glendonald School for the Deaf Auditory Screening Procedure (GASP). (1982). In Erber, N. *Auditory training*. Washington, DC: Alexander Graham Bell Association for the Deaf.

Koch, M. (1998). *Bringing Sound to Life: Principles and Practices of Cochlear Implant Rehabilitation; Word Associations for Syllable Perception (WASP)*. Available from Advanced Bionics, 25129 Rye Canyon Loop, Valencia, CA 91355; (800) 678-2575.

Maxwell, M. J. (1981). *Listening games for elementary grades*. Washington, DC: Acropolis Books.

Moog, J., Biedenstein, J., & Davidson, L. (1995). *Speech Perception Instructional Curriculum and Evaluation (SPICE)*. Available from Central Institute for the Deaf, 818 South Euclid Avenue, St. Louis, MO 63110.

Robbins, A. M., & Osberger, M. J. (1990). *Meaningful Auditory Integration Scale (MAIS)*. Indianapolis: Indiana University School of Medicine. Available from Advanced Bionics, 25129 Rye Canyon Loop, Valencia, CA 91355; (800) 678-2575.

Sound Tracks & Animal Sound Tracks. Lotto Games and Cassettes. Cambridge, UK: Living and Learning.

Stout, G. G., & Windle, J. V. (1992). *Developmental Approach to Successful Listening (DASL)*. Available from: Resource Point, 61 Inverness Drive East, Englewood, CO 80112.

Waddy-Smith, B. (1998). *Kendall School Preschool Auditory and Speechreading Skills Inventory*. Washington, DC: The Laurent Clerc National Deaf Education Center.

Communication Access Resources

RESOURCES

Auditory Processing Disorders

Auditory Processing Disorders in Children. (1999). *Journal of American Academy of Audiology, 10*(6).

Billis, T. J. (2002). *When the brain can't hear.* New York: Pocket Books.

Billis, T. J. (1996). *Assessment and management of central auditory processing disorders in the educational setting.* Clifton Park, NY: Singular.

Chermak, G. D., and Musiek, F. E. (1997). *Central auditory processing disorders: New perspectives.* Clifton Park, NY: Singular.

Foli, K. J. (2002). *Like sound through water: A mother's journey through auditory processing disorder.* New York: Pocket Books.

Masters, G. M. (1998). *Central auditory processing Disorders.* Boston: Allyn & Bacon.

Communication Technologies

Manufacturers of Auditory, Alerting, and Telecommunication Technologies

Ameriphone, Inc.

12082 Western Avenue, Garden Grove, CA 92841

(800) 874-3005

(714) 897-0808

(714) 897-4703 (f)

Email: ameriphone@ameriphone.com

Web: www.ameriphone.com

Auditech
P.O. Box 821105
Vicksburg, MS 39182-1105
(318) 574-8170
(318) 574-8178 (tty)
(318) 574-8173 (f)
Email: info@auditechusa.com
Web: www.auditechusa.com

Audiotech Healthcare Corporation
#760 175 Second Avenue
Kamloops, BC
Canada, V2C 5W1
(250) 372-5847
(888) 590-3555 (250) 372-3859 (f)
Email: info@audiotech.org
Web: www.audiotech.org/index.php

Audex
710 Standard Street
Longview, TX 75601
(800) 237-0716
Email: cbeatty@audex.com
Web: www.audex.com

AVR Sonovation, Inc.
7636 Executive Drive, Eden Prairie, MN 55344
(953) 934-3111
(800) 426-8336
(952) 934-3033 (f)
Email: sono@avrsono.com
Web: www.arvsono.com/

COMTEK Communications Technology, Inc.
357 West 2700 South
Salt Lake City, UT 84115
(801) 466-3463
(800) 496-3463
(801) 484-6906 (f)
Email: service@comtek.com
Web: www.comtek.com/index.html

Effective Communication Consultants, Inc.
1030 Clubhouse Dr.
Independence, KY 41051
(800) 838-1649 (v,tty)

(859) 371-9203 (v,tty)
(859) 371-1363 (f)
Email: custserv@beyondhearingaids.com
Web: www.beyondhearingaids.com

Interactive Solutions
iCommunicator
6448 Parkland Drive
Sarasota FL 34243
(941) 753-5000
(800) 362-4584 (tty)
Web: www.myicommunicator.com

Oval Window Audio
33 Wild Flower Court
Nederland, CO 80466
(303) 447-3607 (v/tty)
Email: paula@ovalwindowaudio.com
Web: www.ovalwindowaudio.com/index.html

Phonak
P.O. Box 3017
Naperville, IL 60566
(800) 777-7333
(888) 777-7316
Web: www.phonak.com

Phone TTY, Inc.
1246 Route 46 West
Parsippany, NJ 07054-2121
(888) 332-3889
(973) 299-6627
(973) 299-6626 (tty)
Email: phonetty@aol.com
Web: www.phone-tty.com

Phonic Ear, Inc.
3880 Cypress Drive
Petaluma, CA 94954-7600
(800) 227-0735
Web: www.phonicear.com

Plantronics/Walker equipment
345 Encinal Street
Santa Cruz, CA 95060

(800) 544-4660
(831) 426-5858
(831) 426-6098
Web: www.plantronics.com

Radio Shack
300 One Tandy Center
Fort Worth, TX 76102
Web: www.radioshack.com

Sennheiser Electronic Corporation
1 Enterprise Drive
Old Lyme, CT 06371
(860) 434-9190
(860) 434-1759 (f)
Web: www.wennheiser.com

Silent Call Corporation
4581 S. Lapeer Road Suite F
Lake Orion, MI 48359
(800) 572-5227 (v/tty)
(248) 377-4700 (v/tty)
(248) 377-4168 (f)
Email: silentcall@ameritech.net
Web: www.silent-call.com

Sonic Alert, Inc.
1050 East Maple Road
Troy, MI 48083
(248) 577-5400 (v/tty)
Email: sonic-info@sonicalert.com
Web: www.sonicalert.com

Telex Communication, Inc.
12000 Portland Avenue South
Burnsville, MN 55337
(952) 884-4051
(952) 884-0043 (f)
Email: info@telex.com
Web: www.telex.com

Ultratec, Inc.
450 Science Drive
Madison, WI 53711
(608) 238-5400

(608) 238-3008 (f)
Email: service@ultratec.com
Web: www.ultratec.com

Unitron Industrues, Inc
2300 Berkshire Lane North
Plymouth, MN 55441
(763) 744-3300
(800) 888-8882
(763) 557-8828 (f)
Email: paul.giffin@unitronhearing.com
Web: www.unitron.com

Wheelock, Inc.
273 Branchport Avenue
Long Branch, NJ 07740
(800) 613-2148
(732) 222-8707
Email: info@wheelockinc.com
Web: www.wheelockinc.com

Whelen Engineering Company
Route 145 Winthrop Road
Chester, CT 06412-0684
(860) 526-9504
(860) 526-4078 (f)
Email: whelen@connix.com
Web: www.whelen.com

Williams Sound Corporation
10399 West 70th Street
Eden Prairie, MN 55344-3459 USA
(800) 328-6190
(952) 943-2252
(952) 943-9675 (tty)
(952) 943-2174 (f)
Web: www.williamssound.com

Wynd Communications Corporation
75 Higuera Street, Suite 240
San Luis Obispo, CA 93401
(800) 549-9800 (v)
(800) 549-2800 (tty)
(805) 781-6001 (f)
Email: wyndtell@wynd.com
Web: www.wyndtell.com

Internet (IP) Telephone Services

AT&T
>http://www.relaycall.com/vrs/

Communication Services of the Deaf (CSD)
>http://www.usavrs.com/USAVRSHome.asp

Sprint
>http://www.sprintbiz.com/government/relay/internet.html

WordCom
>http://www.ip-relay.com/calloptions.html

Internet-based, Live Text Communication

Nextalk.net
>http://www.nextalk.net/index.stm

Online Interpreting

Deaf-Talk
>http://www.deaf-talk.com

Communication Services of the Deaf (CSD)
>http://www.c-s-d.org

Information Resources and National Support Organizations

Laurent Clerc National Deaf Education Center
Gallaudet University
800 Florida Avenue, NE
Washington, D.C. 20002
(202) 651-5000
Web: http://clerccenter.gallaudet.edu

Boys Town National Research Hospital (BTNRH)
555 North 30th Street
Omaha, NE 68131
(402) 498-6511
Email: moeller@boystown.org
Web: www.boystown.org/btnrh

Alexander Graham Bell Association for the Deaf, Inc.
3417 Volta Place, NW
Washington, DC 20007
(202) 337-5220 (v/tty)
(202) 337-8314 (f)
Email: agbell2@aol.com
Web: www.agbell.org

American Academy of Audiology
8201 Greensboro Drive, Suite 300
McLean, VA 22102
(800) 222-2336 (v/tty)
(703) 610-9022 (v/tty)
(703) 610-9005 (f)
Email: molek@audiology.org
Web: www.audiology.com

American Society for Deaf Children
1820 Tribute Road, Suite A
Sacramento, CA 95815
(800) 942-ASDC (v/tty)
(916) 614-6084 (v/tty)
(916) 641-6085 (f)
Email: ASDCI@aol.com
Web: www.deafchildren.org

American Speech-Language-Hearing Association
10801 Rockville Pike
Rockville, MD 20852
(800) 638-8255 (v/tty)
(301) 897-7355 (f)
Email: actioncenter@asha.org
Web: www.asha.org

Auditory-Verbal International, Inc.
2121 Eisenhower Avenue, Suite 402
Alexandria, VA 22314
(703) 739-1049 (v)
(703) 739-0874 (tty)
Email: avi@auditory-verbal.org
Web: www.audiotryverbal.org

BEGINNINGS for Parents of Children Who are Deaf or Hard of Hearing, Inc.
P.O. Box 17646
Raleigh, NC 27619
(800) 541-4327 (v/tty)
Email: info@beginningssvcs.com
Web: http://www.beginningssvcs.com/index.htm

Cochlear Implant Association, Inc.
5335 Wisconsin Avenue, NW Suite 440
Washington, DC 20015-2034
(202) 895-2781 (v/tty)

Email: pwms.cici@worlknet.att.net
Web: www.cici.org

National Association of the Deaf
814 Thayer Avenue
Silver Spring, MD 20910-4500
(301) 587-1788 (v)
(301) 587-1789 (tty)
(301) 587-1791 (f)
Email: nadinfo@nad.org
Web: www.nad.org

National Cued Speech Association
23970 Hermitage Road
Shaker Heights, OH 44122
(800) 459-3529
Web: www.cuedspeech.org

National Information Center for Children and Youth with Disabilities (NICHCY)
P.O. Box 1429
Washington, DC 20013
(800) 695-0285 (v/tty)
(202) 884-8200 (v/tty)
(202) 884-8441 (f)
Email: nichy@aed.org
Web: www.nichcy.org/

National Institute on Deafness and Other Communication Disorders Information Clearinghouse
1 Communication Avenue
Bethesda, MD 20892-3456
(800) 241-1044 (v)
(800) 241-1055 (tty)
(301) 907-8830 (f)
Email: nidcdinfo@nidcd.nih.gov
Web: www.nih.gov.nidcd

Self Help for Hard of Hearing People
7910 Woodmont Avenue, Suite 1200
Bethesda, MD 20814
(301) 657-2248 (v)
(301) 657-2249 (tty)
(301) 913-9413 (f)
Email: national@shhh.org
Web: www.shhh.org

Familiarity and Transparency Ratings for 100 Idioms*

	Familiarity		Transparency	
	Adolescents	*Adults*	*Adolescents*	*Adults*
1. Beat around the bush	1.30	1.15	2.40	2.85
2. Bet one's bottom dollar	1.90	1.90	1.50	2.30
3. Blow off some steam	1.30	1.40	1.85	1.55
4. Blow one's own horn	2.00	1.55	2.25	2.85
5. Blow the cobwebs away	2.80	3.15	2.15	2.55
6. Blow the lid off	2.35	2.10	2.25	2.60
7. Breathe down one's neck	1.50	1.55	1.95	2.05
8. Bring home the bacon	1.35	1.30	2.10	2.20
9. Bring the house down	2.05	1.70	2.30	2.85
10. Cast the first stone	2.65	1.55	1.55	1.70
11. Comes home to roost	2.70	2.85	2.60	2.80
12. Cross swords with someone	3.10	3.35	1.85	2.20

	Familiarity		Transparency	
	Adolescents	*Adults*	*Adolescents*	*Adults*
13. Cut down to size	1.90	1.80	2.25	2.69
14. Draw a long breath	2.90	3.55	1.45	1.05
15. Get away with murder	1.60	1.05	1.55	1.50
16. Get off the ground	2.50	2.00	2.20	2.20
17. Get off the hook	2.00	2.05	1.70	1.85
18. Get the ball rolling	1.95	1.80	1.75	2.15
19. Get the lead out	1.85	1.80	2.75	2.90
20. Gets in one's hair	2.10	1.75	2.05	2.65
21. Gets under one's skin	1.70	1.55	2.15	2.05
22. Give someone enough rope	3.25	2.95	1.85	2.25
23. Give up the ship	3.20	3.30	1.95	1.95
24. Go against the grain	2.69	1.50	2.50	2.65
25. Go around in circles	1.45	1.35	2.05	2.15
26. Go by the board	3.75	4.10	2.70	3.00
27. Go by the book	1.60	1.30	1.15	1.15
28. Go into one's shell	3.05	2.45	1.70	1.70
29. Go through the mill	3.60	3.10	2.60	2.55
30. Go through the motions	2.35	1.70	1.90	1.65
31. Go through the roof	1.75	2.30	2.15	2.70
32. Go to the dogs	2.75	2.55	2.55	3.00
33. Hang by a thread	1.60	1.70	1.60	2.05
34. Hang on one's coat-tails	3.45	2.80	2.35	2.50
35. Haul over the coals	3.45	3.00	2.20	2.35
36. Have a hollow ring	4.00	3.55	2.40	2.60
37. Have a soft spot	1.95	1.25	2.05	2.65
38. Hit below the belt	1.70	1.45	2.05	2.40
39. Hoe one's own row	4.35	3.55	2.65	2.45
40. Hold one's head up	1.95	1.45	1.80	1.85
41. Jump through a hoop	3.30	2.05	2.30	2.65
42. Keep one's chin up	1.45	1.30	1.75	2.05
43. Keep one's nose clean	1.70	1.90	2.30	2.90
44. Keep one's shirt on	1.60	1.65	2.35	2.80
45. Keep the pot boiling	3.40	3.75	2.00	2.20
46. Keep under one's hat	2.35	2.10	1.60	1.80
47. Keep up one's end	2.75	2.20	1.85	1.60
48. Kick up one's heels	1.95	1.55	2.20	2.20
49. Lay at one's door	3.75	3.80	2.35	2.65
50. Lead with one's chin	4.15	3.75	2.65	2.95
51. Leave the door open	2.25	2.30	2.35	2.40

	Familiarity		Transparency	
	Adolescents	Adults	Adolescents	Adults
52. Let one's hair down	1.80	1.20	2.00	2.45
53. Make one's hair curl	2.60	2.10	2.45	2.90
54. Make the fur fly	3.60	3.30	2.35	2.45
55. Paddle one's own canoe	3.45	3.35	1.65	1.75
56. Paint the town red	2.00	1.50	2.50	3.00
57. Paper over the cracks	4.25	4.30	2.00	1.80
58. Pick up the threads	3.70	3.40	2.60	2.80
59. Play one's cards well	2.20	1.85	1.90	2.00
60. Pull in one's belt	3.55	3.60	2.15	2.75
61. Pull up one's socks	3.95	4.20	2.80	2.95
62. Put one's foot down	1.20	1.10	2.10	2.75
63. Put their heads together	1.45	1.35	2.05	2.10
64. Put up the shutters	3.60	4.35	2.50	2.30
65. Read between the lines	1.15	1.35	2.20	2.40
66. Remain in the saddle	3.40	3.45	1.95	2.15
67. Rise to the bait	4.05	3.55	2.30	2.35
68. Roll up one's sleeves	2.55	2.00	1.84	2.25
69. Run circles around someone	1.65	1.80	2.55	2.85
70. Run out of steam	2.05	1.35	1.35	1.40
71. Sail against the wind	2.40	2.70	1.95	1.80
72. See beyond one's nose	3.30	2.95	1.90	2.00
73. Shake in one's shoes	1.75	1.70	1.90	2.00
74. Shoot from the hip	2.45	2.20	2.00	2.35
75. Sing a different tune	2.35	1.75	1.95	1.85
76. Sing for one's supper	3.75	2.45	2.10	2.25
77. Sit on one's hands	3.35	2.90	2.40	2.50
78. Skating on thin ice	1.30	1.30	1.35	1.55
79. Slip through one's fingers	1.85	1.80	2.05	2.45
80. Spread it on thick	1.75	1.85	2.25	2.65
81. Step into one's shoes	2.15	2.10	1.95	2.45
82. Strike the right note	2.95	2.25	1.95	1.90
83. Swear black is white	3.95	3.75	1.45	1.50
84. Swim against the tide	2.40	2.05	1.70	1.90
85. Take a back seat	2.50	1.95	2.40	2.75
86. Take a long view	3.30	3.45	1.85	1.90
87. Take down a peg	4.30	3.30	2.60	2.70
88. Take for a ride	2.30	1.90	2.65	2.90
89. Take under one's wing	2.20	1.55	1.55	1.70
90. Talk the same language	2.20	2.20	1.85	1.80

	Familiarity		Transparency	
	Adolescents	Adults	Adolescents	Adults
91. Talk through one's hat	4.70	3.70	2.70	2.80
92. Throw out of gear	3.20	3.65	2.25	2.50
93. Throw to the wolves	2.65	2.15	1.50	1.75
94. Turn back the clock	1.75	1.50	1.75	1.85
95. Turn the other cheek	1.35	1.20	1.95	1.90
96. Vote with one's feet	4.55	4.35	2.65	2.80
97. Walk the chalk line	3.30	4.35	2.20	2.60
98. Wave a white flag	2.50	2.35	2.20	2.20
99. Whistle in the dark	3.70	3.65	2.30	2.75
100. Wither on the vine	3.65	3.20	2.15	2.05
Mean (M)	2.60	2.38	2.09	2.29
Standard deviation (SD)	.91	.94	.35	.46
Range	1.15–4.70	1.05–4.35	1.15–2.80	1.05–3.00

Source: Reprinted with permission from Nippold, M. (1988). *Later language development: The school age and adolescent years* (pp. 118–120). Austin, TX: Pro-Ed.

Note: Some of the data are from "Familiarity and Transparency in Idiom Explanation: A Developmental Study of Children and Adolescents," by Marilyn A. Nippold and Mishelle Rudzinski, 1993, *Journal of Speech and Hearing Research, 36*, p. 733. Copyright 1993 by the American Speech-Language-Hearing Association. Adapted with permission.

*Familiarity is a measure of how often one has heard or read the idiom before: 1 = many times; 2 = several times; 3 = a few times; 4 = once; 5 = never.

Transparency is a measure of how closely the literal and nonliteral meanings of the idiom compare: 1 = closely related; 2 = somewhat related; 3 = not related.

Familiarity Ratings for 107 Proverbs*

	Adolescents	Adults
1. A bad broom leaves a dirty room.	1.40	1.10
2. A caged bird longs for the clouds.	1.55	1.30
3. A drowning man grabs at a straw.	1.48	2.53
4. A forced kindness deserves no thanks.	1.50	1.38
5. A golden key opens every door.	2.38	1.58
6. A good sailor likes a rough sea.	1.55	1.13
7. A leopard cannot change its spots.	3.20	4.18
8. A little bait catches a large fish.	1.85	1.90
9. A little spark can kindle a great fire.	2.93	2.38
10. A mouse may help a lion.	1.93	1.50
11. A peacock should look at its legs.	1.13	1.03
12. A rolling stone gathers no moss.	2.50	4.75
13. A small leak will sink a great ship.	2.50	2.63
14. A still river never finds the ocean.	1.55	1.18
15. A still tongue makes a wise head.	2.18	1.65

	Adolescents	Adults
16. A tree is known by its fruit.	2.33	3.18
17. A wonder lasts but nine days.	1.13	1.25
18. All bread is not baked in one oven.	1.85	1.20
19. An optimistic attitude is half of success.	1.85	1.95
20. Anger is never without reason.	2.13	1.65
21. Big fish eat little fish.	3.00	2.70
22. Big trees grow from little acorns.	1.85	3.35
23. Blame is safer than praise.	1.20	1.53
24. Blood is thicker than water.	4.48	4.78
25. Cleanliness is next to godliness.	2.93	4.85
26. Clothes do not make the man.	4.08	4.25
27. Courage is always safer than cowardice.	1.95	1.23
28. Crooked logs make a straight fire.	1.18	1.00
29. Democracy is better than tyranny.	2.30	2.30
30. Envy is destroyed by true friendship.	2.00	1.18
31. Even a blind hen sometimes finds a grain.	1.53	1.25
32. Even a monkey will fall from a tree.	1.70	1.13
33. Every bird is known by its feathers.	1.60	1.90
34. Every bird likes its own next best.	1.98	1.75
35. Every bird must hatch its own eggs.	1.78	1.10
36. Every cloud has a silver lining.	3.85	4.90
37. Every horse thinks its own pack heaviest.	1.88	1.30
38. Every oak must be an acorn.	1.75	2.45
39. Expectation is better than realization.	1.85	1.63
40. Falling raindrops will wear through a stone.	1.40	1.33
41. Fine feathers make fine birds.	2.00	1.45
42. Foresight is better than hindsight.	2.78	3.95
43. Forgiveness is better than revenge.	2.63	2.30
44. Gentle persuasion is better than force.	2.25	2.43
45. Gentleness skillfully subdues wrath.	1.63	1.13
46. Good fences make good neighbors	1.88	3.43
47. Goodness is better than beauty.	2.35	2.28
48. Gratitude is a heavy burden.	1.80	1.43
49. Great events have small beginnings.	2.55	2.70
50. Great trees keep down the little trees.	1.40	1.15
51. Half a loaf is better than no bread.	2.18	2.73
52. Harmony seldom makes a headline.	1.65	1.13
53. Humility often gains more than pride.	1.90	1.53
54. In idleness there is perpetual despair.	1.23	1.20
55. Intelligence is worth more than richness.	2.30	1.83

	Adolescents	Adults
56. Knowledge is better than wealth.	3.38	2.15
57. Little by little the bird builds its nest.	1.68	1.68
58. Little pitchers have big ears.	1.50	2.60
59. Little sticks kindle big fires.	2.03	1.78
60. Little streams make mighty rivers.	2.68	2.98
61. Loose teeth are better than no teeth.	1.55	1.25
62. Many eyes are upon the king.	1.65	1.40
63. Misfortunes may come in spite of watchfulness.	1.43	1.18
64. Newborn calves don't fear tigers.	1.10	1.00
65. No garden is without its weeds.	2.40	2.25
66. Of idleness comes no goodness.	1.55	1.83
67. One rotten apple spoils the barrel.	3.60	4.40
68. One saddle is enough for one house.	1.30	1.03
69. One stone does not make a wall.	1.75	1.50
70. Patience is the best virtue.	4.25	4.08
71. Persistence will accomplish more than force.	2.38	2.10
72. Quality is better than quantity.	4.48	4.58
73. Quarreling sparrows do not fear man.	1.10	1.00
74. Scalded cats fear even cold water.	1.75	1.10
75. Shared sorrow is half sorrow.	1.58	1.63
76. Sleeping cats catch no mice.	2.43	2.18
77. Sleeping foxes catch no poultry.	1.58	1.45
78. Small fish mingle with big fish.	1.38	1.30
79. Sorrow is born of excessive joy.	1.25	1.33
80 Sour grapes can never make sweet wine.	2.38	2.00
81. Success is first a dream.	2.48	1.75
82. The apple never falls far from the tree.	3.53	3.53
83. The bad workman always blames his tools.	1.85	2.03
84. The bait hides the hook.	2.18	1.30
85. The cat plays with the mouse.	3.33	2.30
86. The chickens give advice to the hen.	1.33	1.05
87. The crying baby gets the milk.	2.58	2.58
88. The early bird catches the worm.	4.65	4.95
89. The end justifies the means.	3.25	4.88
90. The pen is mightier than the sword.	3.83	4.75
91. The pot calls the kettle black.	2.80	4.43
92. The pretty shoe often pinches the foot.	1.90	1.40
93. The reddest apple has a worm in it.	2.50	1.55
94. The restless sleeper blames the bed.	1.50	1.25
95. The saddest dog sometimes wags its tail.	1.53	1.15

	Adolescents	Adults
96. The squeaking wheel gets the grease.	2.63	4.88
97. The tongue is more powerful than the sword.	2.88	3.35
98. The tongue is sharper than the sword.	3.55	3.63
99. The tongue wounds more than the arrow.	2.53	2.08
100. The truth is mightier than a lie.	4.03	3.43
101. The twigs are rarely better than the trunk.	1.10	1.20
102. There is no glory without sacrifice.	3.13	2.55
103. Tigers and deer do not stroll together.	1.33	1.03
104. Too many cooks spoil the broth.	2.33	4.73
105. Too much bed makes a dull head.	1.95	1.63
106. Two captains will sink a ship.	1.73	1.35
107. Two wrongs don't make a right.	4.95	4.98
Mean (M)	2.22	2.24
Standard deviation (SD)	.88	1.22
Range	1.10–4.95	1.00–4.98

Source: Reprinted with permission from Nippold, M. (1988). *Later language development: The school age and adolescent years* (pp. 134–136). Austin, TX: Pro-Ed.
*Familiarity is a measure of how often one has heard or read the proverb before: 1 = never; 2 = once; 3 = a few times; 4 = several times; 5 = many times. (Note that this scale is the reverse of the idiom familiarity scale in Appendix D.)

Pronunciation Skills Inventory

Directions:
Each item should receive a raw score (RS) indicating number of items correct, a percent score (number right out of total possible) as well as an inventory score (PSI) based on the following scale:

1 = Understands task, scores 85–100%
2 = Stimulated by example(s), score 85–100%
3 = Understands task, scores 21–84%
4 = Stimulated by example(s), scores 21–84%
5 = Does not understand task and/or not stimulable by example, scores 0–20%

Use Client Response Form for items with asterisks (*).

Clinician Note: The clinician should review the Clinician's Guide prior to administering the Pronunciation Skills Inventory. The Guide includes correct responses, protocols for administration, and normative data as well as rehabilitation directives. The Client Stimulus Form should be used to cue responses. The Client Profile Form should be used for clarification of test results.

PRONUNCIATION SKILLS INVENTORY
Clinician's Response Form

Client name: _____ ID/SSN: _____

Clinician name:_____ Date:_____

1. ALPHABET: Instruct client to "say the alphabet." Transcribe responses phonetically.

a/e/ ( )	j/dze/ ( )	s/es/ ( )
b/bi/ ( )	k/ke/ ( )	t/ti/ ( )
c/si/ ( )	l/el/ ( )	u/yu/ ( )
d/di/ ( )	m/em/ ( )	v/vi/ ( )
e/i/ ( )	n/en/ ( )	w/dub l yu/ ( )
f/ef/ ( )	o/o/ ( )	x/eks ( )
g/dzi ( )	p/pi/ ( )	y/wai/ ( )
h/ets/ ( )	q/kyu/ ( )	z/zi/ ( )
i/ai/ ( )	r/ar/ ( )	

1a. RS: /26   %_____   Stim.? Y N   PSI: 1   2   3   4   5
b. RS: /26   %_____   Stim.? Y N   PSI: 1   2   3   4   5

Comments:

2. VOWELS: Instruct the client to "tell me which letters are vowels." Check, if correct. Number responses in order given.

a   e   i   o   u

2. RS: /5   %_____   Stim.? Y N   PSI: 1   3   5

Comments:

*3. a.   VOWEL DESIGNATIONS: Ask the client to "explain the difference between long and short vowels."
Response:

b.   If unable to explain 3a: Indicate number 3 on the Client Stimulus Form. Ask the client to "pronounce each vowel."

1. a_____   6. ā_____
2. e_____   7. ē_____
3. i _____   8. ī_____
4. o_____   9. ō_____
5. u_____   10. ū_____

c.   If unable to produce correct resonses to item 3b: Give client a dictionary and ask client to "use the dictionary to help you tell me how to pronounce the vowels on this list." (Client Stimulus Form Number 3)

1. a_____	6. ā_____
2. e_____	7. ē_____
3. i_____	8. ī_____
4. o_____	9. ō_____
5. u_____	10. ū_____

3a. RS: /1 %_____	Stim.? Y N	PSI: 1	2	3	4	5
b. RS: /10 %_____	Stim.? Y N	PSI: 1	2	3	4	5
c. RS: /10 %_____	Stim.? Y N	PSI: 1	2	3	4	5

Comments:

4. VOWEL FUNCTION

a. *Vowel production:* Indicate number 4 on Client Stimulus Form. Instruct the client to "Say the following 'words'." Score based on the accuracy of vowel production.

b. *Speech decoding:* Ask the client to "tell me the real (or equivalent) word by spelling or signing it" (example: "shue" = "shoe").

	Correct vowel production	ID of "real word"
1. mee (me)	_____	_____
2. boan (bone)	_____	_____
3. rume (room)	_____	_____
4. nou (now)	_____	_____
5. nead (need)	_____	_____
6. shie (shy)	_____	_____
7. lain (lane)	_____	_____
8. tew (to, too, two)	_____	_____
9. tyde (tide, tied)	_____	_____
10. poynt (point)	_____	_____

4a. Rs: /10 %_____	Stim.? Y N	PSI: 1	2	3	4	5
b. Rs: /10 %_____	Stim.? Y N	PSI: 1	2	3	4	5

Comments:

5. CONSONANT IDENTIFICATION: Ask the client, "What are letters that are not vowels called?" (Consonants)

5a. Rs: /1 %_____	Stim.? Y N	PSI: 1	3	5

Comments:

6. CONSONANT/VOWELS: Ask the client to "explain the difference between vowels and consonants." Response:

6. Rs: /1 %_____	Stim.?	Y N	PSI: 1	3	5

Comments:

7. CONSONANT FUNCTION: Indicate the following "words" on Client Stimulus Form Number 7.
   a. *Consonant function:* Tell the client to "Say the 'words'." (Score based on the accuracy of production of underlined consonants).
   b. *Speech decoding:* Ask the client to "Tell me the real (or equivalent) word" by spelling it or signing it. (Example: rase = race)

	Correct consonant production	ID of "real word"
1. cend (send)	_____	_____
2. *bight* (bite)	_____	_____
3. *phat* (fat)	_____	_____
4. brix (bricks)	_____	_____
5. *wrat* (rat)	_____	_____
6. *hamb* (ham)	_____	_____
7. geans (jeans)	_____	_____
8. *gnap* (nap)	_____	_____
9. *djello* (jello)	_____	_____
10. jas (jazz)	_____	_____

7a. RS: /10 %_____	Stim.?	Y N	PSI: 1	2	3	4	5
b. RS: /10 %_____	Stim.?	Y N	PSI: 1	2	3	4	5

Comments:

8. GRAMMATICAL CONSTRUCTS: Indicate the words for part 8 of the Client Stimulus Form. Tell the client to "say the words."
   a. *Possessives/Plurals:* (Note production of word endings)

   1. lips(s) _____ 2. beds(z) _____
   3. buses (∂z) _____ 4. buzzes(∂z) _____
   5. Beth's(s) _____ 6. Bill's(z) _____

8a. RS: /6 %_____	Stim.?	Y N	PSI: 1	2	3	4	5

Comments:

  b. *Contractions:* (Note production of second syllable)
        1. didn't   3. it's
        2. isn't   4. won't

8b. RS: /4 %_____   Stim.? Y N PSI: 1 2 3 4 5

Comments:

  c. *Past tense:* (Note production of word endings)
        1. begged (d) _____   2. dipped (t) _____
        3. faded(∂d)   _____   4. waited(∂d) _____

8c. RS: /4 %_____   Stim.? Y N PSI: 1 2 3 4 5

Comments:

9. PHONEME PRODUCTION: Instruct the client to "tell me what sounds (specific) letters make in words." Transcribe responses. This task may be stimulated with the grapheme "w" by contrasting the grapheme "double u" with the phoneme /w/. Use a blackboard or fingerspelling.

      b ( )   k ( )   s ( )

      *c ( )( )( )   l ( )   *t ( )( )

      d ( )   m ( )   v ( )

      f ( )   n ( )   w ( )

      *g ( )( )   p ( )   x ( )

      h ( )   q ( )   y ( )

      j ( )   r ( )   z ( )
      *items have alternate sounds ("c"=/s/k/sh/, "g"=/g/j/, "t"=/t/ch/)

9. RS: /24 %_____   Stim.? Y N PSI: 1 2 3 4 5

Comments:

10. GRAPHEME/PHONEME: Instruct the client to "look at each of the words" on the Client Response Form, part 10. "Say them aloud, and tell me: (a) the number of letters in each, and (b) the number of sounds in each." If the response to 1b (sounds) is "one" the number of sounds may be *stimulated* by saying to client, "That's the number of syllables. How many sounds does it have?"

	Number of letters	Number of sounds
1) tub	(3)_____	(3)_____
2) wine	(4)_____	(3)_____

3) shop   (4)_____   (3)_____
4) box   (3)_____   (4)_____
5) step   (4)_____   (4)_____

| 10a. RS: /5 %_____ Stim.? Y N PSI: 1 2 3 4 5 |
| b. RS: /10 %_____ Stim.? Y N PSI: 1 2 3 4 5 |

Comments:

11a. DIGRAPH IDENTIFICATION: (Consonants): Ask the client to "tell
me the sounds in which two letters equal one sound." (If client correctly
indicates that the "sh" was a single sound in the previous exercise, use it
as a stimulus and ask client to generate others.)

Responses: _____ _____ _____ _____ _____ _____ _____ _____
                (sh) (ch) (th) (TH) (zh) (ng) (ph) (wh)
Comments:

| 11a. RS: /6 %_____ Stim.? Y N PSI: 1 2 3 4 5 |

11b. DIGRAPH PRODUCTION (Consonants): Instruct the client to say the
following five "words" on the Client Stimulus Form:

        1. shim /_____/   3. chup /_____/   5. phop /____/
        2. lang /_____/   4. thull /_____/

| 11b. RS: /5 %_____ Stim.? Y N PSI: 1 2 3 4 5 |

Comments:

11c. DIGRAPH IDENTIFICATION (Vowels): Instruct client, "Now tell me
the vowel sounds in which two letters equal one sound."

Responses: _____ _____ _____ _____ _____ _____ _____ _____ _____
                ai   au   ay   ea   ee   ei   ey   oa   oe

           _____ _____ _____ _____ _____
                oi   oo   ou   oy   uy

| 11c. RS: /5 %_____ Stim.? Y N PSI: 1 2 3 4 5 |

Comments:

11d. DIGRAPH PRODUCTION (Vowels): Instruct the client to "say the following fourteen words" on the Client Stimulus Form:

1. dail /_____/	6. beil /_____/	11. moop /_____/
2. saud /_____/	7. mey /_____/	12. hout /_____/
3. tay /_____/	8. boad /_____/	13. doy /_____/
4. sead /_____/	9. loe /_____/	14. shuy /_____/
5. reen /_____/	10. poin /_____/	

> 11d. RS: /14 %_____ Stim.? Y N PSI: 1 2 3 4 5

Comments:

12. SILENT LETTERS: Indicate the following words on the Client Stimulus Form, and
   a. Instruct the client to "say each word"
   b. Instruct the client to "tell me which letters are 'silent letter'"

1. bell (l) _____	6. night (gh) _____	11. debt (b) _____
2. time (e) _____	7. knot (k) _____	12. watch (t) _____
3. flop (-) _____	8. comb (b) _____	13. walk (l) _____
4. tree (e) _____	9. duck (c or k) _____	14. feed (e) _____
5. wrap (w) _____	10. tax (-) _____	15. island (s) _____

> 12a. RS: /15 %_____ Stim.? Y N PSI: 1 2 3 4 5
>   b. RS: /15 %_____ Stim.? Y N PSI: 1 2 3 4 5

Comments:

*13. SYLLABIFICATION (Grapheme): Indicate the following words on the Client Stimulus From. Ask the client to "tell me the number of syllables in each word."

	Number of syllables
1. rousemicker	(3)_____
2. audishoble	(4)_____
3. treys	(1)_____
4. coufraine	(2)_____
5. hyphus	(2)_____

> 13. RS: /5 %_____ Stim.? Y N PSI: 1 2 3 4 5

Comments:

14. SYLLABIFICATION (Auditory/Visual): Say the following words twice. Ask the client to "tell me the number of syllables in each word."

                           Number of syllables

    1. cheeroid   (2)_____

    2. omnifutile   (4)_____

    3. kwatz   (1)_____

    4. sergid   (2)_____

    5. reductive   (3)_____

14. RS: /10 %_____   Stim.? Y N   PSI: 1   2   3   4   5

Comments:

*15. STRESS (Grapheme): Indicate the following words on the Client Stimulus Form. Explain, "The words are divided into syllables." Instruct the client to "tell me the syllable of each word that gets the most emphasis or stress.

    1. <u>choc</u> tive
    2. <u>mer</u> i ca
    3. ex <u>train</u>
    4. <u>lip</u> <u>lock</u>
    5. re <u>dib</u> a able

15. RS: /10 %_____   Stim.? Y N   PSI: 1   2   3   4   5

Comments:

16. STRESS (Auditory/Visual): Say the following words twice. Instruct the client to "tell me which syllable has the stress or emphasis."
    1. un <u>pip</u> less
    2. a <u>rout</u>
    3. <u>cob</u> i tant
    4. <u>grump</u> ing
    5. a <u>clop</u> tic

16. RS: /10 %_____   Stim.? Y N   PSI: 1   2   3   4   5

Comments:

*17. SYLLABLE/STRESS: Instruct the client to "look up each of following words; (a) tell me how many syllables are in the word, (b) tell me the syllable that gets the stress, and (c) pronounce the word."

    1. pneumonia (   )
    2. revenue   (   )

PRONUNCIATION SKILLS INVENTORY

Client Stimulus Form

(*Note:* Numbers correspond to numbered items on the Clinician's Response Form.)

3. Say each of the following sounds:

   1. a   6. ā

   2. e   7. ē

   3. i   8. ī

   4. o   9. ō

   5. u   10. ū

4. Study each word. Say it the best you can. Tell the real word that is pronounced the same. (Example "shue = shoe")

1. mee	6. shie
2. boan	7. lain
3. rume	8. tew
4. nou	9. tyde
5. nead	10. poynt

7. Look at each word. Say it the best you can. Tell me the real word that is pronounced the same (Example: "knaime" = "name").

1. cend	6. hamb
2. bight	7. geans
3. phat	8. gnap
4. brix	9. dgello
5. wrat	10. jas

8. Look at each word. Say it the best you can.

   a.
1. lips	4. buzzes
2. beds	5. Beth's
3. buses	6. Bill's

   b.
1. didn't	3. it's
2. isn't	4. won't

   c.
1. begged	3. faded
2. dipped	4. waited

10. Look at each word and say it to yourself. For each word, tell me: (a) how many letters it has and (b) how many sounds it has.
    1. tub
    2. wine
    3. shop
    4. step
    5. box

11b. say the following five words:
    1. shim
    2. lang
    3. chup
    4. thull
    5. phop

11d. Say the following fourteen words:

1. dail	2. saud
3. tay	4. sead
5. reen	6. beil
7. mey	8. boad
9. loe	10. foin
11. moop	12. hout
13. doy	14. shuy

12. Look at each word. Tell me which letters are the silent letters. Say each word.

1. bell	6. night	11. debt
2. time	7. knot	12. watch
3. flop	8. comb	13. walk
4. tree	9. duck	14. feed
5. wrap	10. tax	15. island

17a. locating (dictionary) RS: /2	% _____	Stim.? Y N	PSI: 1 2 3 4 5
b. locating (pron. guide) RS: /2	% _____	Stim.? Y N	PSI: 1 2 3 4 5
c. I.D. number of syllables RS: /2% _____		Stim.? Y N	PSI: 1 2 3 4 5
d. I.D. stress RS: /2	% _____	Stim.? Y N	PSI: 1 2 3 4 5
e. pron. syllables RS: /2	% _____	Stim.? Y N	PSI: 1 2 3 4 5
f. pron. strees RS: /2	% _____	Stim.? Y N	PSI: 1 2 3 4 5

Comments:

18. DICTIONARY SKILLS: Instruct the client to indicate which of the following words are not familiar. When you have found two with which client is unfamiliar, instruct the client to "find the selected words in the dictionary." Then instruct the client to "pronounce the word, tell me the part of speech, define the word, and use the word correctly in a sentence."

1. rhyme	(	)	4. gnu	(	)
2. quiche	(	)	5. aisle	(	)
3. svelte	(	)	6. fatigue	(	)

18a. pronounc. RS: /2	%_____	Stim.? Y N	PSI: 1 2 3 4 5
b. part/speech RS: /2	%_____	Stim.? Y N	PSI: 1 2 3 4 5
c. define RS: /2	%_____	Stim.? Y N	PSI: 1 2 3 4 5
d. use RS: /2	%_____	Stim.? Y N	PSI: 1 2 3 4 5

Comments:

Preliminary Comparative Data:
Mean PSI Scores for Grade Schoolers/Prelingually Deaf Adults

Item (#)	Skill	Grade K (n = 25)	Grade 1 (n = 22)	Grade 2 (n = 22)	Grade 3 (n = 22)	Grade 4 (n = 25)	Deaf Adults (n is denoted by ( ) after mean)
1	Recite ABC's	1–	1–	1–	1–	1–	1.05 (78)
2	Identify vowels	5–	2.14–	1.18=	1.18=	1=	1.21 (78)
3 a,b,c	Long vs. Short Vowel	5–	4.54–	3.73=	3+	2.6+	4.05(a) (52) 3.30(b) (23) 3.5(c) (8)
4,7,8	Pronounce Words	5–	4.84–	3.38+	3.27+	2.2+	4.03(a) (65)
5	Consonants	5–	5–	3.14=	2+	1.56+	3.20 (62)
6	Vowels vs. Consonants	5–	5–	4.73=	4+	2.68+	4.29 (69)
9	Phonemes	5–	3.30=	2.23+	2.82=	2.44+	3.23 (72)
10a	Number of letters	5–	1.45=	1=	1=	1=	1.20 (77)
10b	Number of sounds	5–	3.27+	3.82=	3.09+	2.84+	3.83 (77)
11	Digraphs	5–	4.72–	4.18–	4.27–	3.04+	3.63 (77)
12	Silent letters	5–	4.18–	3=	2.55+	2.52+	3.31 (71)
13	Number of syllables/written word	5–	5–	2.82–	1.36+	1.24+	2.17 (68)
14	Number of syllables/spoken word	5–	5–	2.05=	1.73=	1.16+	1.98 (70)
15	Stress-written word	5–	5–	3.64–	2.82=	2.52+	3.10 (68)
16	Stress-spoken word	5–	5–	3.95–	2.64–	2.6+	3.2 (52)
17a	Word find	5–	5–	3.86–	4.64–	1+	1.8 (51)
17b	Stress	5–	5–	4.14–	4–	1.72+	2.33 (33)

continues

Preliminary Comparative Data (*continued*)

Item (#)	Skill	Grade K (n = 25)	Grade 1 (n = 22)	Grade 2 (n = 22)	Grade 3 (n = 22)	Grade 4 (n = 25)	Deaf Adults (n is denoted by ( ) after mean)
17c	Pronunciation	5–	5–	4.33–	3–	2.2–	1.6 (23)
18a	Locate	5–	5–	5–	1.36=	1+	1.40 (56)
18b	Pronunciation	5–	5–	3.95–	2.55=	3.0=	2.89 (56)

Source: Bally and Marasco 1991.

Note: Number under each grade indicate mean score for each probe area; "–" after number indicates score worse than deaf population; "+" indicates score better than deaf population; "=" indicates score within .5 deaf population.

Recommendations for a Comprehensive Assessment*

PRAGMATICS

1. Assess pragmatic language development through criterion-referenced checklists in a variety of different settings: home, school, self-contained situation, integrated setting, and peer-to-peer interaction. Incorporate parent/teacher/peer reports to determine pragmatic skills used within the home and school setting.
2. Determine if and how students use a variety of conversational strategies, particularly perspective-taking, maintenance of conversation, clarification, revision, appropriateness, conflict resolution, problem solving, critical listening, questioning, answering, and interpersonal negotiation.
3. Through observation and/or appropriate tests, attempt to determine issues related to ability level: (a) vocabulary knowledge, (b) grammar competence, (c) social skills, (d) self-image and self esteem, (e) extent of experience or world knowledge, (f) extent of explicit teaching, (g) ability to acquire information incidentally, (h) expressive communication-intelligibility in speech and/or sign, and (i) interaction style of adult conversational partners.
4. Use more than one method of characterizing abilities such as: report behavioral sampling, and probe techniques.

---

* Reprinted with permission from Yoshinaga-Itano, C. (1997). The challenge of assessing language in children with hearing loss. *Language, Speech and Hearing Services in Schools, 28,* 362–373.

5. Determine whether a functionally appropriate situation will elicit specific pragmatic targets. Determine the extent to which the pragmatic language characteristics of the conversational partner affect the quality of the student's language. The level of language facility should differ according to the conversational partner and/or the situation. Therefore, assessing the student in a variety of different situations with a variety of conversational partners is optimal. These conversational partners may be parents, teachers, siblings, hearing peers, peers who are deaf or adults who are deaf or hearing-impaired.

6. Determine the pragmatic characteristics of the student's language that contribute to optimal semantic language development. An analysis of the questioning strategies of the child may provide this information. How well can the child use questions to obtain information regarding place or location (where), agent (who), means (how), reason (why), time (when), or new information, or to clarify information provided?

7. Determine the pragmatic characteristics of the conversational partner's language that might contribute to optimal semantic language development. Turn-taking strategies: Does the student have an opportunity to ask questions? Questioning strategies: Is the student predominately required to answer questions rather than initiate questions? Expansion: Does the conversational partner expand the student's language, providing new information for the student? Repetition: Does the conversational partner provide repeated information for the student and many opportunities to learn the information?

8. Determine the student's pragmatic characteristics that enhance expressive development. These characteristics may involve the student's desire to master skills, internal motivation to drill and practice, attention to detail, desire to be understood orally or through sign language, and persistence at communication success.

SEMANTICS

In light of the disturbing plateau in the semantic development of children who are deaf as measured by standardized assessments, it is appropriate to examine the nature of language processing and to identify other variables that might be significant in causing or preventing this result.

1. Determine the flexibility of the vocabulary. Flexibility will be evidenced by: (a) the student's ability to assign a vocabulary label to many instances of the word, such as the label of bird to ostrich, penguin, robin, sparrow, and pigeon; (b) the student's ability to determine an antonym or synonym for a vocabulary item; (c) the student's ability to understand and use the vocabulary word in an analogy or association and to mentally manipulate and consider several attributes simultaneously; (d) the student's ability to

group lexical items by category; and (e) the student's ability to extend from a stereotype or one definition of the word to a novel instance.

2. Determine the student's primary mode for expansions of vocabulary: conversation (through oral and/or sign), print and/or literacy events.

3. Determine the student's pragmatic strategies for obtaining novel information and clarifying meaning, thereby enabling the student to enlarge vocabulary.

4. Determine the rate of acquisition of new vocabulary. In the early developmental period, is the student acquiring significantly more vocabulary, such that the developmental growth improves with age? The development of vocabulary proceeds in multiplicative fashion. During the first 1½ years of life, the child acquires vocabulary linearly, adding new words that inventories can easily identify. However, within the next year of life, the child expands from lexicons of approximately 50 words to lexicons of 600 to 700 words—more than a tenfold increase. This "explosion" of language development marks a critical stage that occurs with only a few children with significant hearing losses. From that stage, vocabulary acquisition proceeds at such a pace that exact inventories of the lexicon are virtually impossible to keep. This stage appears to be a transitional one, during which the child assumes the primary responsibility of language learning through pragmatics, and self-initiates the acquisition of new vocabulary.

5. Once acquired, determine the student's cognitive ability to retain the information and retrieve it for later use. Determine the student's ability to generalize the information to novel learning situations. Are difficulties with retrieval due to incomplete information or inadequate comprehension? A key question concerning whether the student is experiencing memory difficulties or storage difficulties is whether the information can eventually be retrieved if enough questions are posed.

6. Determine the student's ability to operate on vocabulary. How many attributes or characteristics is the student able to provide? What types of analogies does the student understand? This information will help determine the elaboration of concepts/schemata in memory.

7. Determine the student's ability to summarize and provide the most important information. The task of outlining a chapter or taking notes relies on a student's ability to summarize. Determine where the student's abilities are on the developmental continuum. Does the student use a knowledge-telling technique?

8. Determine the student's strategies for filling in meaning from context. How many strategies does the student rely on? Determine the student's ability to infer meaning. Can he or she make an educated guess concerning the meaning of a new vocabulary word, given several different contexts for the word?

9. Determine the percentage of words in the spontaneous production of the child in specific word classes: nouns, verbs, prepositions, adverbs,

conjunctions, and pronouns. Very early in language development (by 2½ years of age), children make a transition from predominantly nouns in the vocabulary to predominantly verbs (also including adverbs, prepositions, conjunctions, and pronouns). Children with significant hearing losses sometimes fail to make this transition. They increase vocabulary size, but predominantly in noun categories.

10. Determine what contributes to the development of an optimal style at each stage. At this student's language stage, do the characteristics of the conversational partner enhance or facilitate the acquisition of specific categories of lexical items? If the characteristics of the conversational partner's speech change, are there measurable differences in the student's acquisition of new lexical items or vocabulary words?

11. Determine the role that the emergence of the hearing-impaired child's nonverbal and subsequent verbal requests for information, beginning with "What is that?" have on verbal language development (Yoshinaga-Itano & Stredler-Brown, 1992). How many different types of questioning has the student mastered and does the student initiate? Are the questions semantically appropriate and do they function successfully in providing the student with desired information?

12. Determine whether there are some styles of lexical learning that lead the child astray or cause language learning plateaus. Between 18 months and 24 months, the continued increase of nonverbal "indexical" gestures, such as pointing, showing, commenting, and requesting and the lack of emergence of the first verbal labels during this same time period, are usually evidence for a language plateau in the infant/ toddler who is hearing-impaired (Yoshinaga-Itano & Stredler-Brown, 1992). An increase proportionally in the child's answers and a decrease in the initiation of conversation and requesting may also be a developmentally troubling characteristic. The continued use of elaboration strategies, like telling everything one knows about a topic, may prevent the transition to a higher level of summarization. The increase of questions that do not function to clarify information or to obtain desired information would be an unsuccessful strategy. An increase in echolalia that prevents an increase in spontaneous initiation of conversation could be detrimental to future language development.

13. Determine semantic characteristics within the student's storytelling (Halliday, 1975; Halliday &Hasan, 1976; Hedberg & Westby, 1993; Stein & Glenn, 1979; Yoshinaga-Itano & Downey, 1992). That is, find out if there is evidence of interference, elaboration, sequence, causality, cohesion, and story grammar.

The development of narrative structure has been found to be highly related to reading comprehension ability. Yoshinaga-Itano & Downey (1996) found that several cognitive processes are prerequisite to the mastery of story grammar. Many children with mild to profound hearing loss have difficulty using background knowledge to make inferences, using schema information to elaborate ideas, incorporating time concepts to produce logically and temporally sequenced ideas and incorporating both syntax and semantics to create reference systems within their discourse. Yoshinaga-Itano & Downey (1992) suggest an assessment procedure, the Colorado Process Analysis of Written Language.

Index